Immunological Engineering

Immunological Engineering

EDITED BY

D. W. JIRSCH
Department of Surgery,
St Michael's Hospital,
University of Toronto,
Toronto, Ontario, Canada

MTP

Published by
MTP Press Limited
Falcon House
Lancaster, England

ISBN: 0-85200-174-6

Printed in Great Britain by
Mather Bros (Printers) Limited, Preston

Contents

List of Contributors

M. P. Arala-Chaves
Department of Basic and Clinical Immunology and Microbiology,
Medical University of South Carolina,
Charleston, South Carolina 29401, USA

A. Basten
Immunology Unit,
Department of Bacteriology,
The University of Sydney,
New South Wales 2006, Australia

D. W. van Bekkum
Radiobiological Institute TNO,
Rijswijk, The Netherlands

S. Croft
Immunology Unit,
Department of Bacteriology,
The University of Sydney,
New South Wales 2006, Australia

H. H. Fudenberg
Department of Basic and Clinical Immunology and Microbiology,
Medical University of South Carolina,
Charleston, South Carolina 29401, USA

R. E. Falk
Department of Surgery,
Toronto General Hospital,
University of Toronto,
Toronto, Ontario, Canada

J. M. Goust
Department of Basic and Clinical Immunology and Microbiology,
Medical University of South Carolina,
Charleston, South Carolina 29401, USA

R. D. Guttmann
Transplant Service,
Royal Victoria Hospital and McGill University,
Montreal, Quebec, Canada

R. Hong
Department of Pediatrics and Medical Microbiology,
University of Wisconsin Center for Health Sciences,
Madison, Wisconsin 53706, USA

Maija Horsmanheimo
Department of Basic and Clinical Immunology and Microbiology,
Medical University of South Carolina,
Charleston, South Carolina 29401, USA

D. W. Jirsch
Department of Surgery,
St Michael's Hospital,
University of Toronto,
Toronto, Ontario, Canada

B. Löwenberg
Erasmus University,
Rotterdam, The Netherlands

G. Opelz
Department of Surgery,
School of Medicine,
University of California at Los Angeles,
Los Angeles, California 90024, USA

R. L. Powles
The Hamilton Fairley Leukaemia Research Fund Unit,
The Royal Marsden Hospital,
Sutton, Surrey

C. R. Stiller
Transplantation Unit, University Hospital,
University of Ontario,
London, Ontario, Canada

R. M. Vetto
Department of Surgery,
US Veterans' Hospital,
Portland, Oregon 97207, USA

H. M. Vriesendorp
Radiobiological Institute TNO,
Rijswijk, The Netherlands

Foreword

Immunology has become one of the most important of the life sciences. As research unravels the mystery of the lymphocyte, a central role of the immune system in health preservation has become evident. The paediatric immunodeficiency disorders or 'experiments of nature' have demonstrated the division of cellular and humoral immunity; specific functional defects are now readily identified. The tendency of persons with immune dysfunction to develop neoplasms has suggested that surveillance mechanisms within the immune apparatus prevent tumour development. Malignancies, in fact, do seem to provoke certain immune responses, begging numerous therapeutic questions. Transplantation surgery, or the demand for 'new parts' has led to description of those antigens important in tissue-typing. Genetic loci have been found responsible for transplantation antigen display; as well, they influence clinical resistance or susceptibility to a wide variety of infections, auto-immune or neoplastic diseases.

Clinicians have been quick to recognize the therapeutic implications of laboratory work and to use this knowledge in disease treatment. Precise patient–tissue matching and immunosuppressive treatment make renal allotransplantation safer and more successful than ever before. Both paediatric and adult immune deficiency states are now often recognized; treatment may involve general immune support or specific manipulations with, perhaps, bone marrow or thymus grafts or treatment with lymphocyte transfer factor.

Transplantation of bone marrow has been used not only to correct certain immune defects but to correct marrow failure of diverse origin. Although the early hopes that cancers would melt away with administration of simple immune sera or cells were puerile and unfounded, augmentation of tumour immunity can benefit the cancer patient and is a welcome addition to oncotherapy.

These achievements may be considered examples of 'immunological engineering' in that diverse manipulations or alterations of immune responses are used therapeutically. In this text members of ten outstanding research communities survey these burgeoning fields of activity in depth.

FOREWORD

No attempt has been made to cover the vast interface between immunology and illness, and certain repetition has been considered both valuable and provocative. The submissions document, I think, an extraordinary approach to the therapy of human disease.

Toronto, Canada
December, 1977

D.W.J.

1
A Biological Approach to the Management of Acute Leukaemia in Man

R. L. POWLES

The Hamilton Fairley Leukaemia Research Fund Unit,
The Royal Marsden Hospital, Sutton, Surrey, England

A decade ago it seemed reasonable to suppose that all diseases embraced within the general term 'leukaemia' were variants of the same fundamental pathological process.

Recently, it has become necessary to challenge the universal acceptance of this hypothesis in order to explain differences in the response to treatment of the various types of leukaemia. For example, chemotherapy with agents known to interfere with RNA and DNA (the 'usual' anti-cancer agents) has been able to render approximately 40% of patients with acute lymphoblastic leukaemia (ALL) disease free for a sufficiently prolonged period of time to assume they are now cured. With similar treatment using the same type of agents 50% or more of the patients with acute myelogenous leukaemia (AML) also become apparently disease free according to the methods of detection at present available, but it is a sad fact that all but a very small minority of these patients develop a rapid recurrence of their disease which then proves fatal. This failure to control the disease in seemingly a highly drug-sensitive condition is not only disappointing but also totally unexpected—in the carcinomas, for example, such a good response to initial treatment would be expected to be associated with a reasonable proportion of cured patients (as occurs with ALL).

There are many possible reasons (such as the emergence of a new clone of AML cells) for this failure to control AML with 'anti-nucleic acid' agents and these will be dealt with more fully later, but it is sufficient to say here that a new approach to the management of this disease is clearly required. At present there are no agents (other than perhaps steroids and asparaginase) that are available with an anti-cancer action that do not interfere with nucleic acid function and this is largely due to screening programmes so far devised, which have always involved inhibition of proliferation of cancer cells. The possibility must be explored that regulation rather than proliferation may be the key problem for certain types of cancer (such as AML) and that it is the soil itself that is defective (i.e. the marrow environment) not the malignant clone of cells, which merely represents the end result of the process. This concept has led us to explore the possibility of a biological control of certain types of leukaemia and it is the purpose of this chapter to discuss one such line of endeavour, namely the manipulation of the host immune system to render the patient permanently disease free.

THE EARLY ATTEMPTS AT IMMUNOTHERAPY

Over 60 years ago Tyzzer[1] attempted to treat acute leukaemia in man with immunotherapy and similar anecdotal studies have been conducted for an even longer period for other forms of malignant disease. Much of this work was independent of animal experiments dating from the time of Paul Erhlich and others at the end of the last century, which appeared to show that immunological manipulation could cause the rejection of tumours. Unfortunately, the uncontrolled and largely unrepeatable clinical studies, followed by the realization that transplanted tumour rejection in 'unrelated' animals was the result of transplantation antigens and nothing to do with cancer, led to a feeling of great pessimism and a virtual abandonment of the subject until after the Second World War.

Interest in the field was revived in the mid-1940s when Ludwich Gross[2] took advantage of the recently developed inbred mice colonies produced by Leonell Strong[3] at Yale University. In this first study published by Gross[2], C3H mice were used. These had been bred by continuous brother to sister mating for more than 20 years, and had thus acquired a remarkable genetic uniformity that may for practical purposes be considered autologous. He studied a chemically induced sarcoma originally produced in an animal of the same line which eliminated the possibility that the immunity to tumour inoculation could be caused by genetic differences between the tumour cells and those of the host. He found that after inoculation of tumour-bearing animals with a suspension of this sarcoma, 20% showed tumour regression.

By the late 1950s carefully conducted animal experiments showed that tumour cells which had been induced by chemical carcinogens, by viruses or by physical carcinogens had in their plasma membranes macromolecules which were not present in the plasma membranes of normal cells. The host recognizes these substances as foreign and reacts against them by producing antibodies and developing cell-mediated immunity. These tumour-specific macromolecules present in membranes are generally referred to as 'tumour-specific transplantation-type antigens' (TSTAs). Subsequent attempts in carefully controlled animal systems to treat tumours known to have TSTAs by immunological methods were disappointing until Haddow and Alexander[4] were able to show that primary sarcomas in rats which had been induced by implanting a pellet of the carcinogen 3,4-benzpyrene could be controlled by two types of immunological treatment after the bulk of the tumour had been removed either by surgery or by radiotherapy. The residual tumour cells could be held in check either by active immunization with irradiated tumour cells derived from the tumour to be treated[4], or by injection of lymphocytes obtained from other animals that had been immunized previously with a piece of the tumour to be treated[5]. It was quickly shown that these immunotherapy procedures were also effective against leukaemias in mice[6,7].

It must be stressed that only some experimental tumours respond well to these immunological treatments and that with many tumours, particularly those of spontaneous origin, no effective immunotherapy can be observed even when the tumour load is very small (e.g. spontaneous acute leukaemias in the rat[8]). Primary experimental tumours which give rise to distant metastases also respond badly, if at all, to immunotherapy and immunotherapy has also been very disappointing in the control of metastatic disease in animals. The possible inappropriateness of animal models in which effective immunotherapy has been demonstrated for the clinical situation may explain in part why, in properly conducted clinical trials using contemporaneous controls, immunotherapy has been shown to be virtually ineffective for the treatment of disseminated human malignant disease and reproducible clinical benefit from immunotherapy has so far only been seen in two situations: (1) The treatment of Stage I lung cancer (but not in later stages), where intrapleural injection of BCG appears to be of substantial benefit[9], and (2) acute myelogenous leukaemia, where some prolongation of life but probably no cures have been obtained using immunotherapy in conjunction with chemotherapy (see below).

METHODS OF IMMUNOTHERAPY

Passive immunotherapy

This method refers to the passive transfer of specific immune material into a tumour-bearing host. It has been highly effective in some animal systems but has not been systematically studied in controlled clinical trials for very good reasons. Until we can be much more sure that human tumours have TSTAs and that one can measure the activity of antibodies, cytotoxic cells, or products derived from them, no rational protocol can be designed.

Local immunotherapy

This relies on the destruction of tumour cells by inflammatory cells drawn locally into a tumour by either injection of BCG, *Corynebacterium parvum* or by using a delayed hypersensitivity reaction with tuberculin or dinitrofluorobenzene. This does not bring about systemic effects and there is no convincing evidence that such treatment affects any lesions other than those directly treated. However, unquestionably, BCG may drain into adjacent lesions or affect tumour cells in adjoining lymph nodes.

Active immunotherapy

Almost all carefully conducted trials of clinical immunotherapy and especially those involving leukaemias make use of this type of procedure, which consists of stimulating the existing immunological machinery of the host either specifically with tumour cells (or modified tumour cells) or non-specifically with substances such as BCG or *Corynebacterium parvum*, which cause hyperplasia of the reticuloendothelial system, or by a combination of the two.

CLINICAL STUDIES OF IMMUNOTHERAPY FOR ACUTE LEUKAEMIA IN MAN

Acute lymphoblastic leukaemia (ALL)

Animal experiments had shown that although immunotherapy was effective for 'prophylaxis' it only worked in tumour-bearing animals if the tumour load was very small. This led Mathé[7] to suggest that acute leukaemia might be an equivalent model to test for the effectiveness of immunotherapy in man. In this situation patients could be given conventional chemotherapy until there was no further detectable disease (the so-called remission state) but at a time when it is known that some leukaemia cells still remain because without further treatment relapse inevitably occurs. This remission state seemed to be an ideal moment to give immunotherapy. It is to Mathé's great credit that he selected the remission state of leukaemia to test the efficacy of immunotherapy and, in addition, he was one of the first oncologists to stress the importance of controlled clinical trials in cancer. In Mathé's later study[10] he selected a group of 30 children with ALL, all of whom had been in remission for at least 2 years. For some, all treatment was stopped whilst the rest were given weekly Pasteur BCG, killed allogeneic ALL cells, or both BCG and cells. All 10 of the untreated patients relapsed within 130 days, whereas half of the 20 immunotherapy patients remained in remission for more than 295 days, some of them for many years. The numbers were too small to decide which of the immunological regimes was best.

This study aroused great interest and several attempts have been made to confirm the value of BCG alone in ALL during remission. In Britain the

Medical Research Council arranged a trial[11] which compared the use of twice weekly methotrexate with BCG and no treatment. Figure 1.1 summarizes the results of this study[12] in which it was found that the duration of remission for 18 patients who received no further treatment after an initial 5½ months of chemotherapy was not significantly different from a similar group of 50 patients given weekly Glaxo BCG. Patients who received further chemotherapy (methotrexate) during the period following the initial 5½ months had longer remissions. Further follow-up of these patients 5 years later confirms these initial findings and only one patient in each of the BCG and no treatment arms remain in first remission. Of interest

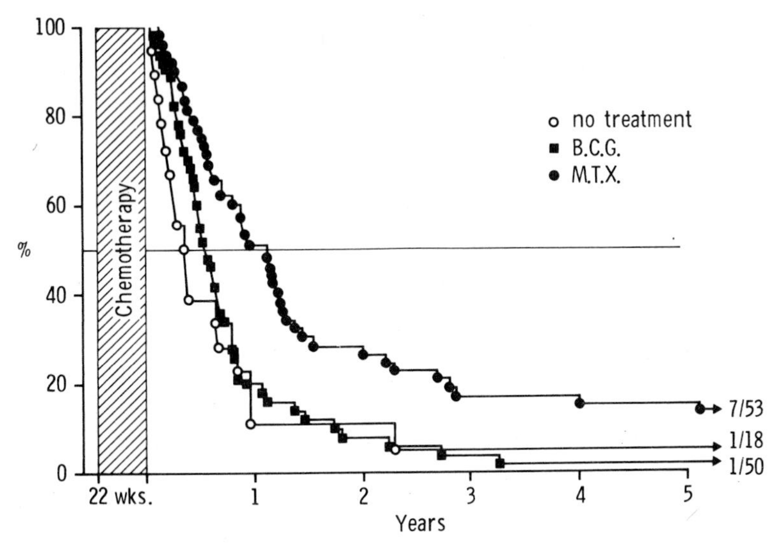

Figure 1.1 Effect of BCG on length of first remission for childhood ALL (MRC Trial 1969–70)

there is no difference in the overall survival curves of these three groups of patients. A similar study in the USA by Leukaemia Study Group A[13] was based upon the same lines as the British study, comparing BCG with no treatment (and with maintenance methotrexate). No difference in remission duration could be detected between those patients receiving Chicago BCG and those untreated although, again, those patients given methotrexate during remission tended to stay longer in remission. In this study the initial randomization was after 3½ months of chemotherapy but the patients receiving maintenance chemotherapy were further randomized after another 8 months into BCG, no treatment, or methotrexate maintenance. This further randomization showed no therapeutic advantage of BCG over no treatment for maintaining remission.

These three studies raise many questions. Table 1.1 summarizes the details and differences of Mathé's study from the two subsequent attempts designed

Table 1.1 Immunotherapy for acute lymphoblastic leukaemia of childhood

Study	*Duration induction chemo-therapy (months)*	*CNS prophylaxis*	*BCG used*	*Number of patients in each treatment group (bracket = median remission lengths in months)*			
				BCG	*BCG + cells*	*No treatment*	*Metho-trexate*
Mathé	24	No	Pasteur	—	20 (7)	10 (2)	—
MRC	5½	No	Glaxo	50 (6)	—	18 (4)	53 (14)
Heyns	3½	No	Chicago	34 (4)	—	31 (4)	285* (8)
,,	11½	No	Chicago	44 (5)	—	52 (6)	57 (14)
Poplack	—	Yes	Pasteur	—	21	—	35

* Patients in this arm still in remission after 8 months further randomized into study below

to test his claim. It can be seen that Mathé's study only included patients who had already been on chemotherapy and in remission for 2 years and this may be a factor in selecting patients with less residual leukaemia than in the other two studies. Animal studies show that immunotherapy is only effective if the mass is very small and recent chemotherapy programmes[14] confirm that chemotherapy of less than 2 years is associated with very early relapse, presumably due to a large number of remaining leukaemia cells. However, this is not the whole answer, because although the control arms in the British and American studies relapsed very quickly (Table 1.1) so did those in Mathé's control arm (median remission duration of the 10 patients was 2 months after 2 years of chemotherapy). Other factors that may be important in explaining the variance between Mathé and the other groups is that the BCG was different for the three studies, and Mathé used cells in addition to BCG for some (and ultimately all) of his patients. Clearly failure to irradiate prophylactically the central nervous system (CNS) is something that should not be allowed to influence possible future studies although careful inspection of the Heyn's Group A and MRC results do not suggest this factor unfavourably biased the results against a possible therapeutic effect of BCG. Many of these objections could have been clarified by a study from the Bethesda group[15] in which Pasteur BCG and (live) allogeneic leukaemia cells were used for immunotherapy for 21 children with chemotherapy-induced remission (including CNS prophylaxis—see Table 1.1). The immunotherapy was given for 2-month periods interspersed with 4 months of chemotherapy and the whole cycle was repeated. Alas, the 35 patients in the control arm were given methotrexate instead of no treatment during the corresponding 2-month period when the treatment group was being immunized. Both arms were indistinguishable for length of first remission and thus a definitive conclusion about the usefulness of immunotherapy in this study is impossible; either immunotherapy is as effective as methotrexate for maintaining remission, or both treatments give no benefit at all.

In a non-randomized study the Houston Group[16] have used Pasteur BCG for the maintenance of remission of all forms of adult leukaemia, and although they report benefit with acute myelogenous leukaemia (see below) there was no evidence that Pasteur BCG prolonged remission in ALL. However, the number of patients studied was small and this was a sequential series of patients using historical controls and is thus open to some criticism. In the related disease Burkitt's lymphoma, Ziegler[17] used Pasteur BCG given to the patients by scarification for 10 weeks after cyclophosphamide induced remission. He reports that 11 of the 21 BCG-treated patients have relapsed which is no different from 11 of the 19 control patients. However, it is always difficult to evaluate negative studies particularly involving small numbers of patients having a disease with many staging parameters. For example, six of the 11 patients that relapsed in the BCG group did so in the CNS compared with only one of the 11 patients in the control group and although this was attributed to an imbalance of the distribution of stage B patients in the original randomization it nevertheless detracts from the significance of the data. It is probably futile to attempt to draw any conclusions from this study concerning BCG, one way or the other.

At present the place of immunotherapy alone for the maintenance of remission in ALL must remain speculative since only Mathé has reported a therapeutic effect and no other study has done exactly as he did in giving Pasteur BCG and cells after two years of chemotherapy. It seems unlikely that it is at present necessary to use immunotherapy alone as the primary method of treatment for ALL in the face of the outstanding results produced by intensive combination chemotherapy with prophylactic treatment of the CNS as developed by Pinkel and his colleagues[14], but the possibility of chemoimmunotherapy as used in adult myelogenous leukaemia deserves careful consideration in properly controlled studies and this has yet to be done.

ACUTE MYELOGENOUS LEUKAEMIA

The Barts/Marsden Study

Towards the end of 1969 recent improvements in chemotherapy had allowed approximately half of all patients with acute myelogenous leukaemia to achieve complete remission[18], but chemotherapy alone was proving disappointing for maintaining these remissions. In consequence a combined study was initiated between St Bartholomew's Hospital in London and The Royal Marsden Hospital, Sutton, Surrey, to see if remission lengths and survival could be increased when immunotherapy was included as part of the remission treatment. In this study remission patients with AML were randomized into two groups, one group receiving chemotherapy alone for the maintenance of remission and the other group receiving the same chemotherapy plus immunotherapy. Any difference between these two groups was attributable only to the immunotherapy. The maintenance chemotherapy was chosen to avoid immunosuppression as far as possible. Laboratory studies had shown that this could be achieved by giving cytotoxic drugs in widely spaced courses of short duration and by avoiding the use of powerfully immunosuppressive agents such as cyclophosphamide. The immunotherapy given was irradiated allogeneic stored myeloblastic leukaemia cells and BCG. Animal data had suggested that BCG and cells given in combination produce a stronger immunotherapeutic response than that seen with either alone[19].

Because of the extremely troublesome logistic problems raised by attempting to include cells as active specific immunotherapy in a therapeutic programme we decided to conduct some preliminary experimental studies to determine if we might expect such treatment to be beneficial. From such studies[20] we learned that the host was able to recognize autologous leukaemia cells as foreign *in vitro* if cultures were set up in a manner similar to the mixed lymphocyte reaction, i.e. in these experiments we found that remission lymphocytes were transformed in the presence of killed autologous leukaemia cells taken when the patient first presented and cryopreserved in a viable state. If, however, remission marrow (not containing leukaemia cells) was handled in a similar manner, then no such stimulation occurred and we concluded that there was something on the surface of the leukaemia cells that behaved as if it was a leukaemia antigen. In addition we found that this host response to leukaemia cells *in vitro* could be enhanced if the patient was immunized with at least 1×10^8 irradiated autologous leukaemia cells, but this effect was transient and so repeated injections were required to obtain a sustained effect. It thus became apparent that large numbers of cells would need to be available for an effective programme to test the efficacy of active specific immunotherapy. In this aspect we were fortunate that the IBM blood cell separator had become available which was capable of removing very large numbers of leukaemia cells from the circulating blood of untreated acute leukaemia patients in a safe and efficient manner[21]. It was this consideration in fact that led us to concentrate our efforts in clinical immunotherapy on AML because this disease primarily affects adults and the use of separators is very much simpler under these circumstances and between 10^{11} and 10^{12} leukaemia cells (a packed volume of several hundred ml) could be removed from a single patient presenting with a high blood count. Cells removed from the patients at presentation were stored in a viable form by freezing in liquid nitrogen[22,23].

It is worth considering in some detail the exact nature of this study because the interpretation of other studies attempting to confirm or refute the results then becomes clearer.

Patient selection

All patients with AML who were first seen at St Bartholomew's Hospital between 10th August 1970 and 31st December 1973 were included in the study. Analysis was made of the data completed to 7th August 1975. Before any treatment was given to induce remission, all patients were allocated into one of two groups on an alternate basis to determine whether they would receive immunotherapy if they achieved remission. The total entry of new patients was 139, 107 of whom were included in the series described by Powles *et al.*[24], and the rest were seen subsequently. The final allocation of patients who attained full remission was 22 to chemotherapy and 31 patients to chemoimmunotherapy. The two groups do not have equal numbers because they were allocated when they first entered hospital, and the number in each group that attained remission happened not to be the same. Of the 31 patients allocated immunotherapy, three were not included in the analysis. One of these patients died of infection after attaining full remission but before immunotherapy was given; one patient was 74 years old and could not tolerate the repeated journey to and from the hospital, and the third patient passed into remission whilst receiving the immunotherapy, so it was felt she was not representative of the group.

Induction treatment

The induction protocol of drugs (for details see ref. 24) consists of daunorubicin and cytosine arabinoside given in slightly modified ways (Studies 2, 3, 4A and 4B in refs. 18 and 25). Fifty-three patients passed into full remission so that the overall remission rate during the trial period now stands at 38%. All patients in remission in Studies 2, 3 and 4A received identical maintenance chemotherapy, as described by Powles *et al.*[24], which consisted of 5-day courses of cytosine arabinoside and daunorubicin alternating with 5 days of cytosine arabinoside and 6-thioguanine. Between every 5 days of treatment there was a 23-day gap, and it was during this period that patients received immunotherapy. The patients in Study 4B were all aged over 60 years, and their maintenance chemotherapy consisted of 3-day courses every 2 weeks. All patients stopped maintenance chemotherapy after 1 year (12 courses) and thereafter the chemoimmunotherapy patients received only immunotherapy and the chemotherapy patients received no further treatment.

Immunotherapy

Immunotherapy was started whenever possible just before complete remission, at a time when the marrow was hypoplastic. In all instances, subsequent marrow biopsies confirmed that these patients had achieved a full remission. The immunotherapy, described in detail previously[24], consisted of weekly BCG (Glaxo) and 10^9 irradiated allogeneic myeloblastic leukaemia cells given i.d. and s.c., and timed to avoid the 5-day courses of chemotherapy. All four limbs received the BCG in turn, once weekly, and the cells were injected into the other three limbs. Individual patients received cells from the same donor for as long as possible.

Treatment after relapse

When patients relapsed, the initial induction treatment with daunorubicin and cytosine arabinoside was repeated whenever possible. If no regression of leukaemia was seen, the treatment was usually changed to a combination of cyclophosphamide and 6-thioguanine. If remission occurred, the maintenance treatment was modified to a single injection of daunorubicin and 3 days of cytosine arabinoside followed 11 days later by 3 days of oral cyclophosphamide and 6-thioguanine. After another 11-day gap the whole cycle was repeated, with maintenance chemotherapy for 3 days every fortnight. Those patients who previously received immunotherapy were given further treatment with BCG and a different population of irradiated AML cells.

Results of the Barts/Marsden Study (As reported by Powles *et al.*[26])

At the time of analysis (August 1975) five of 28 patients in the chemo-immunotherapy arm remained alive, although four of these had relapsed; two of 22 patients on chemotherapy were alive, both still in their first

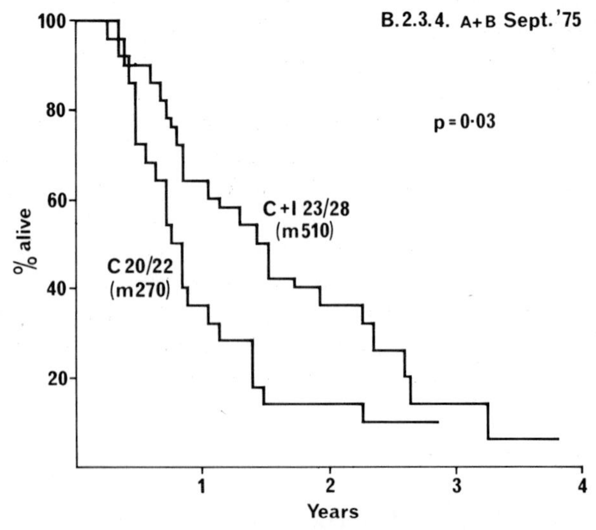

Figure 1.2 Survival following remission of two groups of patients with AML (Barts/Marsden Trial) allocated at presentation: one group receiving maintenance chemotherapy alone (C), the other group chemotherapy plus immunotherapy (C+I). The percentage surviving at different times has been calculated by standard actuarial methods, m = median survival in days. Difference between curves has $p = 0.03$

remission. The actuarial analysis of the duration of survival of these patients after attaining remission is given in Figure 1.2. The median duration of survival of the chemotherapy group is 270 days, and that for the chemo-immunotherapy group 510 days. Statistical analysis of survival data calculated by the 'logrank' non-parametric method[27] gives an overall chi-squared for the differences between these two groups of 4.48; $p = 0.03$. One of the three immunotherapy patients excluded from the analysis died in remission at Day 0, prior to immunotherapy, and the other two patients remained alive at the time of analysis at 465 and 655 days. Their exclusion therefore does not materially affect the analysis.

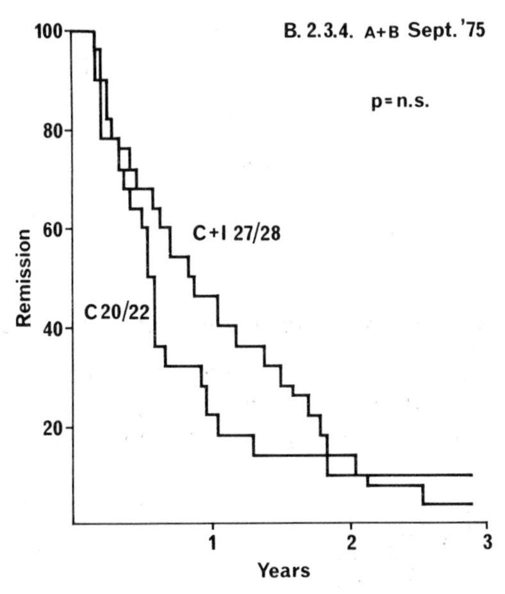

Figure 1.3 Similar analysis to Figure 1.2 of the duration of first remission of the same patients. The difference in length of remission has no statistical significance

Figure 1.3 shows the actuarial analysis for the length of first remission, the median durations being 305 days for the chemoimmunotherapy group and 191 days for the chemotherapy group. However, the overall difference between the two groups was not statistically significant at the 5% level.

The actuarial analysis of the length of survival after relapse for the two groups of patients is shown in Figure 1.4. The median values are 75 days for the chemotherapy patients and 165 days for the chemoimmunotherapy patients, and the difference between the two groups has a very high statistical significance (overall chi-square = 12.24; $p = 0.0005$). One-third of the patients in the chemoimmunotherapy group achieved a second remission, and those who did not receive a full second remission had a prolonged survival when compared with the chemotherapy controls.

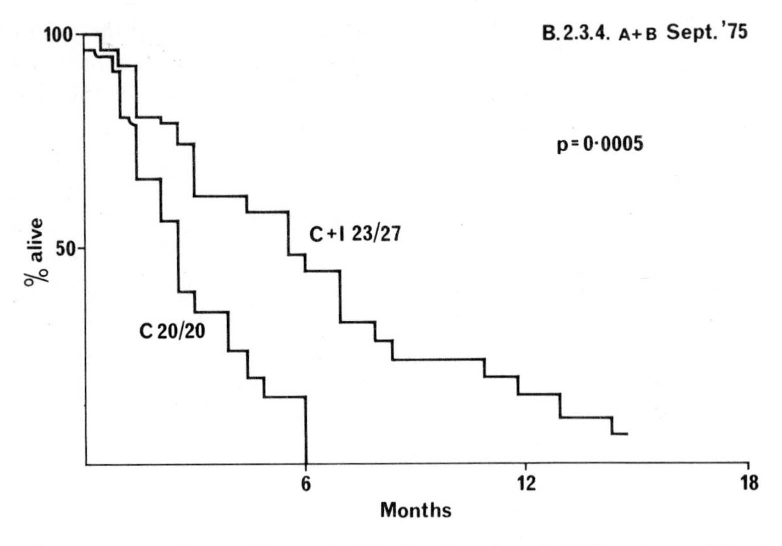

Figure 1.4 Similar analysis to Figure 1.2 of the duration of survival after relapse of the relapse patients shown in Figure 1.3. Difference in survival has $p = 0.0005$

Values and limitations of actuarial analysis of an ongoing trial

The data from this study were analysed at 6-monthly intervals starting in May 1972 (i.e. 18 months after the trial was initiated). The survival of the chemoimmunotherapy group is plotted as raw data without actuarial

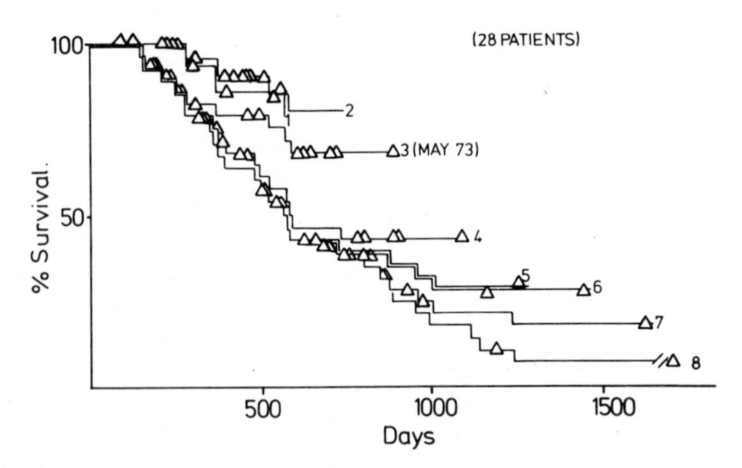

Figure 1.5 Sequential 6-monthly standard fixed interval analysis of the duration of survival (from diagnosis) of the patients in the Barts/Marsden AML trial receiving chemoimmunotherapy. The first analysis (Curve 1) was in May 1972, Curve 3 (May 1973) corresponds to the entry of the last patient in the group, and Curves 4 to 8 are analyses at 6-monthly intervals thereafter. Triangles denote patients remaining alive

correction (i.e. fixed interval) in Figure 1.5 and after actuarial correction in Figure 1.6. Only the actuarial method predicted the median survival. Thus, 6 months before the trial was completed (Curve 2, Figure 1.6) at a time when 80% of the patients were still alive and new patients were still being admitted, the median was accurately predicted. However, it required another 1 year after completion of the study (Curve 5, Figure 1.6) before it became certain, even with actuarial analysis, that the inclusion of immunotherapy in the treatment regime did not lead to a significant deviation of the survival curves from the constant risk pattern in which all patients ultimately die of their disease: i.e. the treatment had not given rise to a subpopulation of patients who had become long-term survivors. Initially the actuarially corrected curves indicated a tail and the possibility of long-term survivors (Curves 3 and 4, Figure 1.6). As time went on, it became clear that the

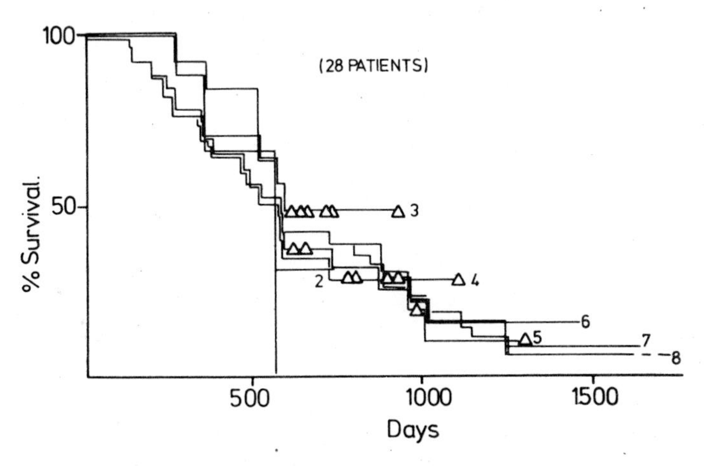

Figure 1.6 Similar analysis to Figure 1.5 for the same data except the standard actuarial method has been used

fraction of patients with the tail progressively decreased (Curves 6–8, Figure 1.6). We must now conclude that while immunotherapy increases the median length of survival by approximately 90%, it does not change the ultimate shape of the survival curve, which is the same for both treatment methods, and indicates that fewer than 5% of patients with AML treated by either of the two procedures in this trial are going to be long-term survivors. Currently (July 1976) only one chemoimmunotherapy and two chemotherapy patients remain alive. Thus, while actuarial analysis reliably predicted the median duration of survival, it did not show whether or not long-term survival was probable for a subpopulation until long after the study was completed. This point will be further discussed in connection with other more recent studies.

Attempts at confirming the Barts/Marsden Study (see Table 1.2)

The encouraging preliminary results of the Barts/Marsden Trial indicated the need for a randomized trial duplicating this study on a larger scale and this was undertaken by the Medical Research Council's Working Party on leukaemia in adults in the United Kingdom which consists of a multicentred group of physicians dealing with this form of leukaemia. When this study was commenced in 1973, there were only three centres in Britain independent of the Barts/Marsden combination with facilities for handling the leukaemia cells for immunotherapy. One of these groups (Manchester) already had some experience of immunotherapy and wanted to randomize their patients between immunotherapy alone and chemotherapy plus immunotherapy. Thus the true MRC study to confirm the Barts/Marsden Study consisted of patients distributed between only two centres, Oxford and Hammersmith, and although a group of six hospitals in the Birmingham region joined in the study from 1974, the total number of AML patients randomized in full remission was unfortunately much smaller than had initially been predicted. Thus, between 1st January 1973 and 30th June 1976, the period during which patients were admitted to this study, 71 patients entered complete remission and were allocated at random to receive maintenance therapy of either chemotherapy alone (24 patients) or chemotherapy with immunotherapy (47 patients). The results of this study were first reported at the Washington immunotherapy meeting in 1976[28] and in terms of remission length the immunotherapy patients fared slightly better than those not receiving such treatment. This difference, like the Barts/Marsden Study, was not significant whether tested directly or after retrospective stratification for the two centres. Likewise, the overall survival curves from the onset of remission for the two groups of patients, although appearing to be consistently better for the immunotherapy group, were nevertheless not statistically secure when tested with the 'logrank' method of analysis. As with the Barts/Marsden Study, by far the most impressive part of the MRC trial was prolongation of survival after relapse. As of September 1976 only 36 of the 71 patients had so far died and it is obvious from our comments concerning our Barts/Marsden Study that definitive conclusions from this trial are not yet possible. However, although it is unlikely that the two curves for the survival after relapse can change markedly as 57 patients had already relapsed, the significance of the difference between the two curves could lie anywhere between the 3% and 10% level.

When comparing the MRC and Barts/Marsden Studies there were some minor differences that need to be considered; in the MRC Study allocation was made randomly at the time when patients were first recorded as having entered remission, whereas in the Barts/Marsden Study they were randomized at presentation and in consequence generally received their immunotherapy earlier during remission at a time when the marrow was hypoplastic.

Table 1.2 Immunotherapy trials for AML

Author	*Duration of initial induction chemotherapy*	*Maintenance chemotherapy*	*BCG used*	*AML cells used*	*Number of patients*		*Duration (weeks)*					
					Chemo-therapy alone	*Chemotherapy plus immunotherapy*	*Remission*		*Survival*		*Survival after relapse*	
							C	C+I	C	C+I	C	C+I
Powles	up to 3/12	yes	Glaxo	irradiated allogeneic	22	28	27	43	39	73	12	23
MRC	up to 3/12	yes	Glaxo	irradiated allogeneic	24	47	21–30	32	44	70	14	22
Reizenstein	up to 3/12	yes	Glaxo	viable allogeneic	14	16	23	36	40	80	—	—
Vogler	at least 5/12	Not during BCG*	Tice (2 × weekly for 4 weeks)	—	33	25	33.5 (13.3)§	40.9 (24.9)§	78.1	93.2	—	—
Hewlett	3/12	OAP	Pasteur Scarified	—	25	20	55	59	74	55+	—	—
Whittaker	3/12	Monthly DNR + ARA-C	Glaxo monthly i.v.	—	19	18	27	34	50	69	—	—
Gutterman‡	3/12	OAP	Pasteur Scarified	—	33	20	50‡	91†	—	—	—	—

* Those patients not receiving BCG received methotrexate
† Sequential study with historical controls
‡ Results 1974
§ From start of immunotherapy

It would appear in consequence that the MRC patients received their immunotherapy 1–4 weeks later than those in the Barts/Marsden Trial and because the definition of remission was a fully cellular marrow and following this a further consolidation course of chemotherapy was given, it might seem that the MRC patients received a more complete induction chemotherapy programme. Other differences between the two studies were that in the MRC Trial bone marrows were examined every month as a routine and relapse was considered when the blast cells rose above 5%, whereas in the Barts/Marsden Study relapse was diagnosed either clinically or when the blood counts began to fall and bone marrow was then used to either confirm or refute the presence of relapse. Further differences were that the MRC Trial included only patients over the age of 19 and undifferentiated leukaemias were also included in the study. Lastly, the randomization in the MRC Trial was adjusted so that twice as many patients were allocated to receive chemotherapy plus immunotherapy rather than chemotherapy as this was hoped to produce the most significant results with the number of patients available. However, in view of only two centres being involved in this study it would now seem more likely that a meaningful result would have been obtained had the distribution been even. This is reinforced by the observation that the 28 chemotherapy-alone patients at other MRC centres who were included in the overall trial (not the control part) and received identical chemotherapy to that given in the control trial were found to die more quickly after relapse than either of the two groups in the randomized study. Overall this reinforces the suggestion that immunotherapy prolongs survival after relapse but obviously the non-randomized comparison should be emphasized.

The Swedish/Austrian Study

The other study to attempt to repeat the Barts/Marsden Study is that by the Swedish group[29]. This study was a combined attempt between a group in Austria and several centres in Sweden. Unfortunately, although many patients were included in this investigation the truly comparative part, which was conducted in Sweden, had only 16 patients in the immunotherapy arm compared with 14 in the control group. The results showed that remission was prolonged by immunotherapy and survival was significantly improved with a doubling of survival time from 40 to 80 weeks. Nevertheless, once again the most important contribution caused by the immunotherapy was prolongation of survival after relapse.

An important variation in this study when compared with that conducted by the Barts/Marsden Group was that live rather than irradiated cells were used for the immunization because of logistic difficulties in obtaining a suitable radiation source. As with the MRC Trial time will need to elapse before the full significance of these results can be interpreted.

THE MECHANISM OF ACTION OF THE IMMUNOTHERAPY

The mechanism of action in these three studies is obscure because for technical reasons it has not been possible to measure the immune reaction of the host directed against the TSTA of AML although tests employing the mixed leukocyte reaction[20,30] indicate that immunization with leukaemia cells increases the ability of AML patients to recognize their own leukaemia cells (which have been kept stored). Two possible mechanisms deserve consideration; the first is an increased immune reaction to TSTAs produced by administration of cells which would account for the prolongation of first remission, and it is not difficult to see how such a mechanism could be involved in the prolongation of survival after relapse. For example, relapse could occur synchronously in immunized and unimmunized patients due to release of AML cells from sanctuary sites; the disease process would then progress more slowly in those patients with the best host reaction against the tumour. A second mechanism which could produce this prolonged survival of immunized patients after relapse is a non-specific stimulation of the bone marrow which permitted these patients to tolerate the high doses of cytotoxic chemotherapy which were then required. Although such an effect has been seen in animal systems[31,32] and could be effective in man because patients who have relapsed usually die due to bone marrow failure, we now feel this mechanism is not operational in our patients. We have found there is no difference in the blood counts between those patients receiving immunotherapy and those not, and there is no difference in the rate of infection between the two groups of patients. Moreover, in mice which were chronically irradiated, immunotherapy, although doubling the number of surviving stem cells in the marrow, afforded no protection against subsequent lethal chemotherapy.

THE RELATIVE CONTRIBUTION OF BCG AND CELLS TO PROLONGING SURVIVAL

An obvious question concerns the relative importance of the BCG and cells and to answer this would require three arms to a trial, i.e. chemotherapy alone, chemotherapy plus BCG, and chemotherapy plus BCG plus cells. This was not possible in our initial study because of the limited number of patients available.

The use of BCG alone without cells for treating patients with AML has been tried by four groups (Table 1.2). The first study was reported initially in 1974[33] when it was seen that patients who had their maintenance chemotherapy stopped after about 5 months of remission and were given Tice BCG twice weekly for 4 weeks and then were put back on chemotherapy, maintained longer remissions than those patients who were given methotrexate instead. However, there are several points difficult to understand in this study. Firstly, only 58 of 351 patients ever reached the maintenance part of the study, secondly the controlled section of the study compared immunotherapy *with* chemotherapy and as has been mentioned

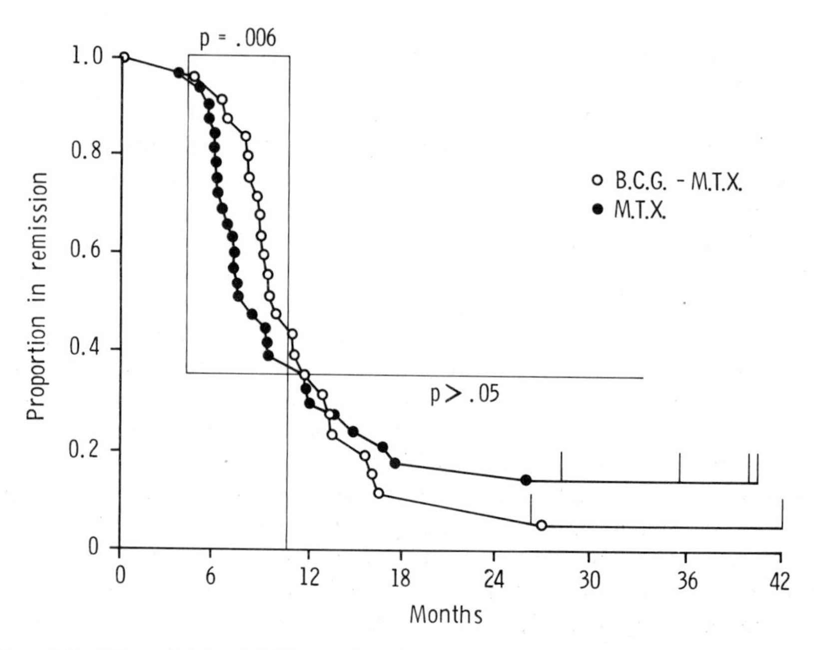

Figure 1.7 Effect of giving BCG intermittently on length of remission of patients with AML (Vogler)

above this is not an interpretable comparison; and lastly in Figure 1.7[34] it can be seen the curves cross over at 10 months and so the statistical interpretation of this must be fraught with hazard. The data concerning survival of patients after relapse is not yet available.

Following this study the Houston Group[16] suggested there was a distinct benefit from the use of immunotherapy in maintaining adult patients with acute leukaemia. This study consisted of 20 consecutive patients who received intermittent chemotherapy (cytarabine, vincristine and prednisolone = OAP) and liquid Pasteur BCG administered weekly by scarification. The duration of remission of these patients was compared with those of a previous group of 33 consecutive patients maintained on OAP alone. Eleven of the 20 OAP plus BCG treated patients remained in remission with an estimated median duration of 91 weeks whereas only 14 of the 33 patients maintained on OAP remained in remission with a median duration of 50 weeks.

Alas, although these results were said to show a significant effect on remission length, subsequent analysis[35] shows this difference to be no longer significant and highlights the pitfalls of using historical controls. When sufficient time has elapsed to rectify the bias of historical controls upon survival data in this study it will be of interest to examine the effect of this immunotherapy programme on survival after relapse.

A more recent study[36] in the same geographical area as the Houston Group (South-west Co-operative Group) attempted to repeat the Gutterman study using OAP and Pasteur BCG but they used randomized controls rather than historically collected patients. Their results, shown in Table 1.2 and published recently[36], showed no advantage for remission length, survival (and presumably survival after relapse) for patients who received BCG in addition to OAP rather than those who received OAP alone.

The fourth of the BCG alone studies for AML has involved giving intravenous BCG to remission patients in conjunction with maintenance chemotherapy[37] (Table 1.2). Although remission length appears to be longer for the 18 patients who received BCG and chemotherapy than for the 19 patients who received only chemotherapy (Figure 1.8), the greatest and most significant effect is upon survival (Figure 1.9) ($p = 0.02$) and we must conclude

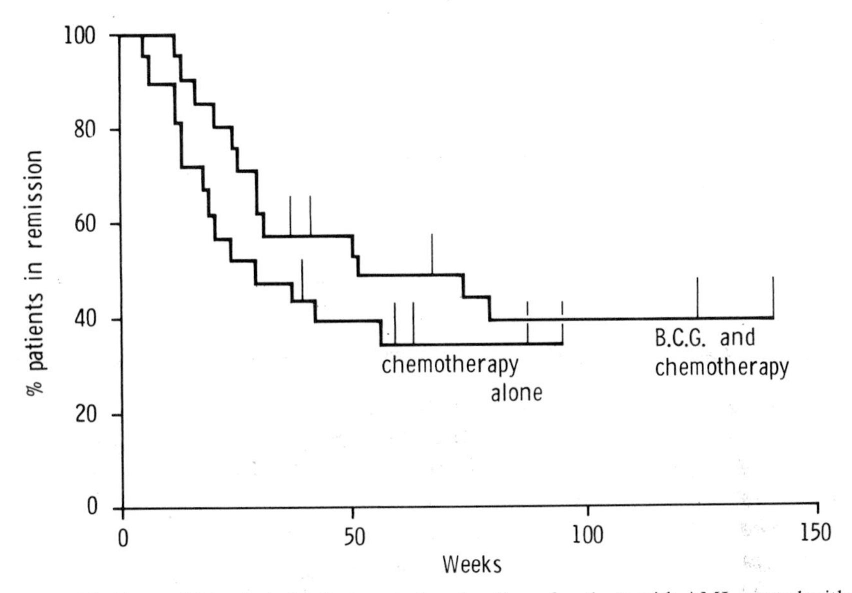

Figure 1.8 Actuarial analysis for first remission duration of patients with AML treated with intravenous BCG (Whittaker)

that this study has produced an effect very similar to that seen in the original Barts/Marsden Study.

Summarizing the seven studies in AML so far described, in all three studies where patients received BCG and cells there was a therapeutic effect seen whereby survival was prolonged, and the major contributory factor to this was prolongation of survival after relapse. In the four studies using BCG alone, only one[37] shows a convincing therapeutic effect and again this was similar to the BCG and cell studies. It must be concluded that the observation that immunotherapy prolongs survival after relapse in patients with AML is a real effect and it seems probable that cells and BCG are better for gaining this effect than BCG alone.

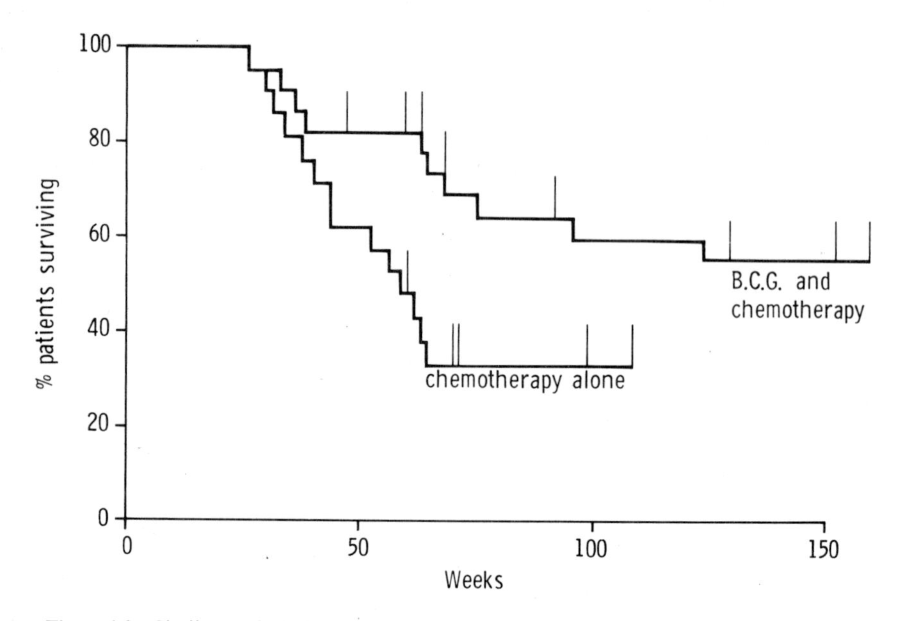

Figure 1.9 Similar analysis for survival of same patients shown in Figure 1.8 (Whittaker)

FURTHER MARSDEN STUDIES OF IMMUNOTHERAPY FOR AML

Our early studies of immunotherapy were conducted on patients given their induction chemotherapy at St Bartholomew's Hospital and then given their immunotherapy at the Royal Marsden Hospital. This arrangement was developed because large numbers of untreated patients were referred to St Bartholomew's Hospital because of the presence of Professor Hamilton Fairley and the central location of the place. However, the Marsden Hospital, which is 16 miles from the centre of London, was better geared for the complicated experimental nature of the treatment, and so patients, once they were in remission, were then immunized at the Royal Marsden Hospital in Sutton, Surrey. As the Leukaemia Unit at the Marsden Hospital developed in its own right, more patients were referred and it was possible to conduct uncontrolled pilot studies in which patients were treated only at this hospital. Starting in 1970 a group of nine consecutive patients in remission were given immunotherapy alone, as in the Barts/Marsden Study, but without maintenance chemotherapy. This study finished in 1972 and the patients were subsequently found to have fared extremely well, an event that often occurs with small pilot studies. The median survival of the whole group was 83 weeks and two patients remain alive at the time of writing[38,39].

This led us to set up a study for the use of immunotherapy for maintaining remission in patients with AML without chemotherapy, but in this instance patients would receive live rather than irradiated cells because it appeared this was more effective in animal studies and the results of the previous two studies made it ethically justifiable. Ultimately, 22 consecutive remission patients were included in this study[40] and although they fared well in spite of receiving no chemotherapy for maintenance, they unfortunately were seen to have no subgroup of cured patients and all ultimately relapsed and died, i.e. they had the constant risk distribution for survival seen in all previous studies. Although this study was not controlled it was clear that, because all patients ultimately died, we could abandon this new method of immunotherapy because we were looking for a treatment that would produce some cured patients.

By the beginning of 1974 we were receiving enough patients at the Marsden Hospital to set up a properly controlled clinical trial (designated title BF3) for immunotherapy given to patients in remission in an attempt to obtain a small group of patients who were long remitters, rather than attempting to prolong median remission length. The exact type of immunotherapy we elected to test was a method based on related work in melanoma patients[41] in which it had been shown that, by using cells mixed with BCG injected intradermally, antitumour immunity was stimulated more effectively than the injection of tumour cells alone. Since BCG and cells given in this way produce skin ulceration we felt that a mixture of BCG and cells could only be given a few times. Thus, in this particular Marsden Study, all AML patients in remission received the same immunotherapy as used in the original Barts/Marsden Study (but without intermittent chemotherapy), and in addition half the patients allocated on an alternate basis were injected with cells mixed with BCG on four separate occasions, early in the course of their first remission. The last patient was entered into this study more than 18 months ago and the results are only reported now to obviate the problems of interpreting survival analysis with inadequate follow-up as mentioned above.

It is worth going into this study in some detail as it opens up many important points for discussion.

PROCEDURE FOR MARSDEN (BF3) STUDY

Patients

Sixty-two patients entered the study between March 1974 and December 1975. They received an infusion of cytosine arabinoside (10 mg/kg) over a period of 24 h; this was immediately followed by an injection of daunorubicin (1.5 mg/kg) and 24 h later by an injection of adriamycin (1.5 mg/kg). This course was repeated 2 weeks later and after a further 2 weeks, three short courses of cytosine arabinoside (2 mg/kg) and 6-thioguanine (2 mg/kg) were given daily for 3 days, 4 days and 5 days respectively with a 5-day gap between each course. Two weeks later cyclophosphamide (2 mg/kg orally daily) was given for 5 days followed by a single dose of daunorubicin (1.5 mg/kg). Those patients who achieved remission usually did so during the first month of this treatment but some remitted on the cytosine arabinoside and 6-thioguanine courses. Thirty patients who achieved a complete remission were available for study. Remission was defined as a cellular marrow with no atypical blast cells present (i.e. less than 1%).

Immunotherapy

All patients received immunotherapy weekly as in the initial Barts/Marsden Study but unlike this earlier study no maintenance chemotherapy was given. Immunotherapy consisted of weekly injections of between 10^8 and 10^9 irradiated allogeneic AML cells which had been collected with a blood cell separator and stored in liquid nitrogen. A single population of cells was used each week for each immunization and any one patient received in rotation four different populations of cells. The contents of a lyophilized ampoule of Glaxo percutaneous BCG was made up to 0.6 ml with distilled water, smeared on the skin and 20 needle punctures to 2 mm were made using a Heaf gun. The estimated dose of BCG was about 10^6 live organisms. One limb received the BCG whilst the other three limbs received the cells. Immunotherapy was given immediately remission had been achieved and frequently this was before or during the three courses of cytosine arabinoside and 6-thioguanine. Those patients allocated to receive cells and BCG mixed together were given four intradermal injections 2 inches apart on each of four occasions. The first of the injections was given 3 weeks after the completion of the cyclophosphamide and daunorubicin and was given instead of the standard immunotherapy. The mixture of BCG and cells was prepared as follows: one ampoule of percutaneous Glaxo BCG was made up to 40 ml and 0.2 ml of this suspension was mixed with 0.6 ml of a suspension of 5×10^7 allogeneic killed AML cells. 0.2 ml of the mixture was injected intradermally into four sites (i.e. approximately 10^6 live BCG organisms and 10^7 AML cells were injected at each site). Three weeks later during which weekly 'standard' immunotherapy was given, a further injection of the mixture was administered, this time in a different limb, and the BCG was diluted a further four times. After another three weeks the third limb was injected but the amount of BCG in the mixture was reduced a further four-fold and 3 weeks after this the last limb was injected with an amount of BCG further reduced by a factor of 4. These increasing dilutions of BCG were given because unacceptable ulceration occurred if the same dose of BCG was given intradermally on subsequent immunizations, presumably due to BCG sensitization. After the fourth injection of cells and BCG mixed together (approximately 3 months after stopping chemotherapy) the patients were maintained on the 'standard' immunotherapy only. Approximately 30% of the patients who received inoculations of BCG and cells mixed together developed ulcers at the site of the inoculation and these could last for as long as 3 to 4 months before healing. The toxicity of the 'standard' immunotherapy was the same as previously described.

Results of the Marsden (BF3) Study

Analysis of the data was performed on 1st August 1977, over 18 months after entry of the last patient to the study[42]. Four patients remain in remission in the group receiving the mixture of BCG and cells and form a plateau at the end of the curve relating the proportion of patients in remission to remission duration; all four have been in remission for longer

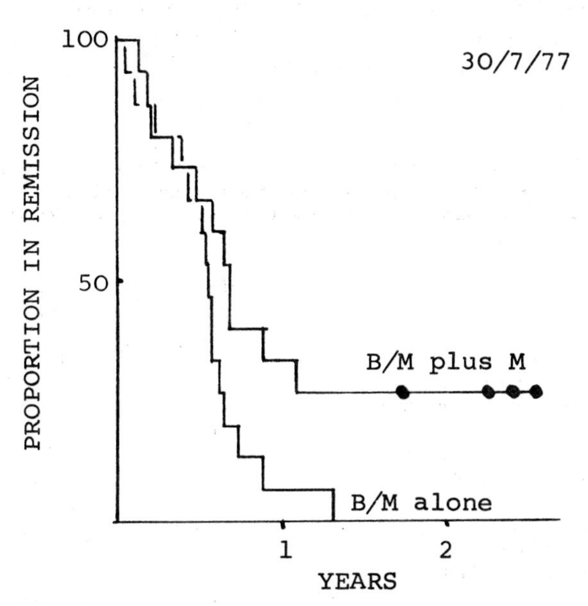

Figure 1.10 The effect of introducing immunization with a mixture of allogeneic leukaemia cells and BCG on length of survival after achieving remission of patients with AML.

Thirty patients who had achieved a complete clinical remission were randomized into two groups of 15 for the following maintenance treatments:

Group 1: Received weekly immunotherapy according to the Barts/Marsden Trial protocol (i.e. irradiated allogeneic leukaemia cells and BCG into a separate site (BM alone)

Group 2: Had the same treatment as Group 1 but received in addition during the first 4 months of their remission treatment four inoculations at monthly intervals of 10^9 irradiated allogeneic cells mixed with 100 μg of BCG (BM plus M)

than 92 weeks (Figure 1.10). None of the patients in the group who received 'standard' immunotherapy remains in remission (maximum length of remission 68 weeks). The median remission durations are 35 weeks for the patients receiving admixed BCG and cells, and 29 weeks for the group who received 'standard' immunotherapy only. Specific analysis shows that the distribution of factors likely to influence prognosis between the two groups of patients was not markedly uneven with the exception of sex and diagnosis. But, while there were more patients of pure myeloblastic type in the group receiving the admixture than in the group receiving 'standard' immunotherapy only, analysis of remission duration by diagnosis (ignoring treatment group) yields no evidence that this contributes to improved remission duration for patients receiving the mixture; indeed, the median remission duration was poorer for patients with the pure myeloblastic type disease. The same is true for female patients, although all four patients remaining in remission are female.

The median survival of the patients who received the mixture was somewhat better than that of those who received the 'standard' immunotherapy only, but this was due almost entirely to the prolongation of remission. In the earlier Barts/Marsden Study 'standard' immunotherapy was found to extend length of survival after relapse but in this investigation both groups had, of course, received 'standard' immunotherapy.

Table 1.3 Median remission length, survival from diagnosis and survival after relapse (in weeks) for those patients receiving 'standard' immunotherapy (B/M) plus the mixture, and those patients receiving 'standard' immunotherapy (B/M) alone

	B/M plus mixture	*B/M alone*
Total number of patients	15	15
Number of patients in remission for more than 92 weeks	4	0
Number of relapsed patients	11	15
Number of dead patients	11	14
Median duration survival from diagnosis	73 weeks	56 weeks*
Median duration remission	35 ,,	29 ,,
Median survival after relapse	15 ,,	17 ,,

* This figure cannot be compared with that reported in the earlier study (1) in which the immunotherapy group also received chemotherapy during remission

Table 1.3 summarizes the median remission, survival and relapse durations for the two groups. While the median remission duration of the group receiving the mixture is greater than that for the group receiving only 'standard' immunotherapy, comparison by means of a 'logrank' test[27], though based on small numbers of patients, suggests that the difference is not significant ($p =$ approximately 0.07). The interpretation of the plateau in Figure 1.10 is discussed below.

Interpretation of the results of the Marsden (BF3) Study

Although the Barts/Marsden Study demonstrated that survival of patients with AML was prolonged by adding 'standard' immunotherapy to maintenance chemotherapy during remission, the overall results were disappointing in that there was no statistically secure prolongation of remission length for these patients, an effect that would show that a host mechanism had been induced which is capable of killing leukaemia cells remaining after induction chemotherapy. In this (and all other) studies of AML immunotherapy all patients ultimately relapsed and died of their disease and the death rate followed a constant risk distribution as described above (although the medians varied). Thus there was not a plateau of long-term remitters who might be considered 'cured'.

At present there is no evidence that intensive maintenance chemotherapy differs in its biological effect from the types of immunotherapy studied[43] and although there is variation of the median duration of remission between treatment groups there appears to be no alteration of the constant risk distribution in which all patients may be expected to succumb to their disease. Consequently, we felt justified in testing a form of immunotherapy which might be more effective than that previously used but which was also more toxic. Because maintenance chemotherapy has not so far produced a plateau of long-term survivors, it was decided not to give maintenance chemotherapy and to employ immunotherapy as the only treatment during remission. The study compared the procedure referred to as 'standard immunotherapy', which had been used in the original Barts/Marsden Study with a regimen which included a novel type of immunotherapy in which cells in admixture with BCG were injected intradermally in addition to 'standard' immunotherapy.

The addition of mixed cells and BCG slightly extended the median duration of remissions and survival but with the small numbers of patients in each arm these differences are not statistically significant when analysed by, for example, the 'logrank' method. Nonetheless, Figure 1.10 reveals a difference in that four of the 15 patients who received the new type of immunotherapy are still in remission (i.e. their remission lengths exceed 92 weeks) while none of the 15 patients who were maintained on 'standard' immunotherapy remains in remission (the maximum remission duration being 68 weeks). This finding leads us to wonder whether the new immunotherapy regimen has genuinely benefited a subgroup of patients (i.e. four out of 15 or 27%) and has produced a true change in the shape of the survival curve so that it is no longer of the constant risk pattern. Alternatively, the present observation that the four patients in long remission are all in the one arm of the study could be a chance event. If the two types of treatments were equally effective then the chance that four of the 30 patients who are long-term remitters will be drawn from the group receiving the mixture is approximately one in 20. This level of significance obviously does not permit a claim that the modified immunotherapy regimen has altered the prognosis of a subgroup of patients with AML. However, a chance of 1:20 clearly justifies testing this procedure in a bigger and more extensive trial and our centre is currently undertaking such an investigation.

Even if it were accepted that the new immunotherapy regimen benefits a fraction of AML patients, we must stress that as yet we can have no indication whether the patients making up such a subgroup are 'cured' or whether the remission is merely prolonged. The problems of using median durations of remission length and life table analysis (with or without 'logrank' analyses) to help recognize and determine the significance of subpopulations of 'cured' patients within treatment groups have already been discussed above[44]. Should a larger study provide a higher level of statistical significance for the presence of a plateau of remission following the modified immunotherapy protocol, then predictive statistical methods perhaps based on assumptions of particular survival distributions[45] may provide the earliest possible indication of the existence of a subgroup of patients who are 'cured'.

OTHER METHODS OF IMMUNOTHERAPY FOR AML

Variations of methods for immunotherapy are now becoming numerous throughout the world and there are under way several excellent studies testing some of the more ambitious approaches. For example, there is evidence to suggest that after sialic acid has been removed from tumour cells using neuraminidase they become more immunogenic[46]. A controlled trial is now under way[47] in which cells so treated are used for immunotherapy, and although some of these patients also received methanol extract residue of BCG (MER) it would appear that the therapeutic effect seen is predominantly upon survival and due largely to the cells. A separate study by Leukaemia Study Group B[48], involving some of the workers in the neuraminidase study, describes over 100 patients in remission, all of whom received maintenance chemotherapy, but 57 of whom also received immunotherapy with MER. Preliminary results suggest those patients receiving the MER have longer remissions than the controls.

Another attempt to increase the specific antigenicity of the immunizing cells comes from the Swiss Group recently reported by Sauter *et al.*[49]. Augmentation of the immunogenicity of tumour-associated antigens by infection with viruses has been claimed by several laboratories[50,51] and an avian influenza A virus (FPV) has been found to be a suitable virus for use with AML cells[52]. In this study 44 patients were randomized to two maintenance arms, 22 for monthly chemotherapy and 22 for monthly chemotherapy plus virus-treated cells. The authors found no difference between the two groups for remission duration and survival, and this study has an average follow-up of 13.5 months.

Two recent studies have attempted to boost the immune system by methods other than cells or BCG. The first of these is from the Sloan-Kettering Institute[53] and follows fascinating observations on a group of untreated AML patients given a vaccine to protect them against *Pseudomonas* infections prior to induction chemotherapy. This study was conducted 8 years ago and in 16 of these patients who subsequently passed into remission, retrospective analysis showed that eight of them became long-term survivors seemingly on a plateau of survival. This group now has a controlled prospective study under way with 25 remission patients already included and it is hoped it will not be long before this mode of treatment can be properly assessed.

The other study not using BCG or cells follows the demonstration in animals that synthetic double-stranded RNA is capable of inducing interferon production and can thus act as a potent immunological adjuvant[54,55]. A pilot study of Poly IC in AML (using historical controls) suggested that some benefit may accrue from this form of treatment[56] so a Leukaemia Study Group B[57] programme has been initiated whereby 20 patients with AML in remission were given a single dose of Poly IC 1 week prior to their third monthly maintenance chemotherapy treatment and their subsequent clinical progress was compared with 35 concurrent control chemotherapy patients. There was no difference between the two groups for remission duration and survival in spite of the Poly IC patients having demonstrably produced interferon.

IMMUNOTHERAPY FOR AML PATIENTS WITH ACTIVE DISEASE

The possibility of treating AML patients whilst they still have detectable disease has also been explored. In a preliminary study Hamilton Fairley[58] collected all patients with acute myelogenous leukaemia who have been admitted to St Bartholomew's Hospital in London in recent years and who were alive three months after starting chemotherapy, regardless of whether they were in remission or not.

The survival data of these patients show that patients given immunotherapy as part of their maintenance survive significantly longer than those receiving only chemotherapy; indeed it made little difference to survival whether the patient is in so-called 'complete remission' or only in partial remission more than 4 months from the onset of treatment. Patients not in complete remission, who had immunotherapy, fared better than those in complete remission who only had chemotherapy. Eleven patients who were not in complete remission more than 4 months after the onset of treatment were given the adjuvant form of immunotherapy (i.e. BCG mixed with allogeneic non-irradiated leukaemia cells) without further chemotherapy. These patients were fit and had only a small number (between 6 and 10%) of blast cells in the marrow. Five patients achieved complete remission from 2 to 6 months after the cessation of chemotherapy and the beginning of the immunotherapy. The duration of these remissions ranged from 6 weeks to 4½ months. This was the first clinical indication of a direct effect of immunotherapy on the malignant cell population.

Three other studies have examined the effect of immunotherapy upon patients either before they enter remission or after they have relapsed. In the study by Guttner[48] described above some patients were given MER prior to passing into remission in an attempt to see if this could influence the remission rate using a standard drug protocol. Of 255 evaluable patients, 25% received MER during induction chemotherapy and of those under 60 years of age 66% obtained complete remission compared with 51% of patients receiving chemotherapy alone. An interesting finding was that 50% of patients receiving MER went into complete remission on their first course of chemotherapy as compared to only 34% of patients receiving chemotherapy alone. The Sloan-Kettering study[53] using *Pseudomonas* vaccine described above is also of interest concerning the effect of immunotherapy upon the results of induction chemotherapy. Twenty-nine patients were randomized, 13 to receive *Pseudomonas aeruginosa* vaccine and 16 to the control group. No difference in remission rate was seen with six of 13 complete remissions in the immunotherapy group and seven of 16 in the control arm. The third study of the effect of immunotherapy upon obtaining chemotherapy remission has been examined by the group reinvestigating the effects of Poly IC upon remission[57] (see above). In this study they also included 51 patients in early relapse, of which 19 received Poly IC (and chemotherapy) and the remaining 32 received only chemotherapy as controls. They found no therapeutic advantage with the use of Poly IC.

NEW BIOLOGICAL APPROACHES TO TREATING AML

Recently there have been several new developments helping to elucidate the biological nature of acute leukaemia. Specific xenogeneic antisera are now available for acute leukaemia cells[59,60] and although this has immediate application for monitoring the disease process, the possibility of using such material for passive serotherapy should be considered as their specificity would overcome many of the problems previously encountered with such methods. Likewise the isolation of RNA sequences in human leukaemia cells[61,62] which appear to have a common identity with Simian RNA virus particles have recently been reported. Once the relevance of these claims to pathogenesis has been established the possibility of an immunological (and/or chemotherapeutic) approach to their presence could be considered. Perhaps the hormone thymosin, effective in rats in bringing about total remission[63], will be found useful when available in larger quantities. However, the most promising procedure at present being explored for the management of acute leukaemia involves the use of allogeneic bone marrow transplantation for some of these patients[64].

Bone marrow transplantation for acute leukaemia

The possibility of 'rescue' of leukaemia patients with a bone marrow graft after deliberately giving sufficient chemotherapy to destroy all their remaining marrow has obvious and sensible appeal because the fatal side-effect of 'excessive' chemotherapy (or total body irradiation) is bone marrow failure. Luckily this 'excessive' drug or X-ray treatment also has the bonus of destroying the immune system of the recipient prior to transplantation, thus making a 'take' of transplanted marrow more likely. Other than the rare instance of an identical twin, the only donors who will not have their marrow rejected even after immunosuppression of the recipient are HLA matched sibs. The Seattle Group[64] have suggested the best conditioning combination is cyclophosphamide given in high doses for 2 days and followed by total body irradiation to 1000 rads. Their results of patients grafted before October 1975, and followed up to 1st February 1977 (thus the survival curves are 'real') show that approximately 17 of 110 patients (i.e. 15%) have survived on a 'plateau' (Figure 1.11) and it must be remembered they were all relapse patients. Of these there are six acute myeloblastic leukaemia patients living longer than 600 days. If it is shown that a subgroup of long-term

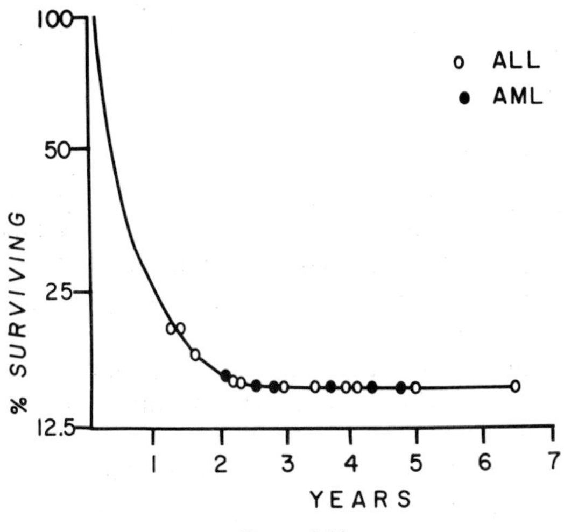

Figure 1.11

survivors with AML exists after allogeneic engraftment, then this would be unlike anything seen previously using conventional chemotherapy. Two possible mechanisms deserve consideration—either the intensive anticancer preparation that is required to immunosuppress the patient prior to grafting has eradicated the leukaemia, or there has been a direct action of the graft against the leukaemia. If these long-term survivors are the result of an antitumour action of the graft then it is vital a definitive test of this mechanism is established *in vitro*. It is now possible to collect and store leukaemia cells in liquid nitrogen such that they can be recovered and grown in proliferative cultures. It therefore seems a relatively simple procedure to use the circulating 'graft' cells and/or serum of the grafted patient to see if there is an antitumour action. Such tests have been used for some time in non-grafted patients and no antitumour action has been clearly established[23], but until these experiments have been repeated for long-term graft survivors we can say little about the possibility of an antitumour action of the graft. If high-dose cytotoxic chemotherapy with or without total body irradiation is responsible for these survivors then we might have more courage to pursue such treatment in ungrafted patients and obviously massive support would be required. If, however, it is due to an antitumour effect of the graft then we might feel more encouraged to explore similar forms of 'immunotherapy' in ungrafted patients. However, it would be misleading to discuss the possible antileukaemic action of the graft without a note of caution concerning the two cases reported from Seattle with leukaemia occurring in the grafted cells of transplanted patients with acute lymphoblastic leukaemia. This raises the very important question of whether the aetiology of acute leukaemia includes a host environmental defect rather than a spontaneous single cell, potentially eradicable, mutation. However, this concept does not counter the possibility that bone marrow transplantation may restore to the host some factor whose absence had contributed to the appearance of leukaemia.

CONCLUDING REMARKS

The present results obtained using intensive chemotherapy with prophylactic irradiation of the central nervous system have so improved the prognosis for childhood patients with ALL that it is difficult at the present time to ethically justify giving these patients immunotherapy instead of this form of treatment. However, it is possible that in the small group of poor-risk patients, particularly adults, it might be worth exploring adjuvant methods of treatment which would include immunotherapy in addition to intensive chemotherapy and radiotherapy.

In AML, however, the situation is different. The realization that conventional chemotherapy, whilst undoubtedly prolonging survival for remission patients with AML, is not producing a subpopulation of patients that are 'cured' clearly comes as a major setback in the understanding and treatment of this disease. Of even greater disappointment is the paradox that AML is a disease highly sensitive to chemotherapy during the induction phase of treatment (i.e. up to 80% remission rates) yet it is virtually drug-resistant during remission. Because of this we must consider that AML may be special among cancers in being a disease of the organ itself, i.e. the marrow environment, rather than the product of a spontaneous mutation of one marrow cell. This is supported by the recent observation[23] that AML cells, when placed in short-term proliferative cultures, are capable of undergoing maturation into polymorphs[65] and subsequent autologous mixed cell cultures shows these polymorphs to be of leukaemic origin. Two distinct scientific approaches are now required; firstly, experiments should be defined to clarify if recurrent AML, which occurs so consistently and rapidly, represents the emergence of a new clone of cells because such a finding would have a profound effect upon our thinking in relation to present methods of treatment; secondly, the biological factors involved in the maturation defect seen in the leukaemic clone of cells must be defined so that the opportunity may be taken for their therapeutic exploitation.

Clinically the emergence of a small but encouraging group of long-term survivors in AML, both for grafted and for some immunotherapy patients encourages specialized units to continue with these methods of treatment. However, we must never forget that at present these methods are highly experimental and if we are to ethically justify the man-made consequences that ensue for many of these patients, then we must include a scientific programme of research to advance the subject so that ultimately the majority will benefit. This will only be possible by understanding the biological nature of the methods we are using.

ACKNOWLEDGEMENTS

I wish to thank the Leukaemia Research Fund of Great Britain for supporting my research; Professor Mathé; Drs Vogler *et al.*, Whittaker *et al.* and Thomas *et al.* and the MRC of Great Britain, and the *British Journal of Cancer* and *British Medical Journal* for permission to publish some of the figures.

References

* *Denotes article to be published in* Immunotherapy of Cancer: Present Status of Trials in Man *(Progress in Cancer Research and Therapy Vol. 5). (D. Windhorst and W. Terry, eds.) (New York: Raven Press) (In press)*

1. Tyzzer, E. E. (1916). Tumour immunity. *J. Cancer Res.*, **1**, 125
2. Gross, L. (1943). Intradermal immunization of C3H mice against a sarcoma that originated in an animal of the same line. *Cancer Res.*, **3**, 326

3. Strong, L. C. (1942). The origin of some inbred mice. *Cancer Res.*, **2**, 531
4. Haddow, A. and Alexander, P. (1964). An immunological method of increasing the sensitivity of primary sarcomas to local irradiation with X-rays. *Lancet*, **i**, 452
5. Delorme, E. J. and Alexander, P. (1964). Treatment of primary fibrosarcoma in the rat with immune lymphocytes. *Lancet*, **ii**, 117
6. Alexander, P., Connell, D. I. and Mikulska, Z. B. (1966). Treatment of a murine leukaemia with spleen cells or sera from allogeneic mice immunized against the tumour. *Cancer Res.*, **26**, 1508
7. Mathé, G. (1968). Immunotherapie active de la leucemie L1210 appliquée après la greffe tumorale. *Rev. Franç. Étud. Clin. Biol.*, **13**, 881
8. Wrathmell, A. and Alexander, P. (1973). V. Immunologic aspects of leukaemia. Growth characteristics and immunological properties of a myeloblastic and lymphoblastic leukaemia in pure line rats. In: *Unifying Concepts of Leukaemia, Bibl. Haematol.* (R. M. Dutcher and L. Chieco-Bianchi, eds.), No. 39, pp. 649–53 (Basel: Karger)
9.*McKneally, M. F., Maver, C. M. and Kausel, H. W. (1977). Regional immunotherapy of lung cancer using postoperative intrapleural BCG
10. Mathé, G. (1969). Approaches to the immunological treatment of cancer in man. *Br. Med. J.*, **4**, 7
11. MRC Report on the treatment of acute lymphoblastic leukaemia (1971). *Br. Med. J.*, **4**, 189
12.*Kay, H. E. M. (1977). Acute lymphoblastic leukaemia: 5-year follow-up of the Concorde trial
13. Heyn, R., Borges, W., Joo, P., Karon, M., Nesbit, M., Shore, N., Breslow, N., Weiner, J. and Hammond, D. (1975). BCG in the treatment of acute lymphocytic leukaemia (ALL). *Blood*, **46**, 3, 431
14. Simone, J. (1974). Acute lymphocytic leukaemia in childhood. *Sem. Haematol.*, **xi**, 25
15.*Poplack, D. G., Leventhal, B. G., Simon, R., Pomeroy, T., Graw, R. G. and Henderson, E. S. (1977). Treatment of acute lymphatic leukaemia with chemotherapy alone or chemotherapy plus immunotherapy
16. Gutterman, J. U., Hersh, E. M., Rodriguez, V., McCredie, K. B., Mavligit, G., Reed, R., Burgess, M. A., Smith, T., Gehan, E., Bodey, G. P. and Freireich, E. J. (1974). Chemotherapy of adult acute leukaemia. Prolongation of remission in myeloblastic leukaemia with BCG. *Lancet*, **ii**, 1405
17. Magrath, I. T. and Ziegler, J. L. (1976). Failure of BCG immunostimulation to affect the clinical course of Burkitt's lymphoma. *Br. Med. J.*, **1**, 615
18. Crowther, D., Bateman, C. J. T., Vartan, C. P., Whitehouse, J. M. A., Malpas, J. S., Hamilton Fairley, G. and Bodley-Scott, R. (1970). Combination chemotherapy using L-asparaginase, daunorubicin and cytosine arabinoside in adults with acute myelogenous leukaemia. *Br. Med. J.*, **4**, 513
19. Parr, I. (1972). Response of syngeneic murine lymphomata to immunotherapy in relation to the autogenicity of the tumour. *Br. J. Cancer*, **26**, 174
20. Powles, R. L., Balchin, L. A., Hamilton Fairley, G. and Alexander, P. (1971). Recognition of leukaemia cells as foreign before and after autoimmunization. *Br. Med. J.*, **i**, 486
21. Powles, R. L., Lister, T. A., Oliver, R. T. D., Russell, J., Smith, C., Kay, H. E. M., McElwain, T. J. and Hamilton Fairley, G. (1974). Safe method of collecting leukaemia cells from patients with acute leukaemia for use as immunotherapy. *Br. Med. J.*, **4**, 375
22. Powles, R. L., Balchin, L. A., Smith, C. and Grant, C. K. (1973a). Some properties of cryopreserved acute leukaemia cells. *Cryobiology*, **10**, 282
23. Chapuis, B., Summersgill, B. M., Cocks, P., Howard, P., Lawler, S. D., Alexander, P. and Powles, R. (1977). A test for cryopreservation efficiency of human acute myelogenous leukaemia cells relevant to clinical requirements. *Cryobiology* (In press)
24. Powles, R. L., Crowther, D., Bateman, C. J. T., Beard, M. E. J., McElwain, T. J., Russell, J., Lister, T. A., Whitehouse, J. M. A., Wrigley, P. F. M., Pike, M., Alexander, P. and

Hamilton Fairley, G. (1973b). Immunotherapy for acute myelogenous leukaemia. *Br. J. Cancer*, **28**, 365
25. Crowther, D., Powles, R. L., Bateman, C. J. T., Beard, M. E. J., Gauci, C. L., Wrigley, P. F. M., Malpas, J. S., Hamilton Fairley, G. and Bodley-Scott, R. (1973). The management of adult acute myelogenous leukaemia. *Br. Med. J.*, **1**, 131
26. Powles, R. L., Russell, J., Lister, T. A., Oliver, T., Whitehouse, J. M. A., Malpas, J., Chapuis, B., Crowther, D. and Alexander, P. (1977a). Immunotherapy for acute myelogenous leukaemia: a controlled clinical study 2½ years after entry of the last patient. *Br. J. Cancer*, **35**, 265
27. Peto, R. and Peto, J. (1972). Asympototically efficient rank invariant test procedures. *J. Roy. Statist. Soc. Ser.* A2, **135**, part II, 185
28.*Peto, R. (1977). Immunotherapy of acute myeloid leukaemia
29.*Reizenstein, P., Brenning, L., Engstedt, L., Franzen, S., Gahrton, G., Gullbring, B., Holm, G., Hocker, P., Hogland, S., Hornsten, P., Hameson, S., Killander, A., Killander, D., Klein, E., Lantz, B., Lindemalm, C. L., Locker, D., Lonnqvist, B., Mellstedt, H., Palmblad, J., Pauli, C., Skarberg, K. O., Uden, A. M., Vanky, F. and Wadman, B. (1977). Effect of immunotherapy on survival and remission duration in acute non-lymphatic leukaemia
30. Powles, R. (1974a). Tumour-associated antigens in acute leukaemia. In: *Advances in Acute Leukaemia* (F. J. Cleton, D. Crowther, and J. S. Malpas, eds.), p. 115 (Amsterdam: North-Holland American Elsevier)
31. Wolmark, N., Levine, M. and Fisher, B. (1974). The effect of a single and repeated administration of *Corynebacterium parvum* on bone marrow macrophage colony production in normal mice. *J. Reticuloendoth. Soc.*, **16**, 252
32. Dimitrov, N. V., Andre, S., Eliopoulos, G. and Halpern, B. (1975). Effect of *Corynebacterium parvum* on bone marrow cultures (38557). *Proc. Soc. Exp. Biol., N.Y.*, **148**, 440
33. Vogler, W. R. and Chan, Y-K. (1974). Prolonging remission in myeloblastic leukaemia by Tice strain Bacillus Calmette-Guerin. *Lancet*, **ii**, 128
34.*Vogler, W. R., Bartolucci, A. A., Omura, G. A., Miller, D., Smalley, R. V., Knospe, W. H. and Goldsmith, A. S. (1977). A randomized clinical trial of BCG in myeloblastic leukaemia. Conducted by the South-eastern Cancer Study Group
35.*Gutterman, J. U., Mavligit, G. M., Rodriguez, V., McCredie, K. B., Bodey, G. T. and Freireich, E. J. (1977). Chemotherapy plus BCG immunotherapy for acute myelogenous leukaemia
36.*Hewlett, J. S., Balcezak, S., Gutterman, J. U., Freireich, E. J., Gehan, E. A. and Kennedy, A. (1977). Remission maintenance in adult leukaemia with and without BCG. A South-west Oncology Group Study
37.*Whittaker, J. A. and Slater, A. J. (1977). The immunotherapy of acute myelogenous leukaemia using intravenous BCG
38. Powles, R. L. (1973). Immunotherapy for acute myelogenous leukaemia. *Br. J. Cancer*, **28**, Suppl. I, 262
39. Powles, R. L. (1974b). Immunotherapy for acute myelogenous leukaemia, using irradiated and unirradiated leukaemia cells. *Cancer*, **34**, 1558
40. Russell, J. A. and Powles, R. L. (1977). The relationship between serum viscosity, hypervolaemia and clinical manifestations associated with circulating paraprotein. *Br. J. Haematol.* (In press)
41. Currie, G. A. and McElwain, T. J. (1975). *Br. J. Cancer*, **31**, 143
42. Powles, R. L., Russell, J. A., Selby, P. J., Jones, D. R., McElwain, T. J. and Alexander, P. (1977). Maintenance of remission for patients with acute myelogenous leukaemia using a mixture of BCG and irradiated leukaemia cells. *Lancet* (In press)
43. Spiers, A. S. D., Goldman, J. M., Catovsky, D., Costello, C., Galton, D. A. G. and Pitcher, C. S. (1977). Prolonged remission maintenance in acute myeloid leukaemia. *Br. Med. J.*, **2**, 544

44. Powles, R. L. (1976). Pitfalls in analysis of survival in clinical trials. *Biomedicine*, **24**, 327
45. Mould, R. F. and Boag, J. W. (1975). *Br. J. Cancer*, **32**, 529
46. Currie, G. A. and Bagshawe, K. D. (1968). The role of sialic acid in antigenic expression: further studies of the Landschütz ascites tumour. *Br. J. Cancer*, **22**, 843
47. Holland, J. (1977). Personal communication
48.*Guttner, J., Glidewell, O. and Holland, J. F. (1977). Chemoimmunotherapy of acute myelocytic leukaemia with MER
49.*Sauter, Chr., Cavalli, F., Lindenmann, J., Gmur, J. P., Bershtold, W., Alberto, P., Obrecht, P. and Senn, H. J. (1977). Viral oncolysis: its application in maintenance treatment of acute myelogenous leukaemia
50. Boone, C. and Blackman, K. (1972). Augmented immunogenicity of tumour cell homogenates infected with influenza virus. *Cancer Res.*, **32**, 1018
51. Lindenmann, J. (1974). Viruses as immunological adjuvants in cancer. *Biochim. Biophys. Acta*, **355**, 49
52. Gerber, A., Sauter, C. and Lindenmann, J. (1973). Fowl plague virus adapted to human epithelial tumour cells and human myeloblasts *in vitro*. I. Characteristics and replication in monolayer cultures. *Arch. ges. Virusforsch.*, **40**, 137
53.*Gee, T. S., Dowling, M. D., Cunningham, I., Oettgen, H. S., Armstrong, D. and Clarkson, B. D. (1977). *Pseudomonas aeruginosa* vaccine with the L-12 protocol for adult patients with acute non-lymphoblastic leukaemia
54. Turner, W., Chan, S. P. and Chirigos, M. A. (1970). Stimulation of humoral and cellular antibody formation in mice by poly Ir:Cr. *Proc. Soc. Exp. Biol. Med.*, **133**, 334
55. Field, A. K., Young, C. W., Krakoff, I. H., Tytell, A. A., Lampson, G. P., Nemes, M. M. and Hilleman, M. R. (1971). Induction of interferon in human subjects by poly IC. *Proc. Soc. Exp. Biol. Med.*, **136**, 1180
56. Cornell, C. J. Jr, Smith, K. A., Cornwell, G. G. III, Burke, G. P. and McIntyre, O. R. (1977). The systemic effects of intravenous polyriboinosinic: polyribocytidylic acid in man. *J. Nat. Cancer Inst.* (In press)
57.*McIntyre, O. R., Rai, K., Glidewell, O. and Holland, J. F. (1977). Polyriboinosinic: polyribocytidylic acid as an adjunct to remission maintenance therapy in acute myelogenous leukaemia
58. Hamilton Fairley, G. (1975). Immunotherapy in the management of leukaemia. *Br. J. Haematol.*, **31** (Suppl.), 181
59. Mohanakumar, T., Metzgar, R. S. and Miller, D. S. (1974). Human leukaemia cell antigens, serological characterizations with xenogeneic antisera. *J. Nat. Cancer Inst.*, **52**, 1435
60. Greaves, M. S., Brown, G., Rapson, N. T. and Lister, T. A. (1975). Antisera to acute lymphoblastic leukaemia cells. *J. Clin. Immunol. Immunopathol.*, **4**, 67
61. Gallo, R. C., Gallagher, R. E., Sarngadharan, M. G., Sarin, P., Reitz, M., Miller, N. and Gillespie, D. H. (1974). The evidence for involvement of Type C, RNA viruses in human adult leukaemia. *Cancer*, **34**, No. 4 (October Supplement) 1398
62. Spiegelman, S., Axel, R., Baxt, W., Kufe, D. and Schlom, J. (1974). Human cancer and animal viral oncology. *Cancer*, October Suppl., **34**, 1406
63. Khaw, B. A. and Rule, A. H. (1973). Immunotherapy of the Dunning leukaemia with thymic extract. *Br. J. Cancer*, **28**, 288
64. Thomas, E. D. (1977). Allogeneic bone marrow grafting for acute leukaemia. *Blood* (In press)
65. Cocks, P., Powles, R. L., Chapuis, B. and Alexander, P. (1977). Further evidence of response by leukaemia patients in remission to antigen(s) related to acute myelogenous leukaemia. *Br. J. Cancer*, **35**, 273

2
Biological and Clinical Aspects of Transfer Factor

M. P. ARALA-CHAVES, MAIJA HORSMANHEIMO, J. M. GOUST and H. HUGH FUDENBERG

Department of Basic and Clinical Immunology and Microbiology,
Medical University of South Carolina, Charleston, South Carolina 29401, USA

According to the Lawrence definition of dialysable transfer factor (TFd) this substance(s) is (are) able to transfer specifically delayed hypersensitivity toward certain antigens to which the donor of TFd has a strong delayed-type hypersensitivity skin reaction. This 'transfer' has been subsequently extended to other parameters of cell-mediated immunity (CMI). Twenty years have passed since this substance was first described[1] and 13 years since it was reported to be dialysable[2], and there are still a number of important questions to be answered regarding this factor or factors, as summarized in Table 2.1.

Table 2.1 Pertinent questions concerning dialysable transfer factor (TFd)

1. Is TFd always or ever specific?
2. What are its cellular sources?
3. What are the target cell(s) for its action(s)?
4. What are the characteristics of its *in vitro* activity?
5. What is its biochemical nature?
6. What are the requirements for an experimental animal model?
7. In what conditions is it useful for therapeutic purposes?

IS TFd ALWAYS OR EVER SPECIFIC?

The question of the specificity of TFd is surely one of the most important questions involving the study of this substance. In fact this question involves

---

Publication No. 178 from the Department of Basic and Clinical Immunology and Microbiology, Medical University of South Carolina. Research supported in part by USPHS Grants HD-09938 and AI-13484.

the existence of TFd as such: if there is no *specific* transfer of a given immunological reaction, then the term is misleading. Therefore in this section we refer to the effects of 'dialysable leukocyte extracts' (DLE), which may or may not contain a substance that can truly *transfer* an immunological reaction rather than induce non-specific reactivity or augment an immunological reactivity present in the recipient, perhaps at a level too low to be detected by current test methods (see Figure 2.1).

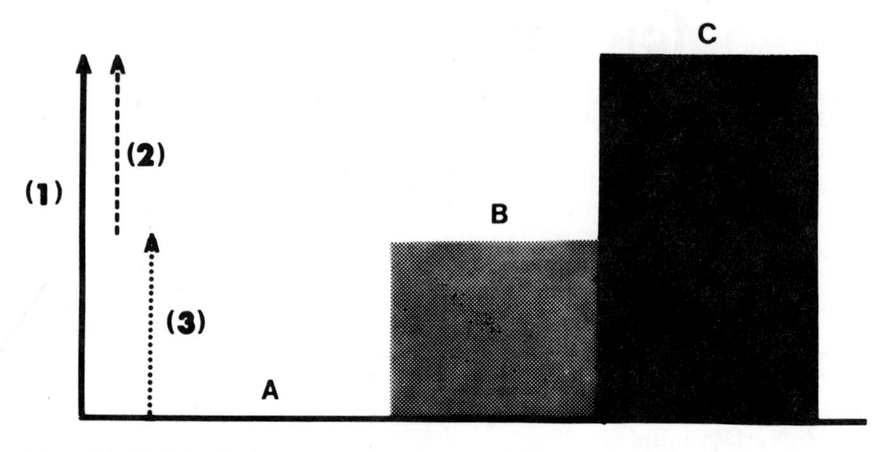

Figure 2.1 DLE is able (1) to convert a status of total absence of sensitivity (A) to a status of apparent sensitivity (B), (2) to convert a status of low-grade sensitivity or (3) to convert a status of total absence of sensitivity into a low-grade non-apparent sensitivity

In the following discussion of specificity of the effects of DLE we will use the terminology indicated in Table 2.2. *Antigen-dependent* effects are those related to a specific antigen; *antigen-independent* effects are those not related to specific antigens. Antigen-dependent effects will be termed *donor-specific* when related to a given status of immunization of the donor and *recipient-specific* when related to a given status of immunization of the recipient. As

Table 2.2 Terminology used in the discussion of specificity of dialysable leukocyte extracts (DLE)

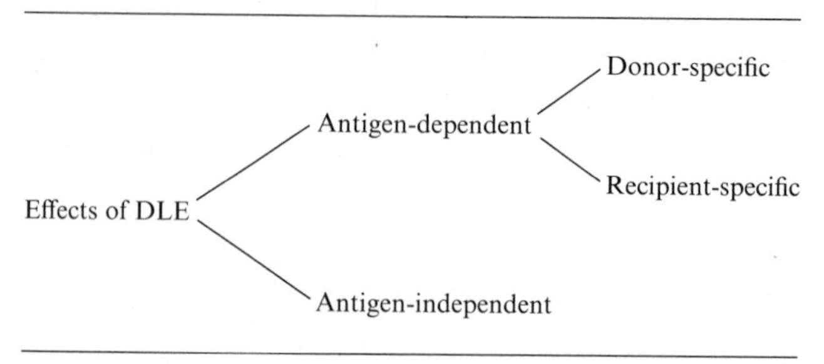

the relationship between the effects of DLE *in vivo* and *in vitro* must also be discussed, in the following paragraphs we will consider only the *in vivo* effects. In addition, since DLE has been demonstrated more consistently in humans than in animals (and until recently only in humans), the following paragraphs deal solely with human studies.

Antigen-dependent effects

Evidence for donor-specific effects

The initial studies on DLE pointed to the existence of a substance in DLE able to transfer CMI specifically. In fact, it was reported that the effects of DLE were seen only if the donor of leukocyte extracts exhibited strong positivity to the antigen for which hypersensitivity was transferred[3,4], and DLE obtained from donors with negative skin-delayed hypersensitivity to a given antigen failed to induce skin reactivity towards the same antigen when injected in negative recipients[3]. Moreover, Lawrence and Pappenheimer[5] observed that when leukocytes from donors with delayed hypersensitivity to both diphtheria toxoid and PPD were incubated with one of these two antigens, the supernatant fluid appeared to contain TFd of the corresponding specificity, whereas the remaining cell population was able to transfer delayed hypersensitivity to the other antigen. Similarly, Rappaport *et al.*[6] observed that the transfer of sensitivity to coccidioidin by sensitized leukocytes was no longer possible when these leukocytes had previously been incubated with the corresponding antigen.

Also pointing to the possibility that DLE contains TFd able to confer a *de novo* sensitivity to the recipient are the following reports. Rappaport *et al.*[6] collected leukocytes from donors sensitive to coccidioidin from an endemic area in California and the leukocyte extracts were given to recipients who were lifelong residents in an area free of coccidioidomycosis. The recipients became positive to coccidioidin and the transferred reaction was correlated quantitatively with the intensity of the coccidioidin reaction of the donors. It was also found by Lawrence *et al.*[7] that skin homograft sensitivity could be specifically transferred by means of DLE obtained from actively sensitized donors. More recently, Zuckerman *et al.*[8] reported that DLE obtained from donors actively sensitized to keyhole limpet haemocyanin (KLH) were able to induce skin test delayed hypersensitivity to this antigen, whereas batches of DLE from non-sensitized donors were not.

In regard to the available data on DLE injected into immunodeficient patients, some authors concluded, after large numbers of injections of DLE in patients, that the immunological reactivity conferred upon the patient was concordant with that of the donor[9]. Others[10,11] reported that the DLE therapy in osteosarcoma patients was successful only when the donor exhibited cellular immunity to the tumour antigens.

Evidence for recipient specificity

Several studies point to the fact that in most cases DLE is not able to confer a *de novo* sensitivity to the recipient but rather enhances a previously in-apparent low-grade sensitivity in the recipient. In fact, attempts to induce sensitivity to artificial antigens or haptens to which the donor is actively sensitized by means of DLE in the recipient have usually been unsuccessful. For example, recipients injected with DLE prepared from donors actively sensitized to dinitrochlorobenzene (DNCB) were not sensitized to this substance[12,13], although a small percentage of recipients were converted to positive for this substance after previously having received low (non-sensitizing) doses of DNCB, which apparently caused low-grade inapparent sensitivity[13]. It has been argued that contact sensitivity, as is the case for DNCB, could be an exceptional situation[3]; however, it is well known that the ability of a given individual to acquire the capacity to be sensitized to DNCB correlates well with the status of his CMI reactivity. There are also several reports of CMI-deficient patients who acquired the capacity to become sensitized to DNCB after being treated with DLE[14,17]. Also DNCB sensitization has been reported to be 'transferred' in animals by means of 'TFd', as pointed out below. Kirkpatrick[18] was unable in five attempts to transfer delayed hypersensitivity to a synthetic antigen, a co-polymer of glutamic acid, lysine, and tyrosine, to non-sensitized patients with muco-cutaneous candidiasis, using DLE from actively sensitized donors. In humans, KLH thus seems to be an exception in regard to the possibility of inducing sensitivity in recipients toward an uncommon antigen. On the other hand, most people eat shellfish and may therefore have a low level of sensitivity to KLH. Furthermore, it has been reported that KLH can cross-react with sheep red blood cells[19,19a], penicillin[19a], and perhaps a wide range of other antigens.

Insofar as the transfer of sensitivity to common antigens is concerned[6,7], enhancement of low-grade sensitivity cannot be excluded on the basis of the results from studies using coccidioidin, as this antigen may cross-react with other antigens[20]. Similarly, low-grade sensitivity in the recipients toward transplantation antigens cannot be excluded in the study of transfer of skin homograft sensitivity.

Other observations also suggest that the sensitivity induced in a given recipient by means of DLE is not always specific in regard to the sensitivities exhibited by the donor. In fact, some authors have observed that the recipient acquired sensitivity toward an antigen to which the donor of DLE was unsensitive[21,22]. In the study of transfer of reactivity to coccidioidin[6], DLE from two negative donors sensitized six of the eight recipients. On the other hand, Dupont *et al.*[23] found that the mixed lymphocyte reaction could be restored in patients who received DLE.

One of us has also observed[17,24] that no matter how strongly positive the donor of DLE was to a given antigen, the particular sensitivity was never acquired by one recipient, who repeatedly acquired sensitivities towards other antigens after DLE injections. Similarly there are reports in the literature of the induction of certain sensitivities exhibited by the donor in the recipient but failure to induce others also present in the same donor.

All these observations indicate an important role of the recipient status in the acquisition of some sensitivities toward a given antigen by means of DLE. It seems in most cases that the existence in the recipient of low-grade sensitivity, and in some patients a defect of genetic or other nature, conditions the effects of DLE. Therefore it is difficult to know, on the basis of the studies presently available, whether DLE contains TFd, i.e. a substance which is donor-specific in its ability to transfer the sensitivities, or whether DLE is merely an adjuvant. Standard preparations of DLE and standard models of assay are required to answer this question.

Antigen-independent effects

To complicate the picture, effects of DLE without relationship to specific antigens have been reported several times. It has been reported that lymphocytes from immunodeficient patients who have received DLE show a considerably increased ability to respond to non-specific mitogens like phytohaemagglutinin (PHA), as assessed by [^{3}H]thymidine uptake[17,25,26]. Wybran *et al.*[27], Valdimarsson *et al.*[25], and Kirkpatrick[18] have also observed that the number of E-rosette-forming cells was increased in immunodeficient patients who received DLE therapy. Moreover, it has been reported that

Table 2.3 Summary of the evidence for donor-specific, recipient-specific, and antigen-independent effects of DLE

Evidence for donor specificity
1. In general the induction of delayed skin sensitivity is correlated with the sensitivity of the donor
2. Induction of delayed skin sensitivity has been possible using antigens for which the recipient has a low probability of being previously sensitized

Evidence for recipient specificity
1. Failure to induce delayed skin sensitivity to a number of artificial antigens
2. Possibility of induction of CMI to these antigens if the recipient has a low-grade non-apparent reactivity
3. Induction of skin-delayed sensitivity towards certain antigen to which the donor is non-sensitive
4. Failure to induce delayed skin reactivity to certain antigens in a given recipient
5. Induction of skin-delayed sensitivity in guinea-pigs by means of DLE is only possible if the animals have been previously primed

Evidence for antigen-independent effects
1. Increased response to PHA
2. Increased number of E rosettes
3. Increased chemotaxis to neutrophils
4. Increased size of rat lymph nodes

DLE contains a chemotactic factor for neutrophils[28]. These effects, which have been considered as side-effects of specific activities of TFd[29], may be due to different substances in DLE (other than TFd) or may be manifestations of the completely non-specific adjuvant activity of DLE, which in that case would not contain TFd.

In summary, DLE *in vivo* and in humans seems to have clearly demonstrable antigen-independent activities. Recipient specificity is an important factor in the activity of DLE, which at least in some cases seems to exclude the possibility of DLE being able to confer a *de novo* sensitivity to the recipient. At present, however, it cannot be excluded that DLE may also contain a donor-specific activity due to the existence of a true TFd. Evidence for donor-specific, recipient-specific, and antigen-independent effects are summarized in Table 2.3.

WHAT ARE THE CELLULAR SOURCES FOR TFd?

It has been claimed on the basis of theoretical considerations, based on the assumption that DLE contains a substance able to transfer CMI (a T-cell-dependent immunological reaction), that the source of DLE activities is the T lymphocyte[3,30]. On the basis of this assumption several authors[31–33] have quantitated DLE in relation to the number of lymphocytes from which the material was extracted.

The matter still remains very unclear. On one hand, as indicated above, it has not been proven that DLE contains a substance able specifically to transfer CMI. On the other hand, methods of purification of different white blood cell populations, which have only recently been developed, have not been used to separate the different cells from which DLE is extracted and therefore to analyse from which cell the activity is produced.

Recent studies of Kirkpatrick's group[34,35] showed that dialysates of granulocytes, and of adherent and non-adherent mononuclear cells (the cells from which DLE is obtained) were able to cause the accumulation of cGMP in monocytes. This effect seems to be due mainly to ascorbate, which is also present in DLE. As cGMP is known to be involved non-specifically in immune reactions, this finding could explain certain antigen-independent effects of DLE.

This substance is thus produced by all the cell types found in the pool of cells from which DLE is obtained. Obviously, the cells that produce the substance(s) responsible for antigen-dependent effects of DLE must also be investigated in the near future.

WHAT IS THE TARGET CELL FOR TFd?

There is still considerable doubt as to the precise nature of the cells on which TFd or DLE exerts its effect. If one considers that TFd is a substance capable of conferring, increasing, or inducing delayed hypersensitivity in previously non-responder recipients, it must be assumed that in the last analysis T lymphocytes and/or monocytes must be involved, since those are the effector cells in delayed hypersensitivity reactions. This problem is most important not only in regard to the biological aspects of DLE effects and the nature of recipient specificity but also with respect to selection of patients to receive DLE therapy (see below).

It is well known that it is more difficult to induce CMI in certain immunodeficient patients than in abnormal controls by means of DLE or even by viable white peripheral blood cells, which are the source of DLE. These include cases of Hodgkin's disease[36,38], sarcoidosis[39,40], and advanced cancers[41]. It has also been reported that in certain immunodeficient patients the transfer of CMI cannot be accomplished by means of DLE unless they have previously received a transplant of an organ source of T cells (i.e. thymus[42–44]); therefore, it seems that DLE needs a reasonably 'intact' T lymphocyte as a target. If the T lymphocytes are too few or too badly 'damaged', induction or transfer of CMI cannot be achieved.

Monocytes also seem to be involved in the response to DLE, as indicated by studies on Wiskott–Aldrich patients[45] (see below). Also, as pointed out above, Sandler *et al.*[34] demonstrated that DLE was able to induce the accumulation of cGMP in monocytes.

Recently we have observed that both *in vitro*[46,47] and *in vivo*[47] DLE is quite ineffective if monocytes are removed from the test cell population or are abnormal in function. Supernatants of cell suspensions containing monocytes can substitute for the function of these cells. This suggests that the target cell for DLE is in fact a T lymphocyte, but that the effect is observed only in the presence of a substance released by monocytes, which by an unknown mechanism enables T lymphocytes to react.

WHAT ARE THE *IN VITRO* EFFECTS OF TFd?

The *in vitro* effects of DLE are summarized in Table 2.4. After several years of unsuccessful or unconvincing attempts[48–50] to set up an *in vitro* assay of DLE, the *in vitro* effects of DLE have been described frequently over the

Table 2.4 ***In vitro* effects of DLE**

Antigen-dependent
Induction of MIF release
Increased [^{3}H]thymidine uptake by lymphocytes in the presence of antigen
Antigen-independent
Increased [^{3}H]thymidine uptake by lymphocytes in the presence of mitogens
Increased response in MLC
Increased number of E rosettes
Chemotactic for neutrophils

past several years. It remains unclear, however, whether these *in vitro* effects of DLE reflect its *in vivo* activity, represent an artifact, or are caused by different molecules present in the same preparation. This problem is posed mainly by the lack of exhaustive work comparing the effects of a given batch of DLE *in vitro* with the effects of the same batch *in vivo*. On the other hand, when the effects of DLE *in vivo* and *in vitro* are compared in a randomized fashion, the *in vitro* activities appear to correlate well with the *in vivo* activities. In fact, DLE has been proven to be chemotactic for neutrophils and poorly chemotactic for monocytes when injected intradermally into Rhesus monkeys[28], and similarly, *in vitro* it has been demonstrated that DLE has chemotactic activity for neutrophils and less chemotactic activity for monocytes[51]. As when injected to humans (see above), DLE is able to increase the number of E-rosette-forming cells *in vitro*[52]. DLE injected into patients was able to induce an increase of the response of the patients' lymphocytes to specific antigens[17,53,54] and to non-specific mitogens[17,25,26] as evaluated by [^{3}H]thymidine uptake, and *in vitro* DLE was able to increase the amount of [^{3}H]thymidine uptake by mononuclear cells stimulated either with specific antigens[55–58] or with non-specific mitogens[59]. Finally DLE is able both *in vitro* and *in vivo* to induce the production of migration inhibition factor (MIF). *In vivo* studies showed that mononuclear cells obtained from immunodeficient patients treated with DLE acquired the capacity to produce MIF when stimulated by specific antigens[17,60,61], and *in vitro* studies demonstrated that DLE was able to induce mononuclear cells to release MIF in the presence of a specific antigen[62–65].

We have obtained a very good correlation between the *in vivo* and *in vitro* effects for the same batch of DLE, using cells obtained from the same recipient for *in vitro* tests. These experiments were performed using enhancement of [^{3}H]thymidine uptake as *in vitro* assay and skin testing as *in vivo* assay. It is evident from Table 2.5 that every batch of DLE capable of increasing the amount of [^{3}H]thymidine uptake by the recipient's lymphocytes in the presence of a given antigen *in vitro* also produced conversion of skin test sensitivity to the same antigen in the same recipient after injection *in vivo*; conversely, when no increase of [^{3}H]thymidine uptake was induced *in vitro* by DLE in the recipient's lymphocytes, no skin test conversion to the same antigen was observed *in vivo*. Thus, the available data suggest rather than exclude a good correlation between *in vitro* and *in vivo* effects of DLE.

A detailed analysis of the *in vitro* effects of DLE suggests also that, as *in vivo*, both antigen-dependent and antigen-independent effects of DLE can be seen and that the antigen-dependent effects can also be analysed on the basis of both donor specificity and recipient specificity. Good examples of *in vitro* antigen-independent effects are the above-described chemotactic activity, increase in E-rosette-forming cells, and increase in the response to PHA.

Regarding the antigen-dependent effects, it has been claimed that DLE produces a greater increase in [^{3}H]thymidine uptake by target cells in the presence of specific antigen than in the absence of antigen[46,47,55,56]. In most cases, however, these effects do not seem to be correlated with the sensitivities exhibited by the donors as evaluated by skin test positivity. In fact, it has been demonstrated that DLE batches obtained from donors skin test negative or positive to a given antigen were able to increase [^{3}H]thymidine uptake by mononuclear cells to the same extent in the presence of the same antigen[57,58]. This observation may be due either to the presence of antigen-independent factors in DLE which can mask possible donor specificity, or to recipient specificity which also can mask the existence of donor specificity.

Table 2.5 Comparison of the effects of DLE *in vivo* (evaluated by skin test) and *in vitro* (evaluated by the increase in [^{3}H]thymidine uptake by the recipient's lymphocytes in the presence of a given antigen prior to *in vivo* administration of DLE)

	Antigens					
	Candidin		*PPD*		*SK-SD*	
	A	*B*	*A*	*B*	*A*	*B*
Patient 1 (first observation)	2+*	+	±	–	3+	2+
Patient 1 (second observation)	+	+	–	–	–	–
Patient 2	+	+	–	–	+	+
Patient 3	+	+	2+	3+	2+	2+
Patient 4	–	–	–	–	–	–
Patient 5	–	–	–	–	–	–

A—Skin test
B—Increase of [^{3}H]thymidine uptake
* The values are ranged between + and 4+

In favour of the existence of recipient specificity are the above-mentioned experiments in which DLE was able to increase [^{3}H]thymidine uptake of some lymphocytes in the presence of a given antigen but not in the presence of another. In addition, some authors have found that the ability of DLE to increase the amount of [^{3}H]thymidine uptake is correlated with the reactivity of the target cells to the antigen[57,58]. The existence of an antigen-dependent effect (which could be recipient- or donor-specific) seems to be confirmed by the fact that the kind of correlation obtained between the effect of DLE and the previous reactivity of recipient cells in the presence of antigen is different from that seen in the absence of antigen[47].

Donor specificity of DLE was strongly suggested in this system in a recent report by Burger *et al.*[66], in which a given fraction of DLE was able to increase specifically the amount of [^{3}H]thymidine uptake of the target cells when cultured in the presence of antigen to which the donor of DLE was skin-test positive. Other fractions of DLE were responsible for antigen-independent enhancing effects. More studies are necessary, however, to confirm this finding.

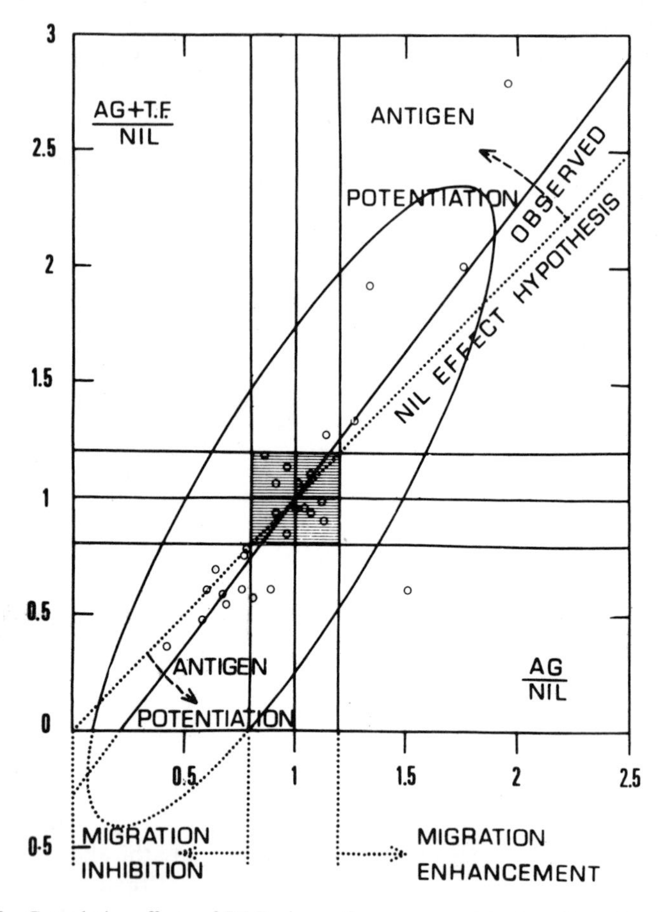

Figure 2.2 Cumulative effects of DLE plus antigen compared to the effect of antigen alone. Migration ratios falling in the hatched area are to be considered, as usual, non-significant and denoting the absence of any effect. Linear regression parameters:

$$Y = Y_0 + bx = -31.43 + 1.33x$$

$$(Y \neq 0)\, t_{27} = 2.02 \quad p < 0.05 \quad (s_{Y_0} = 15.53)$$

$$(b \neq 0)\, t_{27} = 8.85 \quad p < 0.001 \quad (s_b = 0.15)$$

Antigen-dependent donor-specific effects of DLE seem to be more easily demonstrated by MIF assay, as has been reported by others[63–65]. In our hands, however, antigen-dependent recipient specificity of DLE was also clearly demonstrated in this assay (Figure 2.2). In fact, in this experiment DLE was able to increase the release of migration enhancing factor (MEF) or of MIF if the test cells showed a tendency to release MEF or MIF.

It can be concluded that the problem of donor specificity of DLE *in vitro* as well as *in vivo* cannot be solved before standard preparations of DLE and of target cells are available. Also, fractionation of DLE seems to be an important requirement in the study of this problem, since multiple components, each possibly having a different activity (e.g. *de novo* transfer, non-specific adjuvant effect, etc.), are present in DLE.

WHAT IS THE BIOCHEMICAL NATURE OF TFd?

The first question that must be asked concerning this problem is whether the effects of DLE are due to one or to several substances in the dialysate. Most studies on the biochemical characterization of DLE have been based on the concept of a single substance able actually to transfer CMI; indeed, at the time those studies were performed there was little evidence for recipient-specific and antigen-independent effects of DLE. With regard to the characterization of the substance(s) able to transfer or induce CMI in a recipient, most of what is known is summarized in Table 2.6.

Table 2.6 Main biological and biochemical characteristics of dialysable transfer factor

Temperature sensitivity
- Resistant
  - (a) At 25–37 °C for at least 8 h
  - (b) When freeze-dried, to storage at 4 °C, or when frozen, at −20 °C for years
- Destroyed
  - At least partially, at 56–80 °C

Other physical properties
- (a) Dialysable
- (b) Molecular weight ~5000
- (c) Electrophoretic mobility at pH 8.3 similar to most cathodal IgG fraction

Biological properties
- Released *in vitro* in the presence of specific antigen

Resistance to hydrolases
- Resistant to DNase, RNase A, trypsin, and endogenously activated hydrolases
- Destroyed by pronase and RNase T1

Chemical analysis
- Polypeptide?
- Nucleotide?
- Nucleotide–polypeptide?

DLE can be obtained from leukocytes disrupted by repeated freezing and thawing. The material retains its activity for at least 8 h at 25–37 °C[30], indicating that it is not affected by endogenously activated hydrolases. Nor is its activity destroyed by deoxyribonuclease[1,30], pancreatic ribonuclease[1], or trypsin[67]. In contrast, it does seem to be destroyed by pronase[68] and RNase T1 (Wilson and Fudenberg, in preparation). The activity can be maintained for years in the frozen state at −20 °C[3,30]. It is resistant to lyophilization and can be maintained freeze-dried for at least 5 years upon storage at 4 °C. It is inactivated when exposed to temperatures between 56 and 80 °C. As the substance is dialysable, its molecular weight is apparently lower than 10 000. Further analysis of the molecular weight has been performed by several investigators using gel filtration on Sephadex G-10 or G-25 or a combination of both[68,72]. The values reported varied between 700 and 5000. A possible explanation for these discrepancies could reside in the fact that different investigators were dealing with different substances. In addition, since the active substance adheres to Sephadex when distilled water is used as eluent[73,74], it may be that the elution patterns differ according to the kind of buffer used, leading to different estimations of the molecular weight.

Gel filtration has also been used extensively for fractionation of DLE[12,67,69,70,75–79]. The resolving power of these systems is unfortunately poor, and the active fraction(s) eluted by means of gel filtration have turned out to be a rather complex mixture of substances containing nucleotides, polypeptides, hypoxanthine, and uracil.

Several years ago one of us[69] reported that the antigen-dependent activity of DLE *in vivo* was contained in a material that was positively charged at pH 8.3, and that ninhydrin-stainable subfractions were obtained by thin-layer chromatography, suggesting that the substance was mainly a basic polypeptide. More recently it was found that this same fraction was responsible for enhancing [^{3}H]thymidine uptake by non-responder lymphocytes stimulated with specific antigens[80].

Evidence that the induction of skin test sensitivity was due to a polypeptide-like material was also found recently by Kirkpatrick[81]. Others have suggested, however, that this substance was a nucleopolypeptide[82,83], as is the substance responsible for leukocyte migration inhibition in agarose (Wilson and Fudenberg, in preparation). Obviously the question can be resolved only when the substance(s) responsible for the effects of DLE have been completely purified.

EXPERIMENTAL ANIMAL MODELS

The search for an animal model of DLE is sustained by two different needs. The first is to define a system in which human DLE might be tested, giving a clue not only to the possible activities contained in a given human DLE, but also a way to test the protective and/or therapeutic value of this material. In the past, most attempts at 'transfer' in experimental animals were quite unsuccessful; however, Lawrence[3] in 1969 reported that transfer factor does not cross species barriers *in vivo*. The second need was due to the fact that the human is a tedious experimental model, not only in regard to recipient selection but also for donor selection. Therefore it would be interesting to study DLE using material obtained from animals and tested in animals. Here also the first studies were completely ineffective when small rodents were used, as reviewed by Bloom and Chase[84].

In 1971 Burger and Jeter[85] and in 1972 Burger *et al.*[86] reported that 'transfer' of sensitivity to DNCB was easily performed with fluids in which leukocytes from sensitive guinea-pigs to this chemical were incubated. Their results have been confirmed[87], and more recently, DLE (either human or animal) has been described to act in a wide range of animals including primates, small rodents such as guinea-pigs, rats and mice, dogs, and even bovines.

Several studies point to existence of a more easily demonstrable donor specificity of human DLE when animals are used as targets. In fact, Maddison *et al.*[88] reported that Rhesus monkeys acquired sensitivity to PPD but not to *Schistosoma mansonii* after receiving DLE obtained from a donor, human or monkey, sensitive to PPD but not to *S. mansonii*.

Eichberg, *et al.*[89], using gnotobiotic primates (one chimpanzee, *Pan troglodytes*, and two baboons, *Papio cynocephalus*), were able to show that those animals did not have, by *in vitro* assays (lymphocyte stimulation and cytotoxicity against virus-infected cells), any cell-mediated immune reaction to the antigens against which the human donor of DLE was sensitized. This donor, positive to mumps, herpes virus type I, tetanus, monilia, and coccidioidin, did not react against herpes virus type II, PPD, or histoplasmin. Forty-eight hours after DLE injections, the primates exhibited a positive response only to those antigens against which the donor was sensitized, and were still negative to those against which the donor was unsensitized. This *de novo* induction may be due to the particular system used, since immunological differences between non-human primates as well as non-primates are likely.

Trepo and Prince[90] also showed that human DLE is able to convert skin test and induce secretions of mediators, as shown by a leukocyte migration inhibition assay in chimpanzees to HbsAg. However, it is of interest to point out that none of the two chronic carriers exhibited any change in liver functions of HbsAg levels after human DLE injection. Goust *et al.*[91], using dextran sedimented baboon white blood cells incubated with human DLE from PPD-positive donors and PPD, observed an increase in blastogenesis of baboon cells when compared to controls without DLE. Several studies point also to the possibility of obtaining DLE with donor-specific activity in experimental animals.

White cells from various primates have been used as targets for *in vitro* sensitization with transfer factor. Baram and Condoulis[63], using Rhesus monkey DLE, showed that a ribose-containing fraction induced, after *in vitro* incubation with the Rhesus white blood cells, MIF secretion which was apparently antigen specific, since only the sensitizing antigen, KLH, was able to elicit its secretion.

Also Zanelli *et al.*[92] reported that when DLE was prepared from Rhesus monkey leukocytes using gentle shearing forces to disrupt the cells and avoiding lyophilization, an active preparation could be obtained. In fact, DLE obtained from Rhesus monkeys sensitized to BCG was able to transfer skin test reactivity to Cynomoncus monkeys. This conversion was apparent 48 h after injection and lasted for 3 months. Steele *et al.*[93], in the model described above with herpes simplex virus type I, used a leukocyte extract obtained from a sensitized baboon and obtained as good results as with human DLE. The 'life or death' endpoint of this protocol, demonstrating the prophylactic efficiency of this extract in an acute viral disease, represents an opportunity to study in an animal model the possible therapeutic value of DLE.

Although intraspecies transfer in small laboratory rodents by means of DLE or similar material has been difficult, several groups have succeeded in this respect. Liburg *et al.*[93], using DLE from rats sensitized to *Eimeria nieschulzi*, were able to protect the animals, i.e. the oocyst content in their faeces was considerably decreased after injection of DLE, and the animals were completely resistant to a second challenge by the same parasite. Comparable results were obtained by Clinton *et al.*[95] in guinea-pigs. Using white blood cells from guinea-pigs with a strong cell-mediated immune response against *Leishmania enriettii* after natural infection, they protected other guinea-pigs from infection with the same parasite. They also reported that a Sephadex G-25 fraction of this material was also able to induce MIF secretion in non-sensitized guinea-pigs. Dunnick and Bach[82] also found that a small molecular weight fraction of DLE obtained from guinea-pigs sensitized to ovalbumin, when incubated *in vitro* with lymphocytes from non-sensitized animals, enabled that to produce MIF and to incorporate more [^{3}H]thymidine when the sensitizing agent was also present. The increase of [^{3}H]thymidine uptake, however, was small (1.5-fold above the controls), though reportedly significant ($p < 0.001$).

In those experiments where infectious agents were used, whether viral (e.g. herpes simplex virus) or parasitic, the common trait is the prophylactic value of DLE. Therapeutic activity is more difficult to acquire. Basten *et al.*[96] were able to recover a dialysable material from the draining lymph nodes of BALB/c mice sensitized with DNB SO3 which induced sensitized animals to produce MIF in the presence of DNB SO3. This conversion was antigen-specific, since bovine gammaglobulin did not induce MIF secretion in the animals. The production of unlimited quantities of DLE from large mammals now seems possible and could be, in the future, the best source of any DLE. Klesius *et al.*[97,98] used *Eimeria stediai*, a natural parasite of rabbits, and *Eimeria bovis*, a natural parasite of cattle, which cross-react in delayed hypersensitivity reaction, in such a way that sensitization of bovines was demonstrated by lymphoblast transformation in the presence of *E. stediai*. Calves injected with DLE obtained from lymph node lymphocytes of animals sensitized with *E. bovis* exhibited a significantly lower elimination of *E. bovis* eggs in their faeces (40%). DLE in this experiment caused a significant degree of protection and simultaneously elicited antigen-specific response in the recipients, though they were primed 2 to 3 days before injection. Fractionation studies showed that the leukocyte extract transferring activity had a molecular weight around 1200 and was eluted with ribose-containing material. The species specificity of this material was not strict, since the same bovine extracts were able to transfer delayed hypersensitivity to dogs, rabbits, and monkeys. The practical importance of this model in elucidating the nature of this material and its possible use to obtain DLE against tumour antigens makes it very promising. Dogs have also been used as models for the study of DLE[99]. Even in experimental animals, however, there is evidence that recipient specificity is a requirement for the activity of DLE, as well as evidence for the existence of antigen-independent effects.

Evidence for recipient specificity in animals

Welch *et al.*[100] succeeded in converting guinea-pig skin tests using a presensitizing injection of antigen (skin-test dose) 4 weeks before administration of human DLE, together with the antigen. Skin tests performed 1 week later consistently showed antigen-specific conversion in animals given DLE from sensitized donors. The sensitizing schedule must be rigorously followed to give skin-test conversion, demonstrating the inability of DLE to induce *de novo* sensitization of naive, unprimed animals in this system.

Using the same protocol, including priming and simultaneous injection of DLE and small amounts of antigen, Vandenbark *et al.*[101] obtained similar results and further showed that the transfer was long-lasting (at least 98 days after injection) and was associated in four out of ten animals with a significant increase in blast transformation in the presence of PPD. DLE from human donors sensitized to SK/SD but not to PPD failed to convert guinea-pig skin tests to PPD, but significantly increased lymphocyte transformation and converted skin tests to SK/SD. A dose–response study showed that both the number of animals exhibiting conversion and the intensity of the response was dose-related. Goust *et al.*[90], using inbred Lewis rats with human DLE, also obtained skin-test conversion after preliminary skin testing, the cutaneous reaction frequently being stronger 2 weeks after DLE injection.

Evidence for antigen-independent effects in animals

There are also some antigen-independent effects of DLE that have been reported in animals. In fact, Maddison *et al.*[102] concluded that DLE from unsensitized donors was able, in combination with hyperimmune serum or normal serum, to reduce the clinical manifestations and worm burdens in monkeys injected with *S. mansonii*. Ascher *et al.*[103] also observed that within 24 h of injection of Lewis rats, the draining lymph node was four to 10 times larger than the contralateral control. Pathological examination of the lymph node revealed histological features similar to those observed after injection with non-specific immunopotentiator.

CLINICAL EFFECTS OF DLE

Effects of DLE in cancer

In 1973, several investigators dealing with the so-called 'transfer factor' reported[104] that they were obtaining preliminary, very promising results in the treatment of several cases of cancer with DLE. At the present stage of knowledge, however, the matter is rather unclear and it is not known in what kinds of cancer DLE can be useful.

The first study with DLE therapy in cancer patients was reported by Thompson[105] who observed that in seven of 19 patients with advanced disseminated cancer DLE reduced the measurable tumour by more than 50% and produced clinical improvement up to 7 months after treatment. Since then, several authors have reported clinical benefit or increase of CMI in certain patients afflicted with different kinds of cancer by means of DLE therapy, and totally unsuccessful results in other patients afflicted with neoplastic diseases. The results of DLE treatment in cancer patients are summarized in Table 2.7.

Melanoma is a very peculiar kind of cancer which is characterized by an extreme malignancy and by relative resistance to chemotherapy. Because of its major localization, it is also easily approachable. DLE has been used extensively in this kind of neoplastic disease. Melanoma has, however, a somewhat unpredictable evolution and it is well known that in some cases there is a 'spontaneous' cure. This makes the results of therapy difficult to assess. In 1971 Brandes *et al.*[106] reported a preliminary study in which one case of advanced melanoma was treated with DLE obtained from a donor with melanoma who was actively sensitized to the recipient's malignant tissues. The recipient showed a regression of the malignant subcutaneous nodules, including those not injected with DLE. There was some improvement of the patient's immunobiological condition. The patient died, however, after a short period of time.

Spitler *et al.*[107] reported that DLE from donors sensitive to melanoma antigen, consisting of 5–6-year survivors or family members, noted that in one out of five melanoma patients regression of metastatic lesions occurred coincident with DLE therapy. Smith *et al.*[108] reported that DLE obtained from individuals actively sensitized to tumour antigens, combined with

BCG, was able to produce in four out of 10 recipients an erythema followed by necrosis or resolution of dermal subcutaneous lesions of melanoma in four cases, with freedom from recurrent disease for 2 years in an additional patient. Cell-mediated immunity to PPD was converted in one patient.

Table 2.7 DLE in neoplastic diseases

Reference	*Number of patients*	*Increase in cell-mediated immunity*	*Clinical improvement (at least transitory)*
Melanoma (donor-specific DLE)			
Brandes (1971)	1	1	1
Spitler *et al.* (1973)	5	0	1
Smith *et al.* (1973)	10*	1	5
Vetto *et al.* (1976)	11	3	3
Bukowski *et al.* (1976)	6 (stage 4)	3	0
	7 (stage 3)	3	0
Silva *et al.* (1976)	8	8	0
Melanoma (donor-nonspecific DLE)			
Grob *et al.* (1975)	5	ND	0
Khan *et al.* (1976)	4	ND	0
	2*	ND	2
Breast cancer (donor-specific DLE)			
Oettgen (1974)	5	1	1
Smith (1973)	6	1	1
Fudenberg (in preparation)	3	3	2
Breast cancer (donor-nonspecific DLE)			
Khan *et al.* (1976)	2	0	0
Osteogenic sarcoma (donor-specific DLE)			
Levin *et al.* (1972)	1	1	1
Levin *et al.* (1975)	3 (phase I)	3	3
	1 (phase II)	1	1
	3 (phase III)	3	3†
	5 (phase IV)	4	4†
Levin *et al.* (1976)	1	1	1
Bearden *et al.* (1976)	5‡	ND	3
Thor *et al.* (1976)	6‡	4	NE
Vetto *et al.* (1976)	5	1	1
Osteogenic sarcoma (donor-nonspecific DLE)			
Levin *et al.* (1975)	3 (phase I)	0	0
	1 (phase II)	0	0
Acute lymphatic leukaemia (donor-nonspecific DLE)			
Lobuglio and Neidhart (1973)	3	2	2
Hodgkin's disease (donor-specific DLE)			
Khan *et al.* (1975)	8	5	NE
Renal carcinoma (donor-specific DLE)			
Bukowski *et al.* (1976)	3	2	2
Alveolar carcinoma (donor-specific DLE)			
Lobuglio *et al.* (1973)	1	1	NE
Nasopharyngeal carcinoma (donor-specific DLE)			
Goldenberg and Brandes (1972)	2	2	2

* DLE combined with BCG immunotherapy
† Clinical effect was very transitory
‡ DLE combined with chemotherapy

ND—Not done
NE—Not evaluated

Burger *et al.*[109] and Vetto *et al.*[110] also reported promising effects on the treatment of melanoma using household contacts (assumed to be sensitized to tumour antigen) as donors of DLE. In three out of 11 patients a regression of the tumour growth was observed. This observation was correlated with the skin reactivity of the patients; the non-responder patients had no skin reaction to the tumour.

Less promising are the studies of Bukowski *et al.*[111], who reported no effect of DLE therapy in six patients afflicted with stage 4 melanoma, using DLE from individuals sensitized to the tumour antigen. In three instances, there was an increase of 20% in cytotoxic antibodies to the tumour antigens. No clinical improvement was observed, however. In a study performed with seven patients with stage 3 melanoma, an increase of cytotoxicity to the tumour antigens was observed in patients after DLE treatment but not in controls; however, no statistical clinical difference was observed between treated patients and the control group, and there was a demonstrable increase of other CMI parameters in the treated group, such as the number of total or active E-rosette-forming cells or the response to mitogens. Silva *et al.*[112] also reported that DLE therapy was not associated with any detectable therapeutic effect in eight melanoma patients, and only one had doubtful benefit. In general the response to PHA and ConA increased after DLE therapy. Grob *et al.*[113] also were not able to observe any clinical improvement in five cases of melanoma treated with DLE; however, the donors of DLE were not selected on the basis of sensitivity to melanoma antigens. Using DLE from healthy donors not sensitized to tumour antigens, Khan *et al.*[114] failed to observe any clinical benefits in four patients treated with DLE. On the other hand, when DLE and BCG therapy were combined in two patients, a remarkable clinical effect was observed, even though BCG therapy alone seemed to be ineffective in these patients.

Another cancer on which DLE has been used is breast cancer. The first studies were performed by Oettgen *et al.*[115] which were developed and completed later[116]. These investigators used DLE from healthy donors, who were assumed to be sensitive to the tumour antigen since they were women over 45 years of age. In five cases of advanced breast carcinoma, they observed in one case that there was pain at the tumour site 10 h after DLE injection, which was not followed by reduction of tumour growth or clinical improvement. In a second case there was a reduction of tumour growth and clinical improvement during 6 months. No effect was observed whatsoever in the remaining three patients treated. Interestingly, only the patients in whom an effect of DLE was detected showed skin test positivity to one or two antigens following DLE therapy. Smith *et al.*[108], using DLE obtained from actively sensitized donors and combining the DLE therapy with BCG, observed that in five cases treated only one responded to the treatment. Silva *et al.*[112] reported that DLE from donors apparently sensitized to the tumour antigen was able to stabilize 16 metastatic nodules in the mastectomy scar. Khan *et al.*[114] using unrelated healthy donors of DLE, were unable to find any clinical response following DLE therapy. Fudenberg (in preparation) obtained partial remissions in two out of three patients with stage 3 breast cancer, using large amounts of DLE from donors with high cell-mediated cytotoxicity to breast cancer cells.

Of particular interest is the study of DLE therapy in patients afflicted with osteogenic sarcoma, as recently reviewed by Fudenberg[117]. In 1972 Levin *et al.*[118] reported one case of osteogenic sarcoma in which DLE seemed to have some beneficial clinical effect. DLE was obtained from a family contact known to be sensitized to the tumour antigen. Subsequently, Levin *et al.*[10] reported that in 13 patients with osteogenic sarcoma treated with DLE from donors sensitized to the tumour antigen, all increased their immunity against tumour as evaluated by cytotoxicity. Patients who received DLE obtained from donors non-sensitized to tumour antigen showed evidence of declining cell-mediated cytotoxicity. Three patients treated in phase I with 'specific' DLE were free of disease for the time of observation, i.e. from 11 to 15 months, and had increased values of cytotoxicity against tumour. Seven out of seven patients with no demonstrable tumour after resection of the primary tumour (and in two instances, single lung metastases as well) remained free of metastases for 28–29 months after initiation of therapy with DLE from donors with high cell-mediated cytotoxicity to osteosarcoma cell lines. DLE was discontinued 24 months after initiation. At the last report, two patients had relapsed at 40 and 48 months, and five were still disease-free at 48 months. Every time they received DLE from non-immunized donors, the levels of cytotoxicity of the patients against the tumour decreased. Two patients in phase II, one treated with donor-specific DLE had increased values of cytoxicity against tumour tissues and increased numbers of total and active E-rosette-forming cells and had remarkable clinical improvement. The patient not treated with DLE showed no clinical improvement or increase of cytoxicity against tumour tissues. Three patients in phase III treated with DLE from donors sensitized to tumour antigens all showed increased CMI evaluated by cytotoxicity or numbers of active or total E-rosette-forming cells. One was free of disease during the period of observation, but two died. One patient not treated with DLE had consistently low values of cytotoxicity and low numbers of T cells but was normal 11 months after immunization. In stage IV, four out of the five patients treated with DLE obtained from donors sensitized to osteogenic sarcoma antigen, showed increases in CMI parameters which were accompanied by clinical improvement. Only one case seemed to be resistant to DLE therapy.

It is striking that several of the patients described above complained of intensive pain in tumour lesions after DLE therapy, and that most of them had a massive infiltration of mononuclear cells into the tumour after therapy, as shown by biopsies before and after therapy. This is almost never found in patients without treatment, or in patients treated by radiation or chemotherapy. Another interesting observation was reported by Levin *et al.*[119], who observed that one case of osteosarcoma treated with DLE metastasized as giant cell tumours, which is a more benign tumour than osteosarcoma, although the two are closely related. The degeneration of giant cell tumour into malignant sarcoma is common but the reverse situation, which was attributed by the investigators to DLE therapy, is not.

Bearden *et al.*[120] and Thor *et al.*[121] also observed that DLE therapy in combination with chemotherapy could prolong the survival of osteogenic sarcoma patients and induce an increase of CMI. In a recent work, Vetto *et al.*[110] reported clinical benefit in one out of five patients with osteogenic sarcoma treated with DLE obtained from home contacts.

Other neoplastic diseases have also been treated with DLE. Lobuglio and Neidhart[122] reported that in three patients with acute lymphatic leukaemia who had had multiple relapses, DLE from unrelated healthy donors produced a release of MIF against leukaemic blasts in two patients. The third patient relapsed and showed no change in MIF assays. Khan *et al.*[123] reported that skin sensitivity was induced in five out of eight individuals with Hodgkin's disease and that three acquired DNCB hypersensitivity after DLE therapy. DLE was obtained from individuals assumed to be sensitive to the aetiological agent of Hodgkin's disease, as they were household contacts. These patients also showed increased numbers of E-rosette-forming cells.

Bukowski *et al.*[111] reported a study of three patients with renal carcinoma treated with DLE from donors who demonstrated greater than 80% lymphocyte toxicity against cultured renal carcinoma tumour cells. In two of three patients the disease was stable for periods of 4 and 6 months. These two patients had an increase of cytotoxicity against renal carcinoma cells after treatment with DLE.

Lobuglio *et al.*[124] reported a case of alveolar sarcoma who developed MIF to tumour preparations after treatment with DLE obtained from a household contact. Two patients with nasopharyngeal carcinoma have also been treated with DLE obtained from individuals sensitive to Epstein–Barr virus (EBV)[125]. These two patients acquired immunity against tumour tissues and both had clinical improvement. Brandes *et al.*[126] later reported that DLE from EBV-sensitive individuals was able to confer similar reactivity to two out of four patients afflicted with nasopharyngeal carcinoma.

Other neoplastic tumours treated with DLE obtained from household contacts include rhabdomyosarcoma, leiomyosarcoma, Wilm's tumour, renal cell carcinoma, liposarcoma, epidermoid carcinoma, carcinoma of the cervix, adenocarcinoma of the colon, dermal carcinoma and neuroblastoma, lymphosarcoma, synovial sarcoma, basal cell carcinoma, etc. The results are difficult to interpret, as only one case of each kind of tumour has been treated, but in general promising results are reported.

In summary it can be said that DLE of appropriate specificity is able at least to induce in recipients an increase in cellular immunity to tumour antigens. According to the majority of the reports, this can be accomplished only when DLE is obtained from donors with high levels of cellular immunity to tumour antigens. The beneficial therapeutic effect of DLE is somewhat difficult to evaluate, however, due mainly to the fact that most patients who have received DLE have had very advanced forms of cancer. Also, several of these patients have been under treatment with other forms of therapy. Thus there is little evidence that DLE *per se* can 'cure' advanced cancer patients. It appears that DLE provides adjuvant therapy in cancer if used in adequate circumstances, rather than being a major therapeutic agent.

Therapeutic use of DLE in non-malignant diseases

Although the mechanisms of action of DLE are not known, it has been used in a number of patients with immunodeficiencies associated with defective cell-mediated immunity (CMI), beginning in 1969 when Fudenberg's group[22] injected DLE in patients with Wiskott–Aldrich syndrome (for previous reviews see refs. 113, 127 and 128). Resistance to certain organisms (such as *Listeria monocytogenes*, *Salmonella typhimurium*, and *Mycobacterium tuberculosis*) is expressed in mononuclear phagocytes with enhanced bactericidal activity. This activity appears to be induced through the action of chemical 'mediators' of CMI released from sensitized lymphocytes stimulated by microbial antigens[129]. Clinical studies have revealed abnormalities at several steps in this reaction. On the other hand, there is evidence that deficient CMI might in some patient groups be limited to some lymphocyte subpopulations. It has been shown that when cells which are dividing in response to an antigen are killed, the surviving cells are still able to respond to the same antigen by producing migration inhibition factor (MIF)[130]. In fact, in many immunodeficiency diseases there is dissociation between the *in vivo* and *in vitro* expression of CMI. This suggests that in some patients the defect in CMI might be linked to the mediator-producing cell lines, while in other patients the defect may affect both cell lines or a common precursor cell[131].

The differences in the defects of CMI in different diseases and the unknown mechanisms of action of DLE have prompted efforts to treat patients with various infections, with many primary or secondary immunodeficiencies, and with various diseases of unknown aetiology. In patients with combined immunodeficiency diseases bone marrow transplantation has largely been used, and in severe T cell disorders, fetal thymic transplantation has been used alone or in combination with DLE. In this review we have collected only those patients in which crude DLE or its partially purified fractions have been used. In most of these cases it is difficult to determine whether donor-specific DLE is more effective than DLE from random donors; therefore, that aspect is not considered in the following review.

Immunodeficiency diseases

DLE has been used in at least 34 patients with Wiskott–Aldrich syndrome[9,15,22,61,132–139], in eight with ataxia telangiectasia[9,15,113,139,141], in 21 patients with combined immunodeficiency disease[15,26,113,133,134,139,141–146], in six with unclassified immunodeficiency syndrome[17,25,44,54,147–149], in four with Nezelof syndrome[27,43,150], and in five patients with variable a-, hypo-, or dysgammaglobulinaemia[9,15,151].

(a) *Wiskott–Aldrich syndrome (WAS)*—Wiskott–Aldrich syndrome, inherited in an X-linked fashion, consists of eczema, recurrent pyogenic infections, and thrombocytopenia. The diagnosis can be made at birth by demonstration of thrombocytopenia in male infants with positive family history. Patients may have bleeding early in life secondary to thrombocytopenia, and they almost always develop recurrent bacterial infections (e.g. pneumonia, otitis media, and meningitis). Infections early in life are caused by polysaccharide-containing organisms (e.g. pneumococcus, meningococcus, and *Haemophilus influenza*) and later on by other types of microorganisms and viruses. The eczema has similarities with atopic eczema and usually appears by 1 year of age. Splenomegaly is present in 50% of the patients. WAS is progressive, with increasing susceptibility to bacterial and viral infections and lymphomas. Death usually occurs before puberty.

Immunodeficiency in WAS has been reviewed by Blaese *et al.*[152] and by Spitler *et al.*[9]. Briefly, patients with WAS have normal numbers of B lymphocytes and normal or elevated levels of immunoglobulins. The survival of immunoglobulins is shortened and the patients synthesize them at an accelerated rate, but production of specific antibody to all kind of antigens, especially polysaccharide antigens, is very poor.

Decreased CMI is documented in most patients with WAS by skin testing and by *in vitro* tests. Most fail to demonstrate delayed-type hypersensitivity to common microbial antigens and fail more often than controls to develop skin reactivity following sensitization with dinitrochlorbenzene (DNCB) or keyhole limpet haemocyanin (KLH). Lymphocyte DNA synthesis and macrophage migration inhibition factor (MIF) production in response to a number of antigens have been shown to be impaired in these patients. Results for lymphocyte transformation to non-specific mitogens have been variable, and normal in some patients. In addition, mediators of CMI, including MIF, lymphotoxin, and monocyte chemotactic factor, are produced normally in mitogen-stimulated cultures. It has also been reported that cytotoxic effector ('killer') T lymphocyte function *in vitro* is normal. The proportion of circulating T lymphocytes is decreased in some patients but normal in most. Active T cells constitute only 1–3% of the total lymphocytes, however, whereas in normal individuals they average 28% of the total lymphocytes[27]. Thus, based on *in vivo* as well as in many *in vitro* tests, a deficiency of T-cell function has been documented in WAS.

The largest series of WAS patients treated with DLE has been reported by Fudenberg's group from California[9,22,61,132–138]. In the first reports[22,61,134] seven out of 12 patients acquired the same skin reactivities as expressed by the donor of DLE, with the exception of one patient who acquired delayed skin sensitivity toward an antigen to which the donor of DLE was negative. In addition, conversion to MIF production to the same antigens, as well as clinical improvement, was noted in all seven patients, although lymphocyte transformation tests remained negative. Six out of 12 recovered from infection, and regression of splenomegaly was observed. The eczema cleared in five of the 12 patients, and a rise in platelets and decrease in bleeding were seen in three out of 10 patients.

The number of active T cells increased from 1–3% to 10–12%[27]. The clinical and immunological remission lasted for about 6 months, and new injections of DLE prevented clinical recurrence[9,135]. This suggests that the clone of antigen-specific lymphocytes has a limited half-life compared with that in normal individuals, in whom the sensitivity transferred even with very small amounts of DLE persists for 1 to 2 years. All the patients with WAS who responded to DLE were found to be defective in the ability of their monocytes to bind IgG-containing complexes, while the patients with normal IgG receptor capacity have been non-responsive[45,61]. The initial results of DLE therapy in WAS reported by Levin *et al.*[22,134] and Spitler *et al.*[61] have been confirmed by many groups of investigators (see Table 2.8). Griscelli *et al.*[15,139] have reported clinical improvement in two out of four patients with two injections of DLE. In these patients, regression of infections, eczema, splenomegaly, and bleeding lasted for 3 months. Ballow *et al.*[138] reported clearing of eczema, conversion of skin reactivity, and blastogenic response of lymphocytes *in vitro* to a number of donor-specific antigens and reactivity of lymphocytes in mixed leukocyte cultures (MLC) after two injections of DLE in two patients with WAS who had a deficiency of monocyte receptors for IgG.

Grob *et al.*[113,140] have reported therapy of three patients, two of whom showed at least transitory clinical benefit after DLE, and Sellars *et al.*[143] described one patient who developed lymphoma during the DLE therapy. Ammann *et al.*[142] did not find immunological conversion nor clinical benefit in two WAS patients treated with DLE. To conclude, immune conversion has been found in 63% and at least some clinical improvement in 52% of the patients with WAS treated with DLE.

(b) *Ataxia telangiectasia*—Immunodeficiency in ataxia telangiectasia has been reviewed by Biggar and Good[153]. Ataxia telangiectasia involves the neurological, muscular, cutaneous, endocrine, and immune systems and is inherited in an autosomal manner. The complete syndrome consists of ataxia, telangiectasia, and recurrent sinopulmonary infections. Ataxia is usually seen at 1 year of age or later but can be delayed until 9 years of age. Secondary

Table 2.8 DLE in congenital immunodeficiency diseases

Disease	*Number of patients*	*Immune conversion (1–3 of following skin reactivity, blastogenesis, MIF production)*	*Clinical improvement (at least transitory)*	*Reference*
Wiskott–Aldrich syndrome	24	15/24	12/23	Levin *et al.* (1970)
				Spitler *et al.* (1972)
				Hitzig *et al.* (1972)
				Levin *et al.* (1973)
				Fudenberg *et al.* (1974)
				Levin *et al.* (1975)
				Spitler *et al.* (1975)
				Ballow *et al.* (1975)
	4	4/4	2/4	Griscelli *et al.* (1973, 1975)
	3	0/1	2/3	Grob *et al.* (1973, 1975, 1976)
	2	0/2	0/2	Ammann *et al.* (1974)
	1	1/1	1/1	Sellars *et al.* (1975)
Ataxia telangiectasia	5	4/5	3/5	Griscelli *et al.* (1973, 1975)
	2	1/2	1/2	Grob *et al.* (1975, 1976)
	1	0/1	0/1	Spitler *et al.* (1975)
Combined immunodeficiency syndrome	1	1/1	1/1	Hitzig *et al.* (1972)
	1	1/1	1/1	Mogerman *et al.* (1973)
	7	4/7	2/6	Spitler *et al.* (1975) (reviewed)
	1	1/1	0/1	Gelfand *et al.* (1973)
	2	0/2	0/2	Griscelli *et al.* (1973, 1975)
	1	1/1	0/1	Goldblum *et al.* (1973)
	1	1/1	1/1	Montgomery *et al.* (1973)
	7	0/3	3/7	Grob *et al.* (1975, 1976)
	4	3/4	2/4	Ammann *et al.* (1974)
Unclassified immunodeficiency syndrome	1	1/1	1/1	Valdimarsson *et al.* (1974)
	1	1/1	1/1	Arala-Chaves *et al.* (1974)
	1	1/1	1/1	Ballow *et al.* (1975, 1976)
	1	1/1	1/1	Strauss *et al.* (1974)
	1	1/1	—	Criswell *et al.* (1975)
	1	1/1	1/1	Stoop *et al.* (1976)
Nezelof syndrome	1	0/1	0/1	Wybran *et al.* (1973)
	3	2/3	0/3	Lawlor *et al.* (1974)
	4	0/4	0/4	Pachman *et al.* (1974)
Variable hypo-, dys-, or agammaglobulinaemia	2	2/2	0/2	Griscelli *et al.* (1973)
	1	0/1	1/1	Zaldivar *et al.* (1975)
	2	2/2	1/2	Spitler *et al.* (1975)

sexual characteristics are usually lacking and the patients exhibit mental retardation.

Patients with ataxia telangiectasia have abnormalities in both T- and B-cell immunity. Selective IgA deficiency is present in 40% of patients and IgE may be absent. The disorder is progressive, and both neurological and immunological abnormalities become more severe with time. Susceptibility to infection includes both viral and bacterial infections, which in addition to lymphoreticular malignancies are the chief cause of death in these patients.

Various degrees of abnormalities in T-cell immunity have been described.

Lymphopenia may be present. The number of T cells, response of lymphocytes to PHA, allogeneic cells, and antigens, and skin-test reactivity to common antigens can be low or sometimes normal. T-cell deficiency is observed to become more severe with advancing age. The thymus shows morphological characteristics of an embryonic thymus.

Fetal thymus transplantation has provided some benefit in these patients, and DLE has been used in eight cases (Table 2.8). Some immune conversion was reported in five of the eight and clinical benefit in half of the patients.

(c) *Combined immunodeficiency diseases*—This disease has been shown to have many variants and different stages of severity depending on the proliferative stage of the stem cells. Severe combined immunodeficiency disease is associated with complete absence of T- and B-cell immunity. Deficiency in T cells is shown by lymphopenia, absence of thymus shadow, low number of T cells, absence of *in vitro* response to PHA, antigens, and allogeneic cells, and absence of delayed skin reactivity. B-cell deficiency includes hypogammaglobulinaemia, absence of antibody response to immunization, and depressed numbers of B cells.

Onset of symptoms is usually by 6 months of age, and patients are susceptible to recurrent viral, bacterial, fungal, and protozoal infections. The disease occurs in both X-linked and autosomal forms, and many patients die before the diagnosis is made. By bone marrow transplantation the immune system of the patients can be completely restored. Complete improvement of immune response is seen even for 10 years after successful bone marrow transplants; however, graft-versus-host reactions are seen in many of these patients. Therefore, in the absence of a histocompatible bone marrow donor, other forms of therapy have been used, such as fetal liver transplants, fetal thymus transplantation, and DLE. DLE has been applied in at least 21 patients with combined immunodeficiency disease, although it is difficult to establish its clinical effect in these multi-defective immune disorders. Immune conversion has been reported in 57% of the patients following DLE and transitory clinical improvement in 40%.

(d) *Unclassified immunodeficiency syndromes*—Six patients with unclassified immunodeficiency syndromes showing heterogeneous symptoms have been treated with DLE (Table 2.8). All these patients showed some degree of

T-cell deficiency, and in all cases immune conversion and at least transient clinical improvement were observed.

(e) *Nezelof's syndrome*—Patients with Nezelof's syndrome (cellular immunodeficiency with abnormal immunoglobulin synthesis) are susceptible to many kinds of infections, and many die before 18 years of age because of infections or malignancies. It is thought that Nezelof's syndrome is the result of thymus hypoplasia with deficient interactions of T and B cells. The degree of T-cell deficiency varies in these patients. Histocompatible bone marrow transplantation has been curative in these patients, and thymus transplantation has been reported to provide reconstitution of T-cell function and partial restoration of B-cell function. DLE has been used in eight patients with Nezelof's syndrome (Table 2.8). Only transient delayed skin-test reactivity was seen in two of eight patients, and no clinical improvement was seen.

(f) *A-, hypo- and dysgammaglobulinaemia*—Congenital agammaglobulinaemia has been considered a stem-cell deficiency involving only B cells. With increasing knowledge about the regulatory effects of T cells on antibody production by B cells and the binding of B lymphocytes with immunoglobulins and receptors for complement in the peripheral circulation of some patients with agammaglobulinaemia, interest has centred on studies of T-cell function in these patients. Recent studies in man have in fact demonstrated a variable T-lymphocyte deficiency in some patients with congenital agammaglobulinaemia or in late-onset 'acquired' hypogammaglobulinaemia. This suggests that the B-cell dysfunction in this disease may result in some cases from faulty interaction of T and B cells. It has been shown that patients with agammaglobulinaemia and impaired CMI respond to DLE with the activation of long-lived systemic delayed hypersensitivity, suggesting the normal function of T cells in expression of CMI. This suggests that regulatory T-cell function is separate from that of T cells responsible for delayed skin reactivity. Although the effect of DLE on T–B interaction has not been defined, such an effect on T cells has been suggested as the cause of clinical benefits in one patient with agammaglobulinaemia[151] and in some patients with hypo- or dysgammaglobulinaemia[9,15].

DLE in chronic fungal infections

(a) *Chronic mucocutaneous candidiasis (CMCC)—Candida* infection may involve skin, nails, and scalp and buccal, gastrointestinal, respiratory, and vaginal mucous membranes. In severe forms granulomatous lesions occur. Involvement of parenchymatous organs such as liver or kidney is also seen. Patients are usually not susceptible to systemic candidal infections. Familial CMCC can be associated with endocrinopathy. Hypoparathyroidism is common and is associated with hypercalcaemia and tetany. Addison's disease is also common. Ovarian insufficiency, thyroid anomalies and thymoma, diabetes, pernicious anaemia, agranulocytosis, myeloperoxidase deficiency, and/or acute or chronic hepatitis have also been reported in these patients and in their first-degree relatives. B-cell immunity is intact, with normal production of antibody to *Candida*, and in some patients the development of autoantibodies associated with endocrinopathies has been found.

There is a selective defect in CMI to *Candida* antigen in patients with CMCC. Delayed hypersensitivity skin tests to *Candida* are negative in 96% of the patients, and half have an absence of [^{3}H]thymidine uptake by their mononuclear cells when stimulated with *Candida in vitro* (Table 2.9). Absence of MIF release by patients' mononuclear cells in the presence of *Candida* is reported in 83% of the cases[9,45,154,164]. Valdimarsson *et al.*[154] distinguished four immunological patterns in 26 patients with CMCC: (a) 10 out of 26 patients had no significant abnormalities in CMI; (b) nine out of 26 had negative skin reactivity and no MIF production or lymphocyte transformation *in vitro* in response to *Candida* antigen; (c) five of the 26 failed to produce MIF *in vitro*, and four out of five were negative by skin test, although the lymphocytes of all five patients showed increased DNA synthesis after stimulation *in vitro* by *Candida* antigen; and (d) in two of the 26, *Candida* did not induce skin reactivity or lymphocyte activation *in vitro*, although the antigen induced normal MIF production; however, intradermal injection of MIF did not produce a delayed inflammatory response in these two patients as it did in healthy persons, suggesting a defective macrophage function. Therefore, one important defect in cellular immunity in CMCC is likely to be in the cells producing MIF. The presence of a factor in the serum which inhibits lymphocyte [^{3}H]thymidine incorporation in some of these patients has also been observed[154,165,166].

Skin reactivity, activation of lymphocytes *in vitro*, and MIF production in response to antigens other than *Candida* are usually normal. The patients usually also have a normal response of lymphocytes to PHA and allogeneic cells *in vitro*, and T-cell rosettes are present in normal numbers.

Because of the selective absence of CMI to *Candida* antigen, DLE preparations from normal donors with positive skin test to *Candida* have been used in the therapy of CMCC[9,14,15,45,60,113,133,141,155–164,167–170]. At least 65 patients have been treated by different investigators (Table 2.9). Positive skin tests to *Candida* were found in 89%, compared with 4% before DLE therapy. Blastogenesis to *Candida* was also seen more often after DLE than before (71% and 48% respectively). Conversion of MIF production has been found as often as conversion of skin reactivity to *Candida* after DLE therapy (Table 2.9).

A final judgement on the clinical effect of DLE therapy in CMCC is difficult, since many patients received additional treatment and because this is a syndrome rather than a disease. In all cases, patients with CMCC had been pretreated unsuccessfully with mycostatic drugs such as amphotericin B,

Table 2.9 DLE in chronic fungal infections

Reference	*Number of patients*	*Positive response to specific antigen before DLE*			*Positive response to specific antigen after DLE*			*Clinical improvement (at least transitory or combined with antifungal therapy)*
		Skin test	*Blasto-genesis*	*MIF*	*Skin test*	*Blasto-genesis*	*MIF*	
Chronic mucocutaneous candidiasis (donor-specific DLE)								
Kirkpatrick *et al.* (1970)	3	0/3	0/3	ND	0/1	1/1	ND	0/3
Kirkpatrick *et al.* (1972)	5	0/5	1/5	0/5	5/5	3/5	5/5	2/5
Kirkpatrick and Smith (1974)	5	0/5	1/5	0/5	5/5	3/5	5/5	2/5
Kirkpatrick (1975) (reviewed)	5	0/5	1/5	0/5	5/5	3/5	5/5	2/5
Kirkpatrick and Gallin (1975)	1	0/1	ND	0/1	1/1	ND	1/1	0/1
Rocklin *et al.* (1970)	2	0/2	1/2	0/2	1/2	1/2	1/2	0/2
Pabst and Swanson (1972)	1	0/1	0/1	ND	1/1	1/1	ND	1/1
Rocklin *et al.* (1975) (reviewed)	2	0/2	1/2	0/2	2/2	2/2	1/2	1/2
Schulkind *et al.* (1972)	1	0/1	1/1	ND	1/1	1/1	1/1	1/1
Schulkind and Ayoub (1975)	1	0/1	0/1	0/1	1/1	1/1	1/1	1/1
Spitler *et al.* (1973)	7	0/7	4/7	4/7	5/7	4/7	5/6	5/7
Hitzig *et al.* (1972)	3	0/3	3/3	3/3	3/3	3/3	2/2	3/3
Spitler *et al.* (1975) (reviewed)	4	1/4	1/3	0/2	2/3	1/1	1/1	1/3
Valdimarsson *et al.* (1972)	1	0/1	0/1	1/1	1/1	1/1	1/1	1/1
Griscelli *et al.* (1973)	1	0/1	0/1	ND	1/1	1/1	ND	1/1
Blaker *et al.* (1973)	2	0/2	0/2	0/2	2/2	2/2	ND	2/2
Snyderman *et al.* (1973)	1	0/1	1/1	ND	1/1	0/1	ND	1/1
Group *et al.* (1975)	12	0/12	5/10	ND	11/12	8/9	ND	10/12
Group *et al.* (1976)	10	—	—	—	—	—	—	7/10
José (1975)	6	0/6	6/6	0/6	6/6	ND	ND	6/6
Ballow *et al.* (1975)	1	0/1	0/1	ND	0/1	0/1	ND	1/1
De Sousa *et al.* (1976)	1	0/1	0/1	0/1	1/1	0/1	1/1	1/1
Lawton *et al.* (1976)	1	0/1	0/1	ND	1/1	0/1	ND	1/1
Littman *et al.* (1977)	1	0/1	1/1	0/1	1/1	1/1	1/1	1/1
Krohn *et al.* (1977)	7	+	ND	ND	++	ND	ND	7/7
Chronic vaginal candidiasis (donor-specific DLE)								
Grob *et al.* (1974)	1	0/1	0/1	ND	1/1	1/1	ND	1/1
Coccidioidomycosis (donor-specific DLE)								
Graybill *et al.* (1973, 1975), Catanzaro and Spitler (1976)	49	8/44	9/32	3/28	32/44	27/32	24/28	31/49
Stevens *et al.* (1974)	1	0/1	0/1	ND	1/1	0/1	ND	1/1
Steele *et al.* (1976)	1	0/1	0/1	ND	1/1	1/1	ND	1/1
TOTAL	117	10/95 (11%)	30/79 (38%)	8/57 (14%)	77/94 (82%)	54/70 (77%)	42/48 (88%)	84/116 (72%)

5-fluorocytosin, carbinazon, clotrimatzole, or others before DLE was tried. In about 78% some clinical improvement, at least transitory, has been reported (Table 2.9). It seems that one requirement for a clinical effect of DLE is treatment with large and repeated doses. Improvement in most studies was questionable and transitory after the first injection but more pronounced after several injections of DLE. The same transitory or weak response after the first DLE injection has also been seen in skin reactivity and *in vitro* reactivity of lymphocytes to *Candida* in many patients.

Spitler *et al.*[9] reported that patients with granulomatous lesions might respond more successfully than those with other forms of candidiasis. On the other hand, Grob *et al.*[113] could not find any characteristic clinical form of candidiasis nor specific type of immune deficiency which responded better to DLE therapy than others. More studies and long-term observations are needed for a definitive decision about the therapeutic value of DLE in chronic mucocutaneous candidiasis.

(b) *Vaginal candidiasis*—DLE has also been used successfully in the treatment of vaginal candidiasis[171].

(c) *Chronic coccidioidomycosis*—DLE has been used in a number of patients with chronic coccidioidomycosis[172–176] (Table 2.9). In 51 patients reported, responses to coccidioidin were seen in skin tests in 17%, in lymphocyte DNA synthesis tests in 26%, and in MIF production in 11% of the patients. After DLE injections, skin reactivity was seen in 74%, blastogenesis in 82%, and MIF production in 86% of the patients in response to coccidioidin. Clinical improvement was seen in 65%. Thus chronic coccidioidomycosis has many similarities with CMCC pertinent to the effects of DLE.

Viral infections

Cell-mediated immunity is the primary defence against viral infections. In addition, decreased CMI has been documented in many viral diseases. Therefore, several attempts have been made to stimulate the function of T cells in patients with viral infections. DLE has been used in measles[177], neonatal herpes, herpes zoster[178,179], eczema vaccinatum[9,180], human warts[181], papillomatosis of the larynx[138,182], and cytomegalovirus retinitis[179,183] (Table 2.10). In most of these studies only clinical observations have been made, and improvement in the clinical symptoms has been reported in all patients, except in human warts, where because of the high incidence of spontaneous remission, the clinical course is difficult to evaluate. Stevens *et al.*[181] have treated the largest series of patients with warts; they found clinical improvement in seven cases, but this did not differ from patients without DLE therapy.

(a) *Subacute sclerosing panencephalitis (SSPE)*—Briefly, SSPE is a degenerative disease of the central nervous system. The measles virus, or a virus closely associated, plays an important role in the disease and can be seen in the brain and other organs of these patients. Complement deposits in the glomerular basement membrane have been found in many patients. Increased antibody response and decreased CMI response against the viral

Table 2.10 DLE in viral diseases

Reference	*Number of patients*	*Immune conversion*	*Clinical improvement (at least transitory)*
Measles			
Moulias *et al.* (1973)	2	2/2	2/2
Neonatal herpes			
Moulias *et al.* (1973)	1	ND	1/1
Herpes zoster			
Drew *et al.* (1973)	1	ND	1/1
Heim *et al.* (1976)	1	ND	1/1
Human warts			
Stevens *et al.* (1972)	18	ND	7/18*
Spitler *et al.* (1975)	5	ND	1/5
Eczema vaccinatum			
Dahl *et al.* (1975)	1	ND	1/1
Grob *et al.* (1976)	2	ND	2/2
Papillomatosis of the larynx			
Quick *et al.* (1975)	2	2/2	2/2
Ballow *et al.* (1975)	1	ND	1/1
Cytomegalovirus retinitis			
Rytel *et al.* (1975)	1	ND	1/1
Heim *et al.* (1976)	1	ND	1/1
Subacute sclerosing panencephalitis			
Moulias *et al.* (1973)	15	9/15	2/15
Vandvik *et al.* (1973)	1	0/1	1/1
Grob *et al.* (1975), Ter Meulen *et al.* (1975), Kackel *et al.* (1975)	13	0/13	0/13
Pabst *et al.* (1975)	2	1/2	0/2
Blease *et al.* (1975)	6	ND	0/6
Chronic hepatitis B			
Kohler *et al.* (1974)	2	1/2	1/2
Shulman *et al.* (1974, 1976)	6	ND	5/6
Sano *et al.* (1977)	5	3/5	0/5
Grob *et al.* (1975)	1	0/1	0/1
Spitler *et al.* (1975)	1	ND	0/6
Jain *et al.* (1975, 1976)	6	ND	0/6
Tong *et al.* (1976)	1	1/1	0/1
Khan *et al.* (1976)	3	ND	0/3
Multiple sclerosis			
Jersild *et al.* (1973, 1976)	5	4/5	0/5
Zabriskie *et al.* (1975)	16	+	?/15
Grob *et al.* (1975, 1976)	5	5/5	0/5
Platz *et al.* (1976)	12	9/9	2/11
Khan *et al.* (1976)	2	ND	?/2
Behan (1976)	14	ND	1/14
Angers *et al.* (1976)	20	8/14	11/20

* Same as controls

agent have been reported, although generalized defects of CMI are not a typical feature in such patients. Results have been reported for 37 patients with SSPE who received DLE injections[32,13,172,184–187] (Table 2.10). In most cases, large doses have repeatedly been given to these patients. Immune conversion has been reported in only one out of 16 patients, except by Moulias *et al.*[177], who reported conversion in nine of his 15 patients. Their study was the only one in which the donors were tested for CMI against measles virus, which is low or absent in 30% of normal adults, despite the presence of anti-measles antibodies. Some clinical improvement has been reported in three out of 37 patients (8%).

(b) *Chronic hepatitis B*—Chronic active type B hepatitis is caused by the hepatitis B virus and is characterized by progressive hepatocellular damage leading to cirrhosis and portal hypertension. Hepatocellular carcinomas also develop later on in these patients. Since abnormal CMI responses to HBsAg have been found in some of these patients, it has been postulated that decreased CMI may permit the invasion by the hepatitis B virus, or that decreased interferon production in the host may be involved. Several attempts have been made to correct the immune defect by DLE. Twenty-five patients have been given DLE[9,113,114,181–194] (Table 2.10); in five out of nine immune conversion was seen and in only six out of 25 some clinical improvement. It might be that DLE can confer or enhance the recipient's immune response to hepatitis B virus or related antigens, resulting in transient antibody production; on the other hand, it may increase the cytotoxicity to virus-infected hepatocytes and increase the damage in the liver.

(c) *Multiple sclerosis*—Reports of paramyxovirus-like structures in the nuclei of mononuclear cells in lesions of acute multiple sclerosis (MS) have received much attention. Increased antibody titres to measles and other paramyxoviruses and diminished CMI to these antigens as measured by lymphocyte stimulation and MIF production have been reported in MS, as have oligoclonal antibodies to these viruses in spinal fluid; therefore, DLE therapy has been tried in this disease[113,141,195–200]. Except for one non-critical study by Angers *et al.*[200], using an undialysed extract of whole blood which was nevertheless termed 'transfer factor', almost no clinical benefit has been found. However, Platz *et al.*[198] reported immune conversion in all of his nine patients studied and signs of clinical benefit in two out of 11 patients. Angers *et al.*[200] reported immune conversion in eight out of 14 and clinical benefit from DLE in 11 out of 20 patients. The doses of DLE needed for immune conversion seem to vary considerably, and changes in reactivity to measles virus or other virus antigens seem to be only temporary. Systematic and long-term trials, including careful selection of donors and careful monitoring of recipients so that therapy can be given at appropriate intervals, are needed to judge the clinical effects of DLE in this disease.

Other infectious diseases

(a) *Leprosy*—Decreased CMI in lepromatous leprosy has been demonstrated by delayed hypersensitivity skin tests, by lymphocyte transformation tests with various antigens, and by delayed rejection of skin allografts, decreased MIF production, histological study of lymph nodes, and decreased numbers of rosette-forming T cells in the peripheral blood of patients.

DLE has been used in 18 patients with leprosy[201–203], almost all of whom had lepromatous leprosy, in which the decrease of CMI is much more pronounced than in tuberculoid or borderline leprosy. Immune conversion, mainly shown by skin-test reactivity to leprosium, was seen in 63% and clinical benefit in 51% of the patients. Most of the patients continued to receive chemotherapy, assumed to be effective against *Mycobacterium leprosum*, along with DLE therapy, however, and therefore the effect of DLE alone is difficult to evaluate.

(b) *Mycobacterium tuberculosis* and *M. avium*—In certain instances, infection by *M. tuberculosis* is associated with defective CMI. In these cases classic therapeutic procedures frequently fail. In attempting to correct the CMI defect, several investigators have used DLE therapy in their patients[141,160,204]. The results of treatment of various forms of *M. tuberculosis* infections, either pulmonary or cutaneous, are summarized in Table

Table 2.11 DLE in other infectious diseases

Reference	Number of patients	Immunological conversion	Clinical improvement
Leprosy			
Bullock *et al.* (1972)	9	6/7	6/9
Saha *et al.* (1975)	4	2/4	0/4
Hastings *et al.* (1976)	5	4/5	5/5
Mycobacterium tuberculosum			
Graybill *et al.* (1973)	1	1/1	0/1
Rocklin (1975)	1	1/1	1/1
Grob *et al.* (1976)	2	—	2/2
Horsmanheimo *et al.* (1976)	1	1/1	1/1
Miliary lupus of the face			
Grohn *et al.* (1976), Krohn *et al.* (1977)	2	2/2	2/2
Mycobacterium avium			
Thestrup-Pedersen *et al.* (1974)	1	1/1	0/1
Respiratory tract infections			
Dupree (1972)	1	1/1	1/1
Grohn (1977)	5	5/5	4/5
Histoplasmosis			
Graybill *et al.* (1976)	1	1/1	1/1
Schistomiasis			
Warren *et al.* (1975)	6	1/6	0/6
Urinary tract infections			
Anttila *et al.* (1976, 1977)	20	10/15	—

2.11. In all cases in which CMI was tested before and after DLE therapy, increased CMI was observed. Further, eight of the nine patients treated showed clinical improvement. In one case of a patient with *M. avium* infection, CMI was recovered after DLE therapy but there was no observable clinical improvement[53].

(c) *Respiratory tract infections*—Excellent clinical results have also been observed with DLE therapy in respiratory tract infections. All patients treated in two separate reports[207,208] showed improved CMI, and five out of six showed clinical improvement.

(d) *Histoplasmosis and schistosomiasis*—Recovery of CMI and clinical improvement was observed in one case of histoplasmosis[209]. In schistosomiasis[210], the effect was much less impressive; of six patients treated, only one experienced improvement of CMI and none showed clinical improvement.

(e) *Systemic lupus erythematosus*—Grob *et al.*[113] reported skin test conversion in one patient with systemic lupus erythematosus after DLE treatment, but no clinical improvement was observed. The dosage used may have been insufficient to be clinically effective.

(f) *Rheumatoid arthritis and juvenile rheumatoid arthritis*—Results in these cases are controversial. Cozine *et al.*[211] reported recovery of CMI in 16 of 27 patients with rheumatoid arthritis and clinical improvement in 10 patients after DLE therapy. Healey *et al.*[212] reported increase of CMI in one patient out of two but no clinical improvement in either patient. In a double-blind study, Maini *et al.*[213] reported that the effects of DLE and of saline were the same in terms of both apparent recovery of CMI and clinical improvement; however, there was no donor selection by immunological tests. In juvenile rheumatoid arthritis, Frøland *et al.*[214] and Grohn *et al.*[215] reported excellent results with DLE therapy. In all cases there was an increase of CMI; all three cases reported by Frøland *et al.* showed clinical improvement, and five of the eight cases reported by Grohn *et al.* showed clinical improvement.

(g) *Crohn's disease and sarcoidosis*—In Crohn's disease good results have also been reported. In fact, according to Asquith[216], six out of seven patients showed increased CMI and clinical improvement. In sarcoidosis, Horsmanheimo *et al.*[217] observed increased CMI in six out of eight patients, and Platz *et al.*[218] observed increased CMI in the only case treated. Similarly, Krohn *et al.*[179] observed increased CMI in six patients treated. In the past, Lawrence and Zweim[39], using crude non-dialysed leukocyte extract, and Urbach *et al.*[40], using viable leukocytes, had observed little or no effect on the CMI of recipients. No clinical improvement has been reported in any patients with sarcoidosis.

(h) *Behcet's syndrome*—Spitler *et al.*[9] reported unsuccessful DLE therapy in one case of Behcet's syndrome, and Heim *et al.*[179] reported increased CMI in one case tested and clinical improvement in three out of eight patients. More recently, Wolf *et al.*[219] reported clinical improvement in three out of six patients treated with DLE. Whether or not improvement occurred apparently depended on the donor used for preparation of DLE.

(i) *Miscellaneous*—Several other clinical conditions have also been treated with DLE, with variable results[9,171,179,220–223], as summarized in Table

Table 2.12 DLE in other diseases

Reference	*Number of patients*	*Immunological conversion*	*Clinical improvement (at least transitory)*
Systemic lupus erythematosus			
Grob *et al.* (1975)	1	1/1	0/1
Rheumatoid arthritis			
Healey *et al.* (1974)	2	1/2	0/2
Cozine *et al.* (1976)	27	16/27	10/27
Maini *et al.* (1976)	6	Same as placebo	Same as placebo
Juvenile rheumatoid arthritis			
Frøland *et al.* (1974), Kass *et al.* (1974)	3	3/3	3/3
Grohn *et al.* (1976)	8	8/8	5/8
Crohn's disease			
Asquith *et al.* (1975)	7	6/7	6/7
Sarcoidosis			
Lawrence *et al.* (1968)	7	2/7	—
Platz *et al.* (1976)	1	1/1	0/1
Horsmanheimo *et al.* (1976)	8	6/8	0/8
Krohn *et al.* (1977)	6	Increased	0/6
Behcet's syndrome			
Spitler *et al.* (1975)	1	ND	0/1
Heim *et al.* (1976)	8	1/1	3/8
Linear morphea			
Spitler *et al.* (1975)	1	1/1	1/1
Stomatitis aphtosa			
Spitler *et al.* (1975)	3	0/3	1/3
Asthma			
Khan *et al.* (1976)	4	3/4	4/4
Malnutrition and infection			
José *et al.* (1976)	40	ND	+
Malnutrition			
Brown *et al.* (1967)	12	12/12	—
Walker *et al.* (1975)	16	Same as controls	—
Reiter's syndrome			
Heim *et al.* (1976)	2	ND	0/2
Chronic dermatitis			
Heim *et al.* (1976)	2	ND	2/2
Cystic acne			
Krohn *et al.* (1977)	3	0/3	3/3

2.12. Of particular interest is the treatment of malnutrition patients. It is well known that patients with malnutrition exhibit defective CMI. Attempts have been made to correct the CMI defect and to treat subsequent infections in these patients by means of DLE. In 1967, Brown and Katz[221] reported that in 12 children with malnutritional problems treated with crude non-dialysed leukocyte extract, all showed increased CMI. In a double-blind study, however, Walker *et al.*[222] were unable to find any difference between the effects of DLE and placebo on CMI. More recently, José *et al.*[223] reported that patients treated with DLE had better protection against diarrhoea and acute gastroenteritis than untreated patients.

Conclusion: clinical effects of DLE

Side-effects

The question of side-effects is a point on which the enormous majority of investigators agree. DLE is a very innocuous substance. Only one case (an infant with severe combined immunodeficiency) has been reported in which the development of malignant disease apparently was connected with DLE therapy[145]. This report most probably represents a coincidence, as was pointed out by several authors[224–226]. Five unreported cases of reticulum cell sarcoma in patients with WAS who received DLE are known to us; however, among untreated patients, who usually die before puberty, 10% develop malignancies of this type, and it appears that most if not all of those kept alive by immunotherapy eventually develop such malignancies. In fact, even after repeated administration of high doses of DLE[10,115,122,127] no serious side-effects have been attributed to this substance either in normals or patients. Occasionally pain at the injection site or at the site of the pathological lesion, and sometimes transient fever, are observed. An erythematous reaction at the site of pathological lesions is also not uncommon.

Is DLE an effective therapeutic agent?

Clinical improvement and increased CMI have been reported frequently in patients treated with DLE, but there are also a number of reports in which DLE has proven to be quite ineffective. The most important of the latter are the double-blind studies in rheumatoid arthritis and in patients with malnutrition. On the other hand, in regard to the former study, it should be noted that if rheumatoid arthritis is, as has been suggested, caused by a given virus, then selection of individuals with high CMI to that virus as donors of DLE could produce beneficial clinical results. Additional controlled, double-blind studies of the use of DLE to treat different clinical conditions are obviously needed. It is well known that several clinical entities are cyclic in evolution, and clinical improvement is sometimes observed without any treatment. On the other hand, certain observations in these patients are difficult to attribute to spontaneous remission rather than to DLE, as is the case for osteosarcoma, mucocutaneous candidiasis, and certain complex immunodeficiencies which have been treated repeatedly with DLE, with observed increases in CMI being coincident with DLE therapy.

Other factors that make difficult a general conclusion about the efficacy of DLE treatment are the different doses of DLE used by each investigator, different methods of preparation and sources of DLE, and different recipients. The importance of recipient specificity in the effects of DLE has been stressed previously, and in fact it cannot be excluded that two individuals afflicted with the same general kind of disease will respond differently to DLE therapy.

ACKNOWLEDGEMENT

We are indebted to Charles L. Smith for his excellent editorial assistance.

References

1. Lawrence, H. S. (1955). The transfer in humans of delayed skin sensitivity to streptococcal M substance and to tuberculin with disrupted leukocytes. *J. Clin. Invest.*, **34**, 219
2. Lawrence, H. S., Al-Askari, S., David, J., Franklin, E. C. and Zweiman, B. (1963). Transfer of immunological information in humans with dialyzates of leukocyte extracts. *Trans. Assoc. Am. Phys.*, **76**, 84
3. Lawrence, H. S. (1969). Transfer factor. *Adv. Immunol.*, **11**, 195
4. Lawrence, H. S. (1971). Factors and activities produced *in vitro* by lymphocytes. In: In vitro *Methods in Cell-Mediated Immunity* (B. R. Bloom and P. R. Glade, eds.), p. 95 (New York: Academic Press)
5. Lawrence, H. S. and Pappenheimer, A. M. (1957). Effect of specific antigen on release from human leukocytes of the factor concerned in transfer of delayed hypersensitivity. *J. Clin. Invest.*, **36**, 908
6. Rapaport, F. T., Lawrence, H. S., Millar, J. W., Pappagianis, D. and Smith, C. E. (1960). Transfer of delayed hypersensitivity to coccidioidin in man. *J. Immunol.*, **84**, 358
7. Lawrence, H. S., Rapaport, F. T., Converse, J. M. and Tillett, W. S. (1960). Transfer of delayed hypersensitivity to skin homografts with leukocyte extracts in man. *J. Clin. Invest.*, **39**, 185
8. Zuckerman, K. S., Neidhart, J. A., Balcerzak, S. P. and LoBuglio, A. F. (1974). Immunologic specificity of transfer factor. *J. Clin. Invest.*, **54**, 997
9. Spitler, L. E., Levin, A. S. and Fudenberg, H. H. (1975). Transfer factor II: Results of therapy. In: *Immunodeficiency in Man and Animals* (D. Bergsma, R. A. Good, J. Finstad and N. W. Paul, eds.) Birth Defects: Original Article Series. The National Foundation, Sinauer Assoc., Inc., Sunderland, Mass., **Vol. XI,** no. 1, p. 449
10. Levin, A. S., Byers, V. S., Fudenberg, H. H., Wybran, J., Hacket, A. J., Johnston, J. O. and Spitler, L. E. (1975). Osteogenic sarcoma. Immunological parameters before and during immunotherapy with tumor specific transfer factor. *J. Clin. Invest.*, **55**, 487
11. Levin, A. S., Byers, V. S., Fudenberg, H. H., Wybran, J., Hackett, A. J. and Johnston, J. V. (1975). Transfer factor therapy in osteogenic sarcoma. *Perspect. Virol.*, **9**, 153
12. Brandriss, M. W. (1968). Attempt to transfer contact hypersensitivity in man with dialysate of peripheral leukocytes. *J. Clin. Invest.*, **47**, 2152

13. Arala-Chaves, M. P. and Pinto, A. S. (1972). Transfer factor with dinitrochlorobenzene. Several remarks. *Int. Arch. Allerg.*, **43**, 410
14. Schulkind, M. L., Adler, W. H., Altemeier, W. A. and Ayoub, E. M. (1972). Transfer factor in the treatment of a case of chronic mucocutaneous candidiasis. *Cell. Immunol.*, **3**, 606
15. Griscelli, C., Revillard, J. P., Betuel, H., Herzog, C. and Touraine, J. L. (1973). Transfer factor therapy in immunodeficiencies. *Biomedicine*, **18**, 220
16. Khan, A., Hill, J. M., Loeb, E., MacLellan, A. and Hill, N. O. (1973). Management of Chediak-Higashi syndrome with transfer factor. *Am. J. Dis. Child.*, **126**, 797
17. Arala-Chaves, M. P., Proenca, R. and Sousa, M. (1974). Transfer factor therapy in a case of complex immunodeficiency. *Cell Immunol.*, **10**, 371
18. Kirkpatrick, C. H. (1975). Properties and activities of transfer factor. *J. Allerg. Clin. Immunol.*, **55**, 411
19. Fudenberg, H. H., Goust, J. M., Arala-Chaves, M. P. and Wilson, G. B. (1976). Dialysable transfer factor. An analytical review. *Folia Allerg. Immunol. Clin.*, **23**, 1
19a. Frick, O. L. and Shimbor, C. (1970). Cross-reactivity between hemocyanins and erythrocytes. *Fed. Proc.*, **29**, 513 (abst.)
20. Smith, C. E., Saito, M. T., Beard, R. R. *et al.* (1949). Histoplasmin sensitivity and coccidioidal infection. I. Occurrence of cross-reactions. *Am. J. Public Health*, **39**, 722
21. Bloom, B. R. (1973). Does transfer factor act specifically or as an immunologic adjuvant? *N. Engl. J. Med.*, **288**, 908
22. Levin, A. S., Spitler, L. E., Stites, D. P. and Fudenberg, H. H. (1970). Wiskott–Aldrich syndrome—a genetically determined cellular immunologic deficiency: Clinical and laboratory responses to therapy with transfer factor. *Proc. Natl. Acad. Sci. USA*, **67**, 821
23. Dupont, B., Ballow, M., Hansen, J. A., Quick, C., Yunis, E. J. and Good, R. A. (1974). Effect of transfer factor therapy on mixed lymphocyte culture reactivity. *Proc. Nat. Acad. Sci. USA*, **71**, 867
24. Arala-Chaves, M., Ramos, M. T. F. and Rosado, R. M. F. (1974). Evidence for prompt and intense reconstitution of cell-mediated immunity by means of transfer factor in a case of complex immune deficiency. *Cell. Immunol.*, **12**, 160
25. Valdimarsson, H., Hambleton, G., Henry, K. and McConnell, I. (1974). Restoration of T lymphocyte deficiency with dialyzable leukocyte extract. *Clin. Exp. Immunol.*, **10**, 141
26. Goldblum, R. M., Lord, R. A., Dupree, E., Weinberg, A. G. and Goldman, A. S. (1973). Transfer factor induced delayed hypersensitivity in X-linked combined immunodeficiency. *Cell. Immunol.*, **9**, 297
27. Wybran, J., Levin, A. S., Spitler, L. E. and Fudenberg, H. H. (1973). Rosette-forming cells, immunologic deficiency diseases and transfer factor. *N. Engl. J. Med.*, **288**, 710
28. Kirkpatrick, C. H. and Gallin, J. I. (1975). The chemotactic activity of dialyzable transfer factor. II. Further characterization of the activity *in vivo* and *in vitro*. In: *The Phagocytic Cell in Host Resistance* (J. A. Bellanti and D. H. Dayton, eds.), p. 155 (New York: Raven Press)
29. Lawrence, H. S. (1976). Summation. In: *Transfer Factor: Basic Properties and Clinical Applications* (M. S. Ascher, A. A. Gottlieb and C. H. Kirkpatrick, eds.), p. 741 (New York: Academic Press)
30. Lawrence, H. S. and Valentine, F. T. (1970). Transfer factor in delayed hypersensitivity. *Ann. N.Y. Acad. Sci.*, **169**, 269
31. Ascher, M. S., Schneider, W. J., Valentine, F. T. and Lawrence, H. S. (1973). *In vitro* properties of dialysates containing transfer factor. *Fed. Proc.*, **32**, 955a
32. Vandvik, B., Frøland, S. S., Høyeraal, H. M., Stien, R. and Degré, M. (1973). Immunological features in a case of subacute, sclerosing panencephalitis treated with transfer factor. *Scand. J. Immunol.*, **2**, 367

33. Valdimarsson, H., Wood, C. B. S., Hobbs, J. R. and Holt, P. J. L. (1972). Immunological features in a case of chronic granulomatous candidiasis and its treatment with transfer factor. *Clin. Exp. Immunol.*, **11**, 151
34. Sandler, J. A., Smith, T. K., Manganiello, V. and Kirkpatrick, C. (1975). Stimulation of monocytic cGMP by leukocyte dialysates. An antigen property of dialyzable transfer factor. *J. Clin. Invest.*, **56**, 1271
35. Kirkpatrick, C. H. and Smith, T. K. (1976). The nature of transfer factor and its clinical efficacy in the management of cutaneous disorders. *J. Invest. Dermatol.*, **67**, 425
36. Kelly, W. D., Lamb, D. L., Varco, R. L. and Good, R. A. (1960). An investigation of Hodgkin's disease with respect to the problem of homotransplantation. *Ann. N.Y. Acad. Sci.*, **87**, 187
37. Fazio, M. and Calciati, A. (1962). An attempt to transfer tuberculin hypersensitivity in Hodgkin's disease. *Panminerva Med.*, **4**, 164
38. Muftuoglu, A. U. and Balkuv, S. (1967). Passive transfer of tuberculin sensitivity to patients with Hodgkin's disease. *N. Engl. J. Med.*, **277**, 126
39. Lawrence, H. S. and Zweiman, B. (1968). Transfer factor deficiency response. A mechanism of anergy in Boecks sarcoid. *Trans. Assoc. Am. Phys.*, **81**, 240
40. Urbach, F., Sones, M. and Israel, H. J. (1952). Passive transfer of tuberculin sensitivity to patients with sarcoidosis. *N. Engl. J. Med.*, **247**, 794
41. Solowely, A. C., Rapaport, F. T. and Lawrence, H. S. In: *Histocompatibility Testing*, p. 75. (Basel: Karger), cited by Lawrence, H. S. (3)
42. Kirkpatrick, C. H., Ottenson, E. A., Smith, T. K., Wells, S. A. and Burdick, J. F. (1976). Reconstitution of defective cellular immunity with foetal thymus and dialyzable transfer factor. *Clin. Exp. Immunol.*, **23**, 414
43. Pachman, L. M., Kirkpatrick, C. H., Kaufman, D. H. and Rothberg, R. M. (1974). The lack of effect of transfer factor in thymic dysplasia with immunoglobulin synthesis. *J. Pediatr.*, **84**, 681
44. Stoop, J. W., Eijsvoogel, V. P., Legers, B. J. M., Blok-Shut, B., Bekkum, D. W. V. and Balieux, R. E. (1976). Selective severe immunodeficiency. Effect of thymus transplantation and transfer factor administration. *Clin. Immunol. Immunopathol.*, **6**, 289
45. Spitler, L. E., Levin, A. S. and Fudenberg, H. H. (1973). Human lymphocyte transfer factor. In: *Methods in Cancer Research* (H. Bush, ed.), p. 59 (New York and London: Academic Press)
46. Arala-Chaves, M. P., Silva, A., Porto, M. T., Ramos, M. T. F. and Fudenberg, H. H. (1976). *In vitro* characterization of the target cell for transfer factor-dialyzable leukocyte extracts. In: *Transfer Factor: Basic Properties and Clinical Applications* (M. S. Ascher, C. H. Kirkpatrick and A. A. Gottlieb, eds.), p. 99 (New York: Academic Press)
47. Arala-Chaves, M. P., Silva, A., Porto, M. T., Picoto, A., Ramos, M. T. F. and Fudenberg, H. H. (1977). *In vitro* and *in vivo* studies of the target cell for dialyzable leukocyte extracts. Evidence for recipient specificity. *Clin. Immunol. Immunopathol.*, **8**, 430
48. Fireman, P., Boesman, M., Haddad, Z. H. and Gitlin, D. (1967). Passive transfer of tuberculin reactivity *in vitro*. *Science*, **155**, 337
49. Fireman, P., Boesman, M. Haddad, Z. and Gitlin, D. (1968). *In vitro* passive transfer of tuberculin reactivity. *Fed. Proc.*, **27**, 29
50. Baram, P. and Condoulis, W. (1970). The *in vitro* transfer of delayed hypersensitivity to Rhesus monkey and human lymphocytes with transfer factor obtained from Rhesus monkey peripheral white blood cells. *J. Immunol.*, **104**, 769
51. Gallin, J. I. and Kirkpatrick, C. H. (1974). Chemotactic activity in dialyzable transfer factor. *Proc. Nat. Acad. Sci. USA*, **71**, 498
52. Holzman, R. S. and Lawrence, H. S. (1977). *In vitro* augmentation of lymphocyte sheep cell rosette formation by leukocyte dialysates. *J. Immunol.*, **118**, 1672

53. Thestrup-Pedersen, K., Thulin, H. and Zachariae, H. (1974). Transfer factor applied to intensify the cell-mediated immunological reactions against mycobacterium avium. *Acta Allergol.*, **29**, 101
54. Strauss, R. G. and Hake, D. A. (1974). Combined immunodeficiency disease with response to transfer factor. *J. Pediatr.*, **85**, 680
55. Ascher, M. S., Schneider, W. J., Valentine, F. T. and Lawrence, H. S. (1974). *In vitro* properties of leukocyte dialysates containing transfer factor. *Proc. Nat. Acad. Sci. USA*, **71**, 1178
56. Arala-Chaves, M., Ramos, M. T. F., Rosado, R. and Branco, P. (1974). Transfer factor *in vitro*: Additional data concerning a new method. *Int. Arch. Allerg. Appl. Immunol.*, **46**, 612
57. Hamblin, A. S., Maini, R. M. and Dumonde, D. C. (1976). Human transfer factor *in vitro*. I. Augmentation of lymphocyte transformation to tuberculin PPD. *Clin. Exp. Immunol.*, **23**, 290
58. Cohen, L., Holzman, R. S., Valentine, F. T. and Lawrence, H. S. (1976). Requirement of precommitted cells as targets for the augmentation of lymphocyte proliferation by leukocyte dialysates. *J. Exp. Med.*, **143**, 791
59. Hamblin, A. S., Dumonde, D. C. and Maini, R. N. (1976). Human transfer factor *in vitro*. II. Augmentation of lymphocyte transformation to phytohaemagglutinin. *Clin. Exp. Immunol.*, **23**, 303
60. Valdimarsson, H., Wood, C. B. S., Hobbs, J. R. and Holt, P. J. L. (1972). Immunological features in a case of chronic granulomatous candidiasis and its treatment with transfer factor. *Clin. Exp. Immunol.*, **11**, 151
61. Spitler, L. E., Levin, A. S., Stites, D. P., Fudenberg, H. H., Pirofsky, B., August, C. S., Stiehm, E. R., Hitzig, W. H. and Gatti, R. A. (1972). The Wiskott–Aldrich syndrome: Results of transfer factor therapy. *J. Clin. Invest.*, **51**, 3216
62. Untermohlen, V. and Zabriskie, J. B. (1973). Suppressed cellular immunity to measles antigen in multiple sclerosis patients. *Lancet*, **ii**, 1147
63. Baram, P. and Condoulis, W. (1974). Studies on Rhesus monkey non-dialyzable and dialyzable transfer factors. *Transplant. Proc.*, **6**, 209
64. Salaman, M. R. (1974). Studies on the transfer factor of delayed hypersensitivity. Effect of dialyzable leukocyte extracts from people of known tuberculin sensitivity on the migration of normal guinea-pig macrophages in the presence of antigen. *Immunology*, **26**, 1069
65. Dunnick, W. and Bach, F. H. (1975). Guinea-pig transfer factor-like activity detected *in vitro*. *Proc. Nat. Acad. Sci. USA*, **72**, 4573
66. Burger, D. R., Vandenbark, A. A., Finke, P., Nolte, J. E. and Vetto, R. M. (1976). Human transfer factor: Effects on lymphocyte transformation. *J. Immunol.*, **117**, 782
67. Lawrence, H. S. and Pappenheimer, A. M. (1956). Transfer of delayed hypersensitivity to diphtheria toxin in man. *J. Exp. Med.*, **104**, 321
68. Spitler, L. E., Webb, D., Muller, C. V. and Fudenberg, H. H. (1973). Studies on the characterization of transfer factor. *J. Clin. Invest.*, **52**, 80a
69. Arala-Chaves, M. P., Lebacq, E. G. and Heremans, J. F. (1967). Fractionation of human leukocyte extracts transferring delayed hypersensitivity to tuberculin. *Int. Arch. Allerg.*, **31**, 353
70. Haddad, Z. H. (1968). Immunochemical characterization of a low molecular weight cellular factor involved in *in vivo* and *in vitro* transfer of delayed hypersensitivity. *J. Allerg.*, **41**, 112
71. Neidhart, J. A., Schwartz, R. S., Hurtubise, P. E., Murphy, S. G., Metz, E. N., Balcerzak, S. P. and LoBuglio, A. F. (1973). Transfer factor: Isolation of a biologically active component. *Cell. Immunol.*, **9**, 319
72. Gottlieb, A. A., Foster, L. G. and Waldman, S. R. (1973). What is transfer factor? *Lancet*, **ii**, 822

73. Arala-Chaves, M. P. (1975). PhD thesis. Louvain
74. Gottlieb, A. A. (1974). Communication at the Workshop No. 138 (Transfer factor: biological properties), 2nd International Congress of Immunology, Brighton
75. Baram, P. and Mosko, M. M. (1962). Chromatography of the human tuberculin delayed-type hypersensitivity transfer factor. *J. Allerg.*, **33**, 498
76. Baram, P. and Mosko, M. M. (1965). A dialyzable fraction from tuberculin-sensitive human white blood cells capable of inducing tuberculin-delayed hypersensitivity in negative recipients. *Immunology*, **8**, 461
77. Baram, P., Yuan, L. and Mosko, M. M. (1965). Purification and characterization of transfer factor. *J. Allerg.*, **36**, 203
78. Baram, P., Yuan, L. and Mosko, M. M. (1966). Studies on the transfer of human delayed-type hypersensitivity. I. Partial purification and characterization of two active components. *J. Immunol.*, **97**, 407
79. Krohn, K., Notila, A., Grohn, P., Vaisanen, V. and Hiltumen, J. (1976). Studies on the biological and chemical nature of a component in transfer factor with immunologically non-specific activity. In: *Transfer Factor: Basic Properties and Clinical Applications* (M. S. Ascher, A. A. Gottlieb and C. H. Kirkpatrick, eds.), p. 283 (New York: Academic Press)
80. Arala-Chaves, M. P. and Ramos, M. T. F. (1976). *In vitro* assay of partially purified dialyzable leukocyte extracts fraction. *Ricerca*, **6**, 5 Suppl.
81. Kirkpatrick, C. H. and Smith, T. K. (1976). Specific and non-specific activities in dialyzable transfer factor. (Symposium II in 11th Leukocyte Culture Conference, Tucson, Arizona)
82. Dunnick, W. and Bach, F. H. (1975). Guinea-pig 'transfer factor' *in vitro*. Physical and chemical properties and partial purification. In: *Transfer Factor: Basic Properties and Clinical Applications* (M. S. Ascher, A. A. Gottlieb and C. H. Kirkpatrick, eds.), p. 185 (New York: Academic Press)
83. Wilson, G., Welch, T. and Fudenberg, H. H. (1977). Tx: A component in human dialyzable transfer factor that induces delayed hypersensitivity in guinea-pigs. *Clin. Immunol. Immunopathol.*, **7**, 189
84. Bloom, B. R. and Chase, M. W. (1967). Transfer of delayed-type hypersensitivity. A critical review and experimental study in the guinea-pig. *Progr. Allergy*, **10**, 151
85. Burger, D. R. and Jeter, W. S. (1971). Cell-free passive transfer of delayed hypersensitivity to chemicals in guinea-pigs. *Infect. Immun.*, **4**, 575
86. Burger, D. R., Vetto, R. M. and Malley, A. (1972). Transfer factor from guinea-pigs sensitive to dinitrochlorobenzene. *Science*, **175**, 1473
87. Jeter, W. S., Paquet, A., Ferebee, R. N., Olson, G. B. and Rornestad, F. (1976). Correlation of *in vivo* and *in vitro* activity of guinea-pig transfer factor. In: *Transfer Factor: Basic Properties and Clinical Applications* (M. S. Ascher, A. A. Gottlieb and C. H. Kirkpatrick, eds.), p. 75 (New York: Academic Press)
88. Maddison, S. E., Hicrlin, M. D., Conway, P. B. and Kagan, I. G. (1972). Transfer factor: Delayed hypersensitivity to *Schistosoma mansoni* and tuberculin in *Macaca mulatta*. *Science*, **178**, 757
89. Eichberg, J. W., Steele, R. W., Kalter, S. S., Kniker, W. T., Herberling, R. L., Eller, J. J. and Rodriguez, A. R. (1976). Cellular immunity in gnotobiotic primates induced by transfer factor. *Cell. Immunol.*, **26**, 114
90. Trepo, C. G. and Prince, A. M. (1976). Attempted immunotherapy with dialyzable transfer factor in hepatitis B carrier chimpanzees: Induction of delayed hypersensitivity to hepatitis B surface antigen (HBsAg). In: *Transfer Factor: Basic Properties and Clinical Applications* (M. S. Ascher, A. A. Gottlieb and C. H. Kirkpatrick, eds.), p. 449 (New York: Academic Press)
91. Goust, J. M., Marescot, M. R., Lesourd, B., Doumercq, S. and Moulias, R. (1976).

Characterization of human dialyzable transfer factor from normal and chronic lymphoid leukemic sources. *Biomedicine*, **24**, 39

92. Zanelli, J. M. and Adler, W. H. (1975). Transfer factor of tuberculin sensitivity in allogeneic and xenogeneic monkey model. *Cell Immunol.*, **15**, 475
93. Steele, R. W., Eichberg, J. W., Heberling, R. L., Eller, S. S., Kalter, S. S. and Kniker, W. T. (1976). *In vitro* transfer of cellular immunity to primates with transfer factor from human or primate leukocytes. *Cell Immunol.*, **22**, 110
94. Liburd, E. M., Pabst, H. F. and Armstrong, W. D. (1972). Transfer factor in rat coccidiosis. *Cell Immunol.*, **5**, 487
95. Clinton, B. A. and Magoc, T. Y. (1976). *Leshmania enrietti* infections in guinea-pigs and transfer factor obtained from convalescent yet immune animals. In: *Transfer Factor: Basic Properties and Clinical Applications* (M. S. Ascher, A. A. Gottlieb and C. H. Kirkpatrick, eds.), p. 709 (New York: Academic Press)
96. Basten, A., Croft, S. and Edwards, Y. (1976). Experimental studies of transfer factor. In: *Transfer Factor: Basic Properties and Clinical Applications* (M. S. Ascher, A. A. Gottlieb and C. H. Kirkpatrick, eds.), p. 75 (New York: Academic Press)
97. Klesius, P. A., Kristenson, F., Ernst, J. R. and Kramer, T. T. (1976). Bovine transfer factor: Isolation and characteristics. In: *Transfer Factor: Basic Properties and Clinical Applications* (M. S. Ascher, A. A. Gottlieb and C. H. Kirkpatrick, eds.), p. 311 (New York: Academic Press)
98. Klesius, P. A. and Kristensen, F. (1977). Bovine transfer factor: Effect on bovine and rabbit coccidiosis. *Clin. Immunol. Immunopathol.*, **7**, 240
99. Shifrine, M., Thilsted, J. and Pappagianis, D. (1976). Canine transfer factor. In: *Transfer Factor: Basic Properties and Clinical Applications* (M. S. Ascher, A. A. Gottlieb and C. H. Kirkpatrick, eds.), p. 349 (New York: Academic Press)
100. Welch, T. M., Triglia, R., Spitler, L. E. and Fudenberg, H. H. (1976). Preliminary studies of human 'transfer factor' activity in guinea-pigs. Systemic transfer of cutaneous delayed-type hypersensitivity to PPD and SK-SD. *Clin. Immunol. Immunopathol.*, **5**, 407
101. Vandenbark, A. A., Burger, D. R. and Vetto, R. M. (1977). Human transfer factor activity in the guinea-pig: Absence of antigen specificity. *Clin. Immunol. Immunopathol.*, **8**, 7
102. Maddison, S. E., Rocklin, M. D. and Kagan, I. G. (1976). *Schistosoma mansoni*: Reduction in clinical manifestation and in worm burdens conferred by serum and transfer factor from immune or normal Rhesus monkeys. *Exp. Parasitol.*, **39**, 29
103. Ascher, M. S., Anderson, A. O. and Andron, L. A. (1976). Adjuvant properties in human dialyzable leukocyte extracts containing transfer factor. *11th Leukocyte Culture Conference.* (Abst.), 124
104. Medical News. *J. Am. Med. Ass.*, **224**, 9
105. Thompson, R. B. (1971). Lymphocyte transfer factor. *Rev. Eur. Etud. Clin. Biol.*, **26**, 201
106. Brandes, L. Y., Gatton, D. A. G. and Wiltshaw, D. R. (1971). New approach to immunotherapy of melanoma. *Lancet*, **ii**, 293
107. Spitler, L., Wybran, J., Fudenberg, H. H. and Levin, A. S. (1973). Transfer factor therapy of malignant melanoma. *Clin. Res.*, **21**, 221
108. Smith, G. V., Morse, P. A., Deraps, G. D., Seshardi, R. and Hardy, J. D. (1973). Immunotherapy of patients with cancer. *Surgery*, **74**, 59
109. Burger, D. R., Vetto, R. M. and Vandenbark, A. A. (1974). Transfer factor immunotherapy in human cancer. *Surg. Forum*, **25**, 93
110. Vetto, R. M., Burger, D., Wolte, Y. E., Vandenbark, A. A. and Barker, H. W. (1976). Transfer factor therapy in patients with cancer. *Cancer*, **37**, 90
111. Bukowski, R. M., Deodhar, S. and Hewlett, J. S. (1976). Immunotherapy of human neoplasms with transfer factor. In: *Transfer Factor: Basic Properties and Clinical Applications* (M. S. Ascher, A. A. Gottlieb and C. H. Kirkpatrick, eds.), p. 543 (New York: Academic Press)

112. Silva, J., Allen, J., Wheeler, R., Bull, F. and Morley, G. (1976). Transfer factor therapy in disseminated neoplasms. In: *Transfer Factor: Basic Properties and Clinical Applications* (M. S. Ascher, A. A. Gottlieb and C. H. Kirkpatrick, eds.), p. 573 (New York: Academic Press)
113. Grob, P. J., Franke, Ch., Reymond, J. F. and Frei-Weltstein, M. (1975). Therapeutical use of transfer factor. *Eur. J. Clin. Invest.*, **5**, 33
114. Khan, A., Thaxton, S., Hill, J. M., Hill, N. O., Loeb, E. and MacLellan, A. (1976). Clinical trials with transfer factor. In: *Transfer Factor: Basic Properties and Clinical Applications* (M. S. Ascher, A. A. Gottlieb and C. H. Kirkpatrick, eds.), p. 583 (New York: Academic Press)
115. Oettgen, H. F., Old, L. J., Farrow, J. H., Valentine, F., Lawrence, H. S. and Thomas, L. (1971). Effects of transfer factor in cancer patients. *J. Clin. Invest.*, **50**, 71a
116. Oettgen, H. F., Old, L. J., Farrow, J. H., Valentine, F. T., Lawrence, H. S. and Thomas, L. (1974). Effects of dialyzable transfer factor in patients with breast cancer. *Proc. Nat. Acad. Sci. USA*, **71**, 2319
117. Fudenberg, H. H. (1976). Dialyzable transfer factor in the treatment of human osteosarcoma: An analytical review. *Ann. N.Y. Acad. Sci.*, **277**, 545
118. Levin, A. S., Spitler, L. E., Wybran, J., Fudenberg, H. H., Hellstrom, I. and Hellstrom, K. E. (1972). Treatment of osteogenic sarcoma with tumor specific transfer factor. *Clin. Res.*, **20**, 568 (abstract)
119. Levin, A. S., Byers, V. S., LeCam, L. and Johnston, J. O. (1976). An unusual metastic lesion in a patient with osteosarcoma receiving tumor specific transfer factor. In: *Transfer Factor: Basic Properties and Clinical Applications* (M. S. Ascher, A. A. Gottlieb and C. H. Kirkpatrick, eds.), p. 537 (New York: Academic Press)
120. Bearden, D. J., Thor, D. E. and Coltman, C. A. (1976). Adjunctive transfer factor in osteogenic sarcoma. Clinical implications of chemotherapy and immunotherapy. In: *Transfer Factor: Basic Properties and Clinical Applications* (M. S. Ascher, A. A. Gottlieb and C. H. Kirkpatrick, eds.), p. 553 (New York: Academic Press)
121. Thor, D. E., Coltman, C. A., Bearden, J. D., Williams, T. E. and Flippan, J. H. (1976). Adjunctive transfer factor in osteogenic sarcoma. II. Methodology and results of the immunological studies. In: *Transfer Factor: Basic Properties and Clinical Applications* (M. S. Ascher, A. A. Gottlieb and C. H. Kirkpatrick, eds.), p. 563 (New York: Academic Press)
122. Lobuglio, A. F. and Neidhart, J. A. (1974). A review of transfer factor immunotherapy in cancer. *Cancer*, **34**, 1563
123. Khan, A., Hill, J. M., Maclelan, A., Loeb, E., Hill, N. O. and Thaxton, S. (1975). Improvement in delayed hypersensitivity in Hodgkin's disease with transfer factor: Lymphopheresis and cellular immune reactions of normal donors. *Cancer*, **36**, 86
124. Lobuglio, A. F., Neidhart, J. A., Hilberg, R. W., Metz, E. N. and Balceszak, S. P. (1973). The effect of transfer factor therapy on tumor immunity in alveolar soft part sarcoma. *Cell. Immunol.*, **7**, 159
125. Goldenberg, G. J. and Brandes, L. J. (1972). Immunotherapy of nasopharyngeal carcinoma with transfer factor from donors with previous infectious mononucleosis. *Clin. Res.*, **20**, 947 (abstract)
126. Brandes, L. J. and Goldenberg, G. L. (1974). *In vitro* transfer of cellular immunity against nasopharyngeal carcinoma using transfer factor from donors with Epstein–Barr virus antibody activity. *Cancer Res.*, **34**, 3095
127. Lawrence, H. S. (1974). Transfer factor in cellular immunity. *Harvey Lect. Ser.*, **68**, 239
128. Hitzig, W. H. and Grob, P. J. (1975). Therapeutic uses of transfer factor. *Progr. Clin. Immunol.*, **5**, 69
129. David, J. R. (1975). A brief review of macrophage activation by lymphocyte mediators. In: *The Phagocytic Cell in Host Resistance* (J. A. Bellanti and D. H. Dayton, eds.), p. 143 (New York: Raven Press)

130. Rocklin, R. E. (1973). Production of migration inhibitory factor by non-dividing lymphocytes. *J. Immunol.*, **110**, 674
131. Kirkpatrick, C. H., Rich, R. R. and Bennett, J. E. (1971). Chronic mucocutaneous candidiasis: Model-building in cellular immunity. *Ann Int. Med.*, **74**, 955
132. Spitler, L. E., Levin, A. J. and Fudenberg, H. H. (1972). Prediction of results of transfer factor therapy in Wiskott–Aldrich syndrome by monocyte IgG receptors. *Sixth Annual Leukocyte Culture Conference* (M. R. Schwartz, ed.), p. 795 (New York: Academic Press)
133. Hitzig, H., Fontanellaz, H. P., Muntener, U., Paul, S., Spitler, L. E. and Fudenberg, H. H. (1972). Transfer factor. *Schweiz. Med. Wochenschr.*, **102**, 1237
134. Levin, A. S., Spitler, L. E. and Fudenberg, H. H. (1973). Transfer factor therapy in immune deficiency states. *Annu. Rev. Med.*, **24**, 175
135. Fudenberg, H. H., Levin, A. S., Spitler, L. E., Wybran, J. and Byers, V. (1974). The therapeutic uses of transfer factor. *Hosp. Pract.*, **9**, 95
136. Levin, A. S., Spitler, L. E. and Fudenberg, H. H. (1975). Transfer factor I: Methods and therapy. In: *Immunodeficiency in Man and Animals.* (D. Bergsma, R. A. Good, J. Finstad and N. W. Paul, eds.), **Vol. XI**, No. 1, p. 449. Birth Defects: Original Article Series. The National Foundation, Sinauer Assoc., Inc., Sunderland, Mass.
137. Spitler, L. E., Levin, A. S. and Fudenberg, H. H. (1975). Transfer factor. In: *Clinical Immunology* (F. Bach and R. A. Good, eds.), **Vol. II**, p. 153 (New York: Academic Press)
138. Ballow, M., Dupont, B., Hansen, J. A. and Good, R. A. (1975). Transfer factor therapy: Evidence for immunospecificity. In: *Immunodeficiency in Man and Animals* (D. Bergsma, R. A. Good, J. Finstad and N. W. Paul, eds.), **Vol. XI**, No. 1, p. 457. Birth Defects: Original Article Series. The National Foundation, Sinauer Assoc., Inc., Sunderland, Mass.
139. Griscelli, C. (1975). Transfer factor therapy in immunodeficiency. In: *Immunodeficiency in Man and Animals* (D. Bergsma, R. A. Good, J. Finstad and N. W. Paul, eds.), **Vol. XI**, No. 1, p. 462. Birth Defects: Original Article Series. The National Foundation, Sinauer Assoc., Inc., Sunderland, Mass.
140. Grob, P. J., Blaker, F. and Schulz, K. H. (1973). Immunofunction and transfer factor. *Dtsch. Med. Wochenschr.*, **98**, 446
141. Grob, P. J., Reymond, J.-F., Hachi, M. A. and Tracy-Wettstein, M. (1976). Some physico-chemical and biological properties of a transfer factor preparation and its clinical application. In: *Transfer Factor: Basic Properties and Clinical Applications* (M. S. Ascher, A. A. Gottlieb and C. H. Kirkpatrick, eds.), p. 247 (New York: Academic Press)
142. Ammann, A. J., Wara, D. and Salmon, S. (1974). Transfer factor: Therapy in patients with deficient cell-mediated immunity and deficient antibody-mediated immunity. *Cell. Immunol.*, **12**, 94
143. Sellars, W. A. and South, M. A. (1975). Wiskott–Aldrich syndrome with 18-year survival. Treatment with transfer factor. *Am. J. Dis. Child.*, **129**, 622
144. Mogerman, S. N., Levin, A. S., Spitler, L. E., Stites, D. P., Fudenberg, H. H. and Shinefield, H. K. (1973). Transfer factor therapy (TF) in X-linked recessive severe combined dual system immune deficiency disorder (SCID). *Clin. Res.*, **21**, 310
145. Gelfand, E. W., Baumal, R., Huber, J., Crookston, M. C. and Shumak, K. H. (1973). Polyclonal gammopathy and lymphoproliferation after transfer factor in severe combined immunodeficiency disease. *N. Engl. J. Med.*, **289**, 1385
146. Montgomery, J. R., South, M. A., Wilson, R., Richie, E., Heim, L. R., Criswell, S. and Trentin, J. J. (1973). Study of a gnotobiotic child with severe combined immunodeficiency. *Clin. Res.*, **21**, 118
147. Ballow, M. and Good, R. A. (1975). Report of a patient with T-cell deficiency and normal B-cell function: A new immunodeficiency disease with response to transfer factor. *Cell. Immunol.*, **19**, 219
148. Ballow, M. and Good, R. A. (1976). Transfer factor therapy in a patient with an isolated

T-cell deficiency. In: *Transfer Factor: Basic Properties and Clinical Applications* (M. S. Ascher, A. A. Gottlieb and C. H. Kirkpatrick, eds.), p. 623 (New York: Academic Press)
149. Criswell, B. S., South, M. A., Jordan, H. W., Kimzey, S. L., Montgomery, J. R. and Heim, L. R. (1975). Fine structure of lymphocytes from an immune deficient child before and after administration of transfer factor. *Exp. Hematol.*, **3**, 327
150. Lawlor, G. L. Jr., Ammann, A. J., Wright, W. C., LaFranchi, S. H., Bilstrom, D. and Stiehm, E. R. (1974). The syndrome of cellular immunodeficiency with immunoglobulins. *J. Pediatr.*, **84**, 183
151. Zaldivar, N. M., Papageorgiou, P. S., Kafee, S. and Glade, P. R. (1975). The use of transfer factor in a patient with agammaglobulinemia. *Pediatr. Res.*, **9**, 541
152. Blaese, R. M., Strober, W. and Waldmann, T. A. (1975). Immunodeficiency in the Wiskott–Aldrich syndrome. In: *Immunodeficiency in Man and Animals* (D. Bergsma, R. A. Good, J. Finstad and N. W. Paul, eds.), **Vol. XI**, No. 1, p. 250. Birth Defects: Original Article Series. The National Foundation, Sinauer Assoc., Inc., Sunderland, Mass.
153. Biggar, W. D. and Good, R. A. (1975). Immunodeficiency in ataxia-telangiectasia. In: *Immunodeficiency in Man and Animals* (D. Bergsma, R. A. Good, J. Finstad and N. W. Paul, eds.), **Vol. XI**, No. 1, p. 271. Birth Defects: Original Article Series. The National Foundation, Sinauer Assoc., Inc., Sunderland, Mass.
154. Valdimarsson, H., Higgs, J. M., Wells, R. S., Yamamura, M., Hobbs, J. R. and Holt, P. J. L. (1973). Immune abnormalities associated with chronic mucocutaneous candidiasis. *Cell. Immunol.*, **6**, 348
155. Kirkpatrick, C. H., Rich, R. R. and Smith, T. K. (1972). Effect of transfer factor on lymphocyte function in anergic patients. *J. Clin. Invest.*, **51**, 2948
156. Kirkpatrick, C. H. and Smith, T. K. (1974). Chronic mucocutaneous candidiasis. Immunologic and antibiotic therapy. *Ann. Int. Med.*, **80**, 310
157. Kirkpatrick, C. H. (1975). Restoration of cell-mediated immune response with transfer factor. In: *Immunodeficiency in Man and Animals* (D. Bergsma, R. A. Good, J. Finstad and N. W. Paul, eds.), **Vol. XI**, No. 1, p. 441. Birth Defects: Original Article Series. The National Foundation, Sinauer Assoc., Inc., Sunderland, Mass.
158. Kirkpatrick, C. H. and Gallin, J. I. (1975). Suppression of cellular immune responses following transfer factor. Report of a case. *Cell. Immunol.*, **15**, 470
159. Rocklin, R. E., Chilgren, R. A., Hong, R. and David, J. R. (1970). Transfer of cellular hypersensitivity in chronic mucocutaneous candidiasis monitored *in vivo* and *in vitro*. *Cell. Immunol.*, **1**, 290
160. Rocklin, R. E. (1975). Use of transfer factor in patients with depressed cellular immunity and chronic infection. In: *Immunodeficiency in Man and Animals* (D. Bergsma, R. A. Good, J. Finstad and N. W. Paul, eds.), **Vol. XI**, No. 1, p. 431. Birth Defects: Original Article Series. The National Foundation, Sinauer Assoc., Inc., Sunderland, Mass.
161. Schulkind, M. L. and Ayoub, E. M. (1975). Transfer factor in patients with depressed cellular immunity and chronic infection. In: *Immunodeficiency in Man and Animals* (D. Bergsma, R. A. Good, J. Finstad and N. W. Paul, eds.), **Vol. XI**, No. 1, p. 436. Birth Defects: Original Article Series. The National Foundation, Sinauer Assoc., Inc., Sunderland, Mass.
162. Blaker, F., Grob, P. J., Hellwege, H. H. and Schulz, K. H. (1973). Immunabuehr und Transfer-Factor-Therapie bei chronischer granulomatoser Candidiasis. *Dtsch. Med. Wochenschr.*, **98**, 415
163. José, D. G. (1975). Treatment of chronic mucocutaneous candidiasis by lymphocyte transfer factor. *Aust. N.Z. J. Med.*, **5**, 318
164. De Sousa, M., Cochran, R., Mackie, R., Parratt, D. and Arala-Chaves, M. (1976). Chronic mucocutaneous candidiasis treated with transfer factor. *Br. J. Dermatol.*, **94**, 79
165. Canales, L., Louro, J. M. and Middlemas, R. O. (1969). Immunological observations in chronic mucocutaneous candidiasis. *Lancet*, **ii**, 567

166. Paterson, P. Y., Semo, R. and Blumenschein, C. (1971). Mucocutaneous candidiasis, anergy, and a plasma inhibitor of cellular immunity; reversal after amphotericin B therapy. *Clin. Exp. Immunol.*, **9**, 595
167. Kirkpatrick, C. H., Chandler, J. W. and Schmike, R. N. (1970). Chronic mucocutaneous moniliasis with impaired delayed hypersensitivity. *Clin. Exp. Immunol.*, **6**, 375
168. Pabst, H. F. and Swanson, R. (1972). Successful treatment of candidiasis with transfer factor. *Br. Med. J.*, **2**, 442
169. Snyderman, R. Altman, L. C., Frankel, A. and Blaese, R. M. (1973). Defective mononuclear leukocyte chemotaxis: A previously unrecognized immune dysfunction. Studies in a patient with chronic mucocutaneous candidiasis. *Ann. Int. Med.*, **78**, 509
170. Lawton, J. W. M., Costello, C., Barclay, G. R., Urbaniak, S. J., Darz, C., Raeburn, J. A., Uttley, W. S. and Kay, A. B. (1976). The effect of transfer factor on neutrophil function in chronic mucocutaneous candidiasis. *Br. J. Haematol.*, **33**, 137
171. Grob, P. J. and Withrich, B. (1974). Transfer factor therapy in a patient with chronic vaginal candidiasis. *J. Obstet. Gynecol.*, **81**, 812
172. Graybill, J. R., Silva, J. Jr., Alford, R. H. and Thor, D. E. (1973). Immunological and clinical improvement of progressive coccidioidomycosis following administration of transfer factor. *Cell. Immunol.*, **8**, 120
173. Graybill, J. R. (1975). Transfer factor in coccidioidomycosis. *Clin. Res.*, **23**, 304
174. Catanzaro, A. and Spitler, L. (1976). The coccidiodomycosis co-operative treatment group (CCTG). Clinical and immunological results of transfer factor therapy in coccidioidomycosis. In: *Transfer Factor: Basic Properties and Clinical Applications* (M. S. Ascher, A. A. Gottlieb and C. H. Kirkpatrick, eds.), p. 477 (New York: Academic Press)
175. Stevens, D. A., Pappagionis, D., Marinkovich, V. A. and Waddell, T. F. (1974). Immunotherapy in recurrent coccidioidomycosis. *Cell. Immunol.*, **12**, 37
176. Steele, R. W., Sieger, B. E., McNitt, T. R., Gentry, L. O. and Moore, W. L. Jr. (1976). Therapy for disseminated coccidioidomycosis with transfer factor from a related donor. *Am. J. Med.*, **61**, 283
177. Moulias, R., Goust, J.-M., Reinert, Ph., Tournel, J.-J., Deville-Chabrolle, A., Duong, N., Muller-Berat, C. N. and Berthaux, P. (1973). Facteur de transfert de l'immunite cellulaire. *Nouv. Presse Med.*, **2**, 1341
178. Drew, W. L., Blume, M. R., Miner, R., Silverberg, J. and Rosenblaum, E. H. (1973). Herpes Zoster: Transfer factor therapy. *Ann. Int. Med.*, **79**, 747
179. Heim, L. R., Bernhard, G., Goldman, A. L., Dorff, G. and Rytel, M. (1976). Transfer factor treatment of viral diseases in Milwaukee. In: *Transfer Factor: Basic Properties and Clinical Applications* (M. S. Ascher, A. A. Gottlieb and C. H. Kirkpatrick, eds.), p. 457 (New York: Academic Press)
180. Dahl, B., Thestrup-Pedersen, K., Ellegaard, J. and Zachariae, H. (1975). Lymphocyte transformation, IgE, and T-cell in eczema vaccinatum treated with transfer factor. *Acta Dermatovener.*, **55**, 187
181. Stevens, D. A., Ferrington, R. A., Merigon, T. C. and Marinkovich, V. A. (1975). Randomized trial of transfer factor treatment of human warts. *Clin. Exp. Immunol.*, **21**, 520
182. Quick, C. A., Behrens, H. W., Brinton-Darnell, M. and Good, R. A. (1975). Treatment of papriclomatosis of the larynx with transfer factor. *Am. Otol. Rhinol. Laryngol.*, **84**, 607
183. Rytel, M. W., Haberg, T. M., Dee, T. H. and Heim, L. H. (1975). Therapy of cytomegalovirus retinitis with transfer factor. *Cell. Immunol.*, **19**, 8
184. Ter Meulen, V., Grob, P. J., Kreth, W. H., Kackell, Y. M. and Kibler, R. (1975). Transfer factor therapy in patients with SSPE. *Arch. Neurol.*, **32**, 501A
185. Kackell, Y. M., Grob, P. J., Kreth, W. H., Kibler, R. and Ter Meulen, V. (1975). Transfer factor therapy in patients with subacute sclerosing panencephalitis. *J. Neurol.*, **211**, 39

186. Pabst, H. F. and Cumming, J. D. A. (1975). Simultaneous immunotherapy of two acute cases of SSPE. *Arch. Neurol.*, **32**, 503
187. Bleare, R. M., Hofstrand, H., Krebs, H. and Stever, J. (1975). Evaluation of transfer factor in the therapy of SSPE. *Arch. Neurol.*, **32**, 502A
188. Kohler, P. F., Trembath, J., Merrill, D. A., Singleton, J. W. and Dubois, R. S. (1974). Immunotherapy with antibody lymphocytes and transfer factor in chronic hepatitis B. *Clin. Immunol. Immunopathol.*, **2**, 465
189. Shulman, S. T., Schulkind, M. and Ayoub, E. (1974). Transfer factor therapy of chronic active hepatitis. *Lancet*, **ii**, 650
190. Shulman, S. T., Hutto, J. H., Scott, B., Ayoub, E. M. and McGuigan, J. E. (1976). Transfer factor therapy of chronic aggressive hepatitis. In: *Transfer Factor: Basic Properties and Clinical Applications* (M. S. Ascher, A. A. Gottlieb and C. H. Kirkpatrick, eds.), p. 439 (New York: Academic Press)
191. Sano, M., Tabeuchi, T., Adachi, M., Tamai, Y. and Ho, K. (1977). Transfer factor in treating hepatitis B. *N. Engl. J. Med.*, **296**, 53
192. Jain, S., Thomas, H. C. and Sherlock, S. (1975). The effect of lymphocytic transfer factor on hepatitis B surface antigen-positive chronic liver disease. *Gut*, **16**, 836
193. Jain, S., Thomas, H. and Sherlock, S. (1976). Failure of transfer factor therapy in chronic active type B hepatitis. *N. Engl. J. Med.*, **295**, 504
194. Tong, M. J., Nystrom, J. S., Redefer, A. G. and Marshall, G. J. (1976). Failure of transfer factor therapy in chronic active type B hepatitis. *N. Engl. J. Med.*, **295**, 209
195. Jersild, C., Paltz, P., Thomsen, M., Hansen, G. S., Svejgaard, A., Dupont, B., Fog, T. and Ciongoli, A. K. (1973). Transfer factor therapy in multiple sclerosis. *Lancet*, **ii**, 1381
196. Jersild, C., Paltz, P., Thomsen, M., Dupont, B., Svejgaard, A., Ciongoli, A. K., Fog, T. and Grob, P. J. (1976). Transfer factor treatment of patients with multiple sclerosis. I. Preliminary report of changes in immunological parameters. *Scand. J. Immunol.*, **5**, 141
197. Zabriskie, J. B., Untermohlen, V., Espinoza, L. R., Plank, C. R. and Collins, R. C. (1975). Immunological studies with transfer factor in multiple sclerosis patients. *Neurology*, **25**, 490
198. Platz, P., Jersild, C., Thomsen, M., Svejgaard, A., Fog, T., Midholm, S., Rauri, N., Hansen, S. K. and Grob, P. (1976). Transfer factor treatment of patients with multiple sclerosis. II. Immunological parameters in a long-term clinical trial. In: *Transfer Factor: Basic Properties and Clinical Applications* (M. S. Ascher, A. A. Gottlieb and C. H. Kirkpatrick, eds.), p. 649 (New York: Academic Press)
199. Behan, P. O., Melville, J. D., Durward, W. F., McGeorge, A. P. and Behan, W. M. H. (1976). Transfer factor therapy in multiple sclerosis. *Lancet*, **i**, 988
200. Angers, J. W., Reid, W. E., Urbania, C., Angres, A. H. and Arron, A. S. (1976). Clinical evaluation of the effects of transfer factor on multiple sclerosis. In: *Transfer Factor: Basic Properties and Clinical Applications* (M. S. Ascher, A. A. Gottlieb and C. H. Kirkpatrick, eds.), p. 715 (New York: Academic Press)
201. Bullock, W. E., Fields, J. P. and Brandries, M. W. (1972). An evaluation of transfer factor as immunotherapy for patients with lepromatous leprosy. *N. Engl. J. Med.*, **287**, 1053
202. Saha, K., Mittal, M. M. and Maheshwari, H. B. (1975). Passive transfer of immunity into leprosy patients by transfusion of lymphocytes and by transfusion of Lawrence's transfer factor. *J. Clin. Microbiol.*, **1**, 279
203. Hastings, R. C., Morales, M. J., Shannon, E. J. and Jacobson, R. R. (1976). Preliminary results on the safety and efficacy of transfer factor in leprosy. In: *Transfer Factor: Basic Properties and Clinical Applications* (M. S. Ascher, A. A. Gottlieb and C. H. Kirkpatrick, eds.), p. 465 (New York: Academic Press)
204. Graybill, J. R., Silva, J., Fraser, D. and Thor, D. E. (1973). Disseminated mycobacteriosis in immunosuppressed patients. *Clin. Res.*, **21**, 62

205. Horsmanheimo, M., Krohn, K. and Virolainen, M. (1977). Clinical study of a patient with lupus vulgaris before and after injection of dialyzable transfer factor. *J. Invest. Dermatol.*, **68**, 10
206. Grohn, P., Kuokkanen, K. and Krohn, K. (1976). The effect of non-specifically acting transfer factor component on acnitis type of lupus miliaris faciei. *Acta Dermatovener.*, **56**, 449
207. Grohn, P. (1977). Transfer factor in chronic and recurrent respiratory tract infections in children. *Acta Paediatr. Scand.*, **66**, 211
208. Duprée, E., Smith, C. W. and Goldman, A. S. (1972). Lymphoid interstitial pneumonia, deficient cell-mediated immunity and lymphocyte dysfunction. *Clin. Res.*, **20**, 100
209. Graybill, J. R., Ellenbogen, C., Drossman, D., Kaplan, P. and Thor, D. E. (1976). Transfer factor therapy of disseminated histoplasmosis. In: *Transfer Factor: Basic Properties and Clinical Applications* (M. S. Ascher, A. A. Gottlieb and C. H. Kirkpatrick, eds.), p. 509 (New York: Academic Press)
210. Warren, K. S., Cook, J. A., David, J. R. and Jordan, P. (1975). Passive transfer of immunity in human *Schistosomiasis mansoni*: Effect of transfer factor on early established infections. *Trans. R. Soc. Trop. Med. Hyg.*, **69**, 488
211. Cozine, W. S., Stanfield, A. B., Stephens, C. A. L., Parsons, J. L., Holbrook, J. P., Strong, J. S., Wongsri, C., Mazur, M. T. and Raymond, L. N. (1976). Transfer factor immunotherapy of rheumatoid arthritis. In: *Transfer Factor: Basic Properties and Clinical Applications* (M. S. Ascher, A. A. Gottlieb and C. H. Kirkpatrick, eds.), p. 617 (New York: Academic Press)
212. Healey, L. A., Wetske, K. R., Webb, D. R. and Sumida, S. S. (1974). Transfer factor in adult rheumatoid arthritis. *Lancet*, **ii**, 160
213. Maini, R. N., Scott, J. T., Hamblin, A., Lindsay, R. and Dumonde, D. C. (1976). Is the clinical benefit from transfer factor in rheumatoid arthritis a placebo effect? In: *Transfer Factor: Basic Properties and Clinical Applications* (M. S. Ascher, A. A. Gottlieb and C. H. Kirkpatrick, eds.), p. 601 (New York: Academic Press)
214. Frøland, S. S., Natvig, J. B., Høyeraal, H. M. and Kass, E. (1974). The principle of immunopotentiation in treatment of rheumatoid arthritis: Effect of transfer factor. *Scand. J. Immunol.*, **3**, 223
215. Grohn, P., Anttila, R. and Krohn, K. (1976). The effect of a non-specifically acting transfer factor component on cellular immunity in juvenile rheumatoid arthritis. *Scand. J. Rheumatol.*, **5**, 151
216. Asquith, P., Mallas, E., Ross, J., Montgomery, R. D., Cooke, W. T. and Thomson, R. A. (1975). Transfer factor in the treatment of Crohn's disease. *Gut*, **16**, 832
217. Horsmanheimo, M. and Virolainen, M. (1976). Transfer of tuberculin sensitivity by transfer factor in sarcoidosis. *Clin. Immunol. Immunopathol.*, **6**, 231
218. Platz, P., Grob, P. J., Jønsson, V., Lorenzen, T. and Thomsen, M. (1976). Transfer factor, sarcoidosis and cellular immunity. *Acta Pathol. Microbiol. Scand., Sect. C*, **84**, 689
219. Wolf, R. E., Fudenberg, H. H., Welch, T. M., Spitler, L. E. and Ziff, M. (1977). Treatment of Behcet's syndrome with transfer factor. *J. Am. Med. Assoc.*, **238**, 869
220. Kahn, A., Sellars, W. A., Pflanzer, J., Hill, H. M., Thometz, D. and Haenke, J. (1976). Asthma and T-cell immunodeficiency: Improvement with transfer factor and immunopeptide I. *Ann. Allerg.*, **37**, 267
221. Brown, R. E. and Katz, M. (1967). Passive transfer of delayed hypersensitivity reaction to tuberculin in children with protein calorie malnutrition. *J. Pediatr.*, **70**, 126
222. Walker, A. M., Garcia, R., Pate, P., Mata, L. J. and David, J. R. (1975). Transfer factor in the immune deficiency of protein-calorie malnutrition: A controlled study with 32 cases. *Cell. Immunol.*, **15**, 372
223. José, D. G., Ford, G. W. and Welch, T. S. (1976). Therapy with parent's lymphocyte transfer factor in children with infection and malnutrition. *Lancet*, **i**, 263

224. Spitler, L. E. (1974). Letter to the Editor: Problems with transfer factor. *N. Engl. J. Med.*, **290**, 1022

225. Arala-Chaves, M. P. and Ramos, M. T. F. (1974). Letter to the Editor: Problems with transfer factor. *N. Engl. J. Med.*, **290**, 1023

226. Cowdrey, S. C. (1974). Letter to the Editor: Problems with transfer factor. *N. Engl. J. Med.*, **290**, 1023

3
Transfer Factor: Clinical Usage and Experimental Studies

A. BASTEN and S. CROFT

Immunology Unit, Department of Bacteriology, The University of Sydney, New South Wales 2006, Australia

---

INTRODUCTION

Transfer factor (TF) is defined as a dialysable cell-free leukocyte extract with the capacity to transfer delayed-type hypersensitivity (DTH) from an immune to a non-immune individual in a specific manner. It was originally described by Lawrence[1,2] in a classical series of experiments in which DTH to the PPD and streptococcal M substance was transferred to naive recipients as judged by conversion of skin test reactivity. Despite the potential value of TF as a therapeutic tool, Lawrence's observations were regarded with scepticism or ignored for many years. It was not until 1970 that TF was first used in treatment of human disease[3]. Since then it has been given with various degrees of success to patients with a wide range of immunological problems including immunodeficiency states, recurrent or disseminated infections and malignancy. This has resulted in intense interest in its properties and mode of action, in accumulation of a substantial literature and in the holding of two international workshops (1973, 1976).

Despite all this activity, considerable controversy still surrounds TF. For example, can it really transfer specific reactivity to a naive host or does it only boost subliminal responses to ubiquitous antigens? How can a substance of such low molecular weight apparently transfer immunity and what could be its mode of action? Is there any evidence from properly controlled trials to suggest that it has a beneficial effect in a clinical situation where DTH reactivity is known to be defective or important? The purpose of this chapter is to attempt to answer these questions by summarizing in a critical and selective manner the available information on TF in the light of current immunological concepts. It is not intended to be a comprehensive review particularly of the earlier literature since several extensive reviews already exist[4–6].

At the outset, the point should be emphasized in fairness to Lawrence that TF as he and his colleagues defined it has a number of characteristic features: it is a dialysable material prepared by freeze thawing of mononuclear cells from human peripheral blood which is apparently capable of transferring DTH reactivity to naive individuals as measured by skin-test conversion or an equivalent *in vitro* test. In other words, certain criteria need to be met before investigators can claim to be working on TF *per se*. Many studies, although of considerable interest and potential therapeutic importance do not meet these criteria and therefore need to be interpreted accordingly. For example, the production of 'TF' by B cells from lymphoblastoid cell lines[7] or the modulation by TF of receptors on E-rosette-forming cells after its administration[8] are intriguing as are attempts to influence the production of cytotoxic T cells against tumours[9], but none of them conform to the strict criteria originally laid down by Lawrence.

MECHANISM OF DELAYED-TYPE HYPERSENSITIVITY

DTH is generally accepted as the prototype of cell-mediated immune responses. Since the effects of TF are measured by transfer of DTH reactivity, an outline of current concepts of its components and mechanism (Figure 3.1)

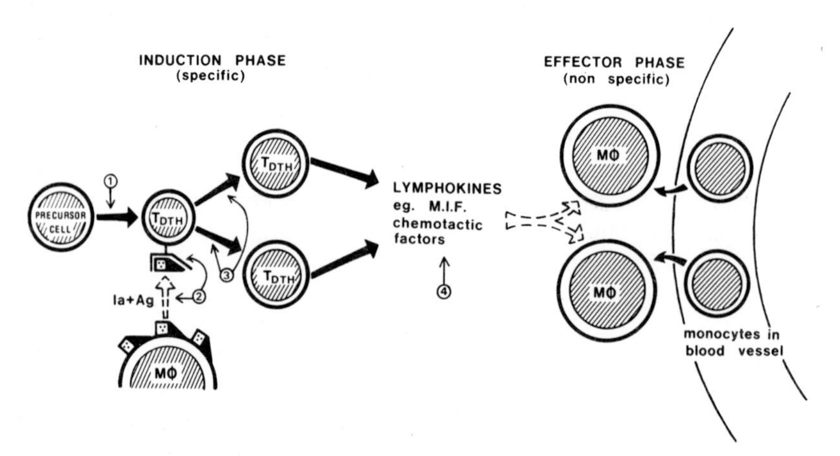

Figure 3.1 Schematic diagram of mechanism of delayed type hypersensitivity. A role for Ia antigens is based on experimental studies in the mouse, but may well apply to man as well. Ringed numbers indicate possible sites at which TF might act (see section of mode of action). In view of the multiplicity of components, more than one site of action is likely

is a prerequisite for any discussion on TF. The induction of DTH depends on activation of T cells by antigen. In the mouse, a subpopulation of T cells distinct from helper T cells and cytotoxic T cells and bearing the phenotype Ia^-, $Ly\text{-}1^+$, $Ly\text{-}2^-$ is responsible for mediating DTH[10] (Vadas *et al.*, 1976). T cell triggering requires antigen presentation by histocompatible macrophages sharing the same I region of the major histocompatibility complex, i.e. the T cell receives two signals, antigen and Ia, possibly in the form of a complex. As a result of activation, T cells release a number of mediators (lymphokines) including chemotactic factors for monocytes and macrophage migration inhibition factor (MIF). These attract and trap macrophages or their precursors at the site of antigen localization (e.g. in the skin) and mediate the effector phase of DTH. TF could, in theory, influence either the induction or effector phases of the response (see section on mode of action).

PHYSICOCHEMICAL PROPERTIES OF TF

Basic properties

The basic physicochemical properties of TF have been well defined[15,11] and are summarized in Table 3.1. It is dialysable and passes through filters of equivalent pore size such as Amicon Diaflo which have considerable technical

Table 3.1 Basic physicochemical properties of TF

1. Dialysable, i.e. MW < 14 000 daltons
2. Stable after freeze thawing and lyophilizing
3. Inactivated at 56 °C for 30 min
4. Resistant to treatment with trypsin, DNase and pancreatic RNase
5. Sensitive to treatment with pronase

advantages for production of large quantities of material for clinical usage[12,13], since they allow rapid concentration of low molecular weight material (see section on production of TF for clinical usage). TF is stable indefinitely at −20 °C, inactivated at 56 °C for 30 min and resistant to treatment with trypsin, DNase and RNase.

Components

The components of TF with defined biological activity have proved difficult to analyse. There are two main reasons for this: first, the multiplicity of components present in the crude cell-free extracts, and secondly the difficulty of isolating an active fraction using conventional biochemical techniques. Early analytical work suggested that TF is composed of polypeptides and polynucleotides containing ribose sugars[14]. Its activity is lost after treatment with pronase[15] indicating involvement of peptides with the active site. RNA is probably associated with the peptides. There is, however, no evidence that it is necessary for activity since treatment of TF with pancreatic RNase or T_1 RNase has no effect on its function[15]. Extracts of RNA with similar properties to TF have been reported to transfer immunological reactivity to naive mice, but like TF, their potency was pronase sensitive[16].

Table 3.2 Components of TF

1. Polypeptides and polynucleotides (ratio 2:1)
2. Hypoxanthine
3. Chemotactic factors
4. Low molecular weight factors such as ascorbate and serotonin which increase intracellular cGMP levels
5. Nicotinamide
6. Uracil
7. Ia-like molecules

More recently TF preparations have been found to contain a number of other components (Table 3.2). These include: hypoxanthine, for which there is no known immunological activity[17]; uracil[18]; chemotactic factors[19]; components such as ascorbate and serotonin which increase intracellular levels of cGMP[20]; nicotinamide which exerts an inhibitory effect on *in vitro* tests of T cell reactivity[21] (Burger *et al.*, 1976c) and Ia-like molecules (Croft, Parish and Basten, unpublished observations). The latter finding is of particular interest in view of the established role of Ia–antigen complexes in induction of T-cell triggering[10,22].

TF does not appear to contain albumin, nor immunoglobulin fragments[5]. Antigen is likewise said to be absent[23] although very few studies exist which formally exclude this. In view of the presence of Ia molecules, the possibility of contamination with antigen fragments needs reappraisal.

The existence of multiple components in TF raises the question of which is/are responsible for transfer of DTH. In an attempt to answer this TF has been subject to extensive chromatographic analysis. When it is passed over Sephadex G-25, for example, five to six peaks are obtained (Figure 3.2). One of these, usually the third, is associated with transfer of skin-test reactivity, but there is controversy over whether this peak elutes after the total volume of the column[24,25] or before[26]. The active peak has a high 260:280 nm ratio and contains hypoxanthine[17] and uracil[18] which has a non-specific stimulatory effect. The nature of the active component in this peak awaits a definitive answer. Analysis of the peaks in *in vitro* assays of DTH has been unrewarding. For example, positive MIF and lymphocyte transformation responses have been obtained not only with the third peak, but others as well[27] (Croft and Basten, in preparation). Consequently it is difficult to equate any biologically active component of TF, specific or non-specific, with a single peak and therefore with defined polypeptide or polynucleotide molecules. On the other hand, carbohydrate-containing material such as Ia antigens[28] would not be expected to separate readily on Sephadex chromatography.

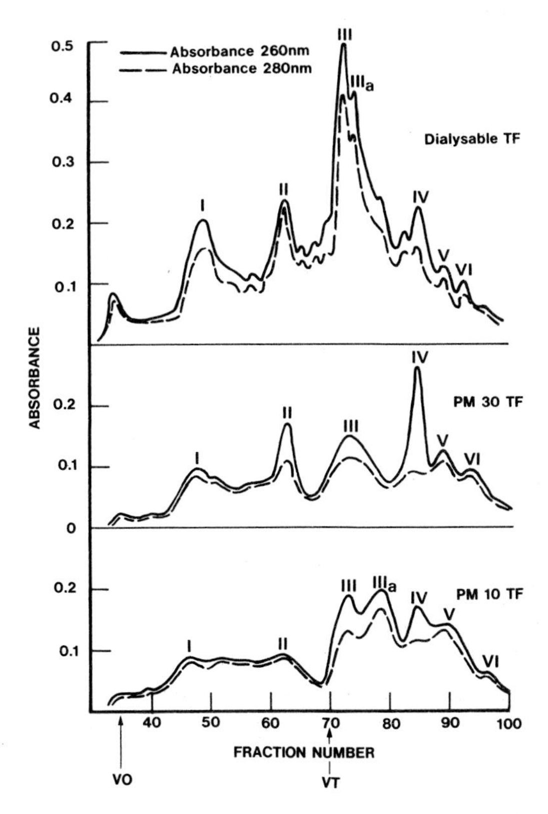

Figure 3.2 G-25 Sephadex chromatography of TF prepared by dialysis or by ultrafiltration through PM30 or PM10 diaflo membranes. Note that the profiles are similar, although the heights of the peaks following PM10 filtration are lower. Key to activities of peaks may be summarized as follows:

skin-test reactivity, peak III
LT, peaks I, II, III
MIF production, peaks I, III, IV

BIOLOGICAL PROPERTIES OF TF

In vivo studies

The original series of experiments of Lawrence on TF[1,2] were all carried out *in vivo*, using skin testing to demonstrate transfer of DTH. The four striking features of these studies were the rapidity of sensitization of recipients, long duration of reactivity following transfer (12 months or more), apparent specificity and selectivity of the effect on cell-mediated immunity[5] (Table 3.3).

Table 3.3 Biological properties of TF

In vivo effects
Confers DTH reactivity within a few hours
Confers DTH reactivity which is long-lasting
Acts specifically
Exerts a relatively selective effect on DTH
Increases number of E-rosette-forming cells if low
Augments MLC reactivity } in immunodeficient recipients
Augments PHA reactivity } in immunodeficient recipients
Augments cytotoxicity against tumours (e.g. osteogenic sarcoma)
In vitro effects
Augments lymphocyte transformation non-specifically
Stimulates MIF production specifically
Exerts variable effects on PHA responses
Target of action is immunologically competent T cell
Inactive in bone marrow colony cultures

Rapidity of action

After injection of TF, the development of skin induration to simultaneous challenge with the appropriate antigen followed the same time course as a conventional DTH skin reaction. Thus TF appeared to trigger immune reactivity in the host within a remarkably short period of time, perhaps no more than 2–3 hours. If the target of TF is assumed to be a naive clone of T cells present at very low frequency, it is difficult to envisage how TF, whatever its nature, could affect the clone in such a way that its T cells were so rapidly induced to behave like memory cells. There is too little time for cell differentiation to occur which might result in expansion of the number of antigen reactive T cells. On the other hand, if the recipients had undergone subliminal sensitization due to prior exposure to antigen naturally or by skin testing, a secondary response might occur. This explanation has some appeal and has formed the basis of several experimental studies to be reported later (see sections on *in vitro* assays and animal models).

Long duration of transferred reactivity

DTH reactivity transferred by TF was found by Lawrence to last for over a year[1]. The antigen used in these studies was, however, PPD and it could therefore be argued that the long duration of the effect was due not to TF but to natural immunity acquired during the course of the experiment. Two other studies in particular have been used as arguments against this possibility. In the first, TF against *Coccidioidis immitis* was extracted from the leukocytes of blood donors from the San Joaquin Valley in California where the fungus is endemic. Following injection into healthy individuals from a New York hospital who could not have been exposed to the fungus, prolonged transfer of skin-test reactivity was observed[29]. In the second study, synthetic antigens prepared by ethylene oxide treatment of serum were used to sensitize medical students. TF from these donors induced reactivity in naive recipients which was as long-lasting as that induced by natural antigens[30]. Although the latter study in particular excludes the possibility of naturally acquired immunity during the course of the experiments, it should be pointed out that both antigens used were complex, consisting of many different determinants. The chance of cross-reactivity with other ubiquitous antigens to which the recipients might have been sensitized is therefore very real. In other words, the problem of subliminal sensitization cannot be readily resolved by assaying with complex multideterminant antigens and highlights the need for studies with simple antigens such as the synthetic copolymers or contact sensitizing agents (see section on animal models).

Specificity

The most controversial and potentially most significant therapeutic property of TF is its specificity. When measured *in vivo* by transfer of DTH skin reactivity, TF appears to be specific[5]. For example, TF prepared from PPD-negative coccidioidin-positive leukocytes has been reported to confer reactivity to the latter but not the former[29]. The conventional technique for testing its efficacy does, however, rely on repeated skin testing of recipients both before as well as after administration of TF. As mentioned previously, this form of repeated challenge may recall subliminal reactivity or may itself cause *de novo* sensitization[31]. One particularly good example of the problem is illustrated by reports of recipients developing new skin test sensitivities after injection of TF of another specificity[11,32]. Furthermore, the interpretation of specific conversion of skin reactivity in recipients undergoing treatment can be rendered difficult by the use of conventional therapy in conjunction with TF. For instance, patients with chronic mucocutaneous candidiasis[33], histoplasmosis[34] or leprosy[35] possess serum inhibitors of lymphocyte activity which may disappear after adequate antimicrobial treatment giving 'false' positive conversions of DTH reactions.

The difficulty in trying to resolve the issue of specificity by working exclusively *in vivo* in man with relatively crude extracts has led investigators to develop new approaches for the study of TF including isolation of individual components by chemical analysis and creation of *in vitro* assays and animal models. The latter two lines of investigation will be discussed later.

Chemical analysis of TF (see previous section) has done little, as yet, to clarify the problem of specificity. Many of the more recently defined components have been found to exert non-specific rather than specific effects, or have no effect at all. In addition, it remains difficult to envisage how any component, including RNA or Ia antigens even if complexed with antigen (Figure 3.1) could trigger a specific response so rapidly (within a few hours) in a truly naive recipient.

Selectivity of effect on DTH

In the great majority of studies, human and experimental alike, no evidence for transfer of humoral immunity by TF has been obtained. The selectivity of its effect is surprising in the light of the known importance of T cells in generation of optimal IgG and IgE antibody responses. There are several possible explanations: first, DTH skin testing may be a more sensitive indicator of reactivity than measurement of serum antibodies by conventional techniques; secondly the threshold of T cell triggering is thought to be lower than that required for B cells[36]; thirdly it is possible that the active component in TF may exert a selective effect on the subclass of T cells mediating DTH rather than helper T cells required for antibody production. This is, however, unlikely since other T cell subpopulations such as cytotoxic T cells appear to be activated by TF[9] and DTH T cells bear the same phenotype as helper T cells[10]. Fourthly, TF might induce suppressor T cells rather than helper T cells for antibody production at the same time as triggering DTH reactive T cells. Indeed a dichotomy of this kind has been reported[37]. On the other hand, the possible presence in TF of Ia antigens would favour activation of helper rather than suppressor cells[22]. These alternatives are now amenable to analysis with the recent development of anti-Ly sera.

Isolated instances exist in the literature where TF has been claimed to boost IgG synthesis[38,39]. Clearly the issue will remain in doubt until the problem of specificity is resolved and the active components of TF are fully identified.

Effects on other parameters of cell-mediated immunity

The potential value of using TF in immunodeficiency states or malignancy has resulted in a study of parameters of cell-mediated immunity other than DTH. These include PHA responses, mixed lymphocyte cultures (MLC), E-rosette numbers and cytotoxicity against tumours. Augmentation of the first three parameters has been reported in patients with immunodeficiency states such as the Wiskott–Aldrich syndrome and a variety of malignant diseases (reviewed by Lawrence[5]). In view of the multiplicity of components in TF, it is possible that these non-specific effects are mediated by different components from those responsible for transferring DTH *in vivo*. Whether this is true or not, the capacity of TF to boost immune responsiveness, albeit non-specifically, gives encouragement for its continued use in clinical situations where the immune system is compromised.

Stimulation of cytotoxic cells has been reported by both Levin *et al.*[9] and

Thor *et al.*[40] in patients with osteogenic sarcomas. These studies are interesting for two reasons in particular: first the cells mediating cytotoxicity were shown to be T lymphocytes[41], and secondly, TF apparently exerted a specific effect in the sense that it had to be produced from donors with reactivity to that particular tumour. Unfortunately basic work with TF in other solid tumour systems has been less rewarding in view of the difficulty in identifying the cytotoxic mechanisms involved and in establishing their specificity (see section on clinical applications).

In vitro studies

DTH assays

The difficulty of working with TF exclusively *in vivo* has already been mentioned. On the other hand, the use of *in vitro* assays can likewise be misleading. Thus it is essential, particularly when studying specificity, to work with test systems which show a good correlation with *in vivo* DTH reactivity. The great majority of *in vitro* studies on TF has utilized one or more of the following three assays: macrophage migration inhibition (MMI), leukocyte migration inhibition (LMI), or lymphocyte transformation (LT). Of these the indirect[42] and direct[43] MMI tests appear to correlate well with DTH skin reactivity, as does LT[44] which is thought to be a good indicator of T cell memory. By contrast, conflicting data have been obtained with the LMI test. For example, using the capillary tube system Søberg and Bendixen[45] found a good correlation with skin tests for *Brucella* antigen. Subsequent studies in which other antigens such as PPD were used in either the capillary or agarose test systems have, however, failed to yield consistent

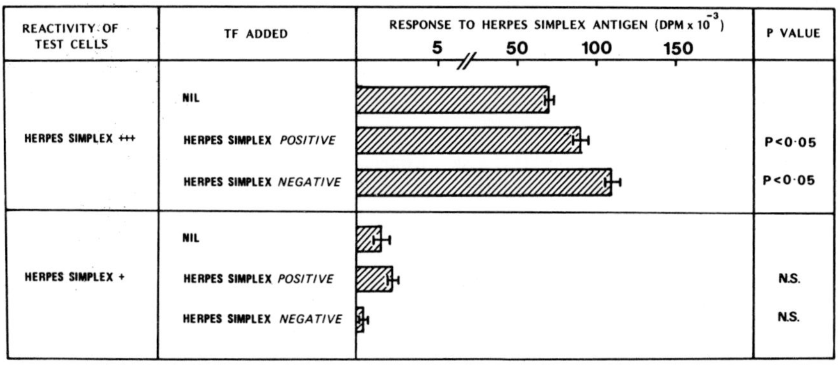

REACTIVITY OF TEST CELLS	TF ADDED	RESPONSE TO HERPES SIMPLEX ANTIGEN (DPM x 10^{-3}) 5 // 50 100 150	P VALUE
HERPES SIMPLEX +++	NIL		
	HERPES SIMPLEX *POSITIVE*		P<0·05
	HERPES SIMPLEX *NEGATIVE*		P<0·05
HERPES SIMPLEX +	NIL		
	HERPES SIMPLEX *POSITIVE*		N.S.
	HERPES SIMPLEX *NEGATIVE*		N.S.

Figure 3.3 Effect of human TF on lymphocyte transformation. Significant augmentation is observed only when the target cells are primed to the test antigen (herpes simplex). TF activity is non-specific in the sense that augmentation of responses occur with TF from herpes simplex negative as well as positive donors

results (reviewed by Fleer *et al.*[44]). Interpretation of studies of TF which have employed the latter technique must therefore be guarded.

The effect of TF in the LT assay has proved variable. Its addition to lymphocyte cultures has been reported to augment the response to antigen[46,47], to have no effect[48], or to have a suppressive action[49]. The reasons for this variability are not entirely clear, although some preparations have been found to be toxic *in vitro* probably on the basis of hypertonicity or hypotonicity. Dialysis against tissue culture medium instead of water has been shown to overcome this problem[46] but is not the entire answer[48]. In those situations where TF has been stimulatory, the effect appears to be antigen-dependent but not antigen-specific. If the target cells display some reactivity to antigens, their response is augmented by addition of TF of relevant or irrelevant specificities. On the other hand, TF does not boost the response of target cells which lack detectable reactivity to antigen. In other words, stimulation is proportional to the degree of reactivity of the test cells rather than that of the TF donors (Figure 3.3). This implies that the stimulatory effect of TF in the LT assay depends on the presence of precommitted antigen reactive cells[127]. Consistent with this are the findings of Cohen *et al.*[50] of abolition of the proliferative response to TF plus antigen by 'suicide' with that antigen, but not an irrelevant antigen. Presumably the components of TF mediating this effect are the same as those responsible for *in vivo* augmentation of PHA and MLC reactivity and E-rosette counts. The presence of TF of such non-specific activity is underlined by the recent findings of Littman *et al.*[51] of augmentation of LT responses with dialysates prepared from polymorphs.

Less information is available about the effect of TF on MIF production *in vitro*: our group therefore decided to examine this using the direct MMI test[12]. When TF was added to cultures of cells from non-reactive donors, migration inhibition was observed in the presence of the relevant, but not of a control antigen (Table 3.4). A similar result was obtained with other antigen combinations. In other words, TF was acting in an apparently specific manner. The TF used was shown to transfer the same reactivity

Table 3.4 Activity of TF in the MMI assay. Evidence for specificity

*Test cells**	*Reactivity of TF donor*	*Antigen*	*MI†*	p *value‡*
PPD−	No TF	PPD	0.94	n.s.
PPD−	PPD+, Mumps+	PPD	0.81	$p < 0.05$
PPD−	PPD−, Mumps+	PPD	1.06	n.s.
Mumps±	No TF	Mumps	0.85	n.s.
Mumps±	PPD−, Mumps+	Mumps	0.75	$p < 0.005$
G.P. PEC§ only	PPD+, Mumps+	PPD	1.09	n.s.

* Reactivity of cells in LT: negative, ± weakly positive, + positive
† Data from a representative experiment, others gave similar results
‡ *p* value for difference of migration with antigen from migration without antigen. n.s. = not significant
§ Guinea-pig peritoneal exudate cells

in vivo as measured by skin test conversion. Furthermore, non-reactivity of cell donors was confirmed, initially *in vitro* and after use in the assays by skin testing. The latter precaution was taken to minimize the possibility of subliminal sensitization. These results are intriguing but why TF should exert a specific effect in one *in vitro* assay for DTH and a non-specific effect in another is puzzling. The suggestion that the two assays measure the activity of different T-cell populations provides one possible explanation. Thus MIF production may be an exclusive property of DTH T cells, whereas other cells as well as DTH reactive cells may be stimulated into DNA synthesis by TF and antigen. The net result could be masking of specificity. It is, however, equally plausible to argue in favour of overall non-specificity by invoking a role for the Ia antigen component of TF. The presence of Ia antigens with multiple specificities can readily explain the non-specificity of the augmentation of LT. Furthermore, if Ia is coupled with trace amounts of antigen fragments which could serve as a 'superantigen', the net result of addition of TF to a shorter term (18 h) assay such as MMI might be apparent specificity. The correct explanation must await further studies on the components of TF and the cells responding to it. In the meantime, it can only be said that *in vitro* assays clearly establish the existence in TF of components with non-specific activity but have not provided a definitive answer to the question of whether a specific component is present as well.

Assays of other parameters of cell-mediated immunity

The finding that TF administered *in vivo* stimulates a variety of cell-mediated responses other than DTH (e.g. PHA and MLC responses, E-rosette-forming cells) has led to attempts to analyse these effects *in vitro*. When the PHA response was studied, variable results were obtained. For example, Hamblin *et al.*[52] reported an augmentation with TF, while Ascher *et al.*[46] and our own group observed little or no effect. Since studies of this kind do not deal with the key issue of specificity and at best confirm the presence of non-specific components in TF, they are of doubtful value. By contrast, the *in vitro* studies on E-rosette formation are of interest. Trypsinized lymphocytes which can no longer undergo E-rosette formation rapidly reacquire their receptors on culture with TF[53]. Similar findings have been reported by Khan *et al.*[54] using thymosin, implying that TF may, like thymosin, contain a factor capable of influencing T-cell differentiation (see section on mode of action).

Source

It is intriguing that the cellular source of TF received little or no attention at the recent International Workshop (1976). Indeed no precise information about the cell of origin (i.e. lymphocyte or phagocyte) has yet been forthcoming with two notable exceptions. First, Pizza *et al.*[7] showed that the B cell component of human lymphoblastoid cell lines can apparently secrete TF-like activity. Secondly, Littman *et al.*[51] (1977) were able to prepare a dialysable extract from polymorphs which exerted a non-specific stimulatory effect in the *in vitro* LT assay. The existence in TF of multiple components does, however, make the question of its origin difficult or even unnecessary to answer until such time as a specific fraction can be positively identified.

Target of action

The capacity of TF to induce rapid transfer of cell-mediated reactivity *in vivo* implies that the target of action is likely to be an immunocompetent lymphocyte. To study this in more detail, our group examined the effect of TF on lymphoid cells from thymus and cord blood as well as adult blood in the MMI and LT assays[12]. Although control cells from peripheral blood responded well, negative results were obtained with immature cells from both the above sources. The finding by Cohen *et al.*[50] of abrogation of the proliferative response to TF plus antigen by the suicide technique is consistent with the need for a differentiated target cell. Since MMI and LT assays have been shown to be a measure of T-cell function[44], it is probable that the T cell is the target of action of TF. In other words, specific and non-specific effects of TF require the presence of immunologically competent T cells.

Animal models

The potential value of animal models for analysis of the nature and mechanism of action of TF is self-evident and is reflected by the substantial number of papers on this subject which have appeared in the past few years. This approach is based on the reasonable assumption that any immunological phenomenon of potential importance should be demonstrable in lower species with comparable immune systems to man. An overall picture of the current status of work in animal models can be obtained by summarizing the key findings of articles published in the Proceedings of the Second International Workshop on TF (1976) (Table 3.5). Examination of the contents of Table 3.5 reveals a striking variation but despite this, a number of interesting points emerge. First, TF was found to transfer DTH reactivity specifically *in vivo* in a number of animals as measured by acceptable test systems. The timing of collection of cells for production of TF and of assaying for its effects was shown to be critical[55]. For example, TF prepared from memory cells (analogous to the human situation) proved to be active, but when cells taken at the peak of a response were used, it had the reverse, i.e. suppressive effect[12]. Secondly, there was one report of protection against

Table 3.5 Summary of essential features of animal models presented at Second International Workshop on TF

TF donors					Test system used	TF recipients						Investigators
Species	*Cell source for TF*	*Cell type*	*Methods of sensitization*	*Detection of sensitization*		*Species*	*Tests used for TF effects*	*Mode of TF administration*	*Cells*	*Results of transfer*	*Specificity of effects claimed*	
Rhesus monkey	PBL	?	KLH in CFA	?	KLH response	Rhesus monkey	Indirect MMI	*In vitro*	PBL	+ve with fractions, not whole TF	Unproven	Baram and Condoulis[115]
Outbred dog	PBL	Memory	*C. immitis* ± CFA	Skin tests or nil	*C. immitus*, PPD response	Dog	Skin test and LT	*In vitro* for LT	PBL	Variable	?	Shifrine *et al.*
Human	PBL	Not relevant	Nil	—	Mitogen responses	Mouse	LT	*In vivo*	Spleen cells	Stimulation and infiltration inhibition	Non-specific	Huard and Baram[116]
Human	PBL	Memory	Natural	Skin tests and LT	Day 3 responses to multiple antigens	Primate	Skin test, LT	*In vivo*	PBL	+ve LT better than skin tests	Specific	Steele *et al.*
Primate	PBL	?	Variable (No CFA)	Skin tests and LT	Day 3 responses to multiple antigens	Primate	Skin test, LT	*In vivo*	PBL	+ve LT better than skin tests	Specific	Steele *et al.*[117]
Human	PBL	Memory	Natural	Cytotoxicity LMI, LT	Protection against herpes virus infection	Marmoset	Survival	*In vivo*	Not relevant	Protection if TF given before infection	Specific	Steele *et al.*[56]
Human	PBL	Memory	Natural	Skin test, LT	*C. immitus*, *Candida*, PPD recipients	Mouse	Skin test	*In vivo*	Not relevant	Positive	Specific	Petersen *et al.*[118]
Human	PBL	Memory	Natural	Skin test	Response to multiple antigens in subliminally primed recipients	Guinea-pig (subliminally sensitized)	Skin test	*In vivo*	Not relevant	Positive	Specific	Welch *et al.*[57]
Human	PBL	Memory	Natural	Skin test	Response to PPD, SK/SD	Guinea-pig	Skin test, LT	*In vivo*	PBL	+ve but only if recipients pre skin tested	Probably specific	Vandenbark *et al.*[119]
Outbred guinea-pig	PEC, lymph nodes, plasma from ALG-treated GP	Memory and peak	Variable (No CFA)	Skin test	Response to multiple antigens using TF or plasma from ALS-treated donors	Guinea-pig	Skin test, MMI, LT	*In vitro* for MMI and LT	PBL	+ve with TF and plasma from ALS-treated donors	?	Jeter *et al.*[120]
Human	PBL	Memory	Previous hepatitis B virus infection	Skin test, LMI	Termination of HBsAg carrier status	Chimpanzee (HBsAg) carriers	Skin test, LMI, HBsAg level	*In vivo*	PBL	+ve for skin tests and LMI. No effect on HBsAg level or liver function	?	Trepo and Prince[121]
Mouse	Lymph node spleen thymus	Memory and peak	DNFB skin sensitization	Skin test, MMI, LT	DNFB, BCG responses	Syngeneic mouse	MMI, LT	*In vivo* and *in vitro*	Lymph node	+ve with memory but not peak TF from lymph nodes – ve with TF from spleen and thymus	LT effect non-specific MMI effect apparently specific	Basten *et al.*[122]
Human	PBL	Memory	? natural	? skin test	Response to streptococcal cell membranes	Mouse	LMI	*In vitro*	Spleen, thymus	+ve with both cell sources	Possibly specific	Read *et al.*[123]
Guinea-pig	Pool of PEC lymph node, spleen	?	Antigens in CFA	?	Response to multiple antigens	Guinea-pig	MMI, LT	*In vitro*	PEC, lymph node	+ve even at very high dilutions	Possibly specific	Dunnick and Bach[59]
Human	PBL	Memory	Natural	Skin test	Responses to PPD and SK/SD	Guinea-pig (presensitized)	Skin test	*In vivo*	Not relevant	Positive	Possibly specific	Triglia and Spitler[55]
Guinea-pig	? pool of lymphoid cells	?	*L. enriettii* infection	Skin test	Protection against *L. enriettii* infection	Guinea-pig	MMI, LT	*In vivo*	PEC	+ve *in vitro* tests. No protection	Specific effect in *in vitro* tests	Clinton and Magoc[124]

MMI = macrophage migration inhibition, LMI = leukocyte migration inhibition, LT = lymphocyte transformation fatal infection with herpes virus[56]. This is clearly of great potential value clinically and needs urgent confirmation with larger numbers of animals and in other systems. Thirdly, human TF was found to work in animals which provides the basis for better analysis and potency testing of material used in treatment of patients[57,58]. The presence of Ia antigens in it does, however, need to be taken into consideration in view of their established role in modulating T-cell interactions including DTH and of their possible importance in conferring specificity. Thus, if Ia antigens do contribute to the activity of TF one might not expect it to function optimally across histocompatibility antigen barriers. Fourthly, it was encouraging to note the similarity of chromatography profiles of human and animal TF preparations (e.g. refs. 12, 59).

Certain key issues were not resolved at the workshop. Perhaps the most important was the immune status of the recipients. For example, an absolute requirement for priming of recipients was found by some groups[55,57,58] but not by others[56]. Furthermore, prior skin testing was used in the majority of models, with its inherent risk of inducing subliminal sensitization. The subsequent studies of Eichberg *et al.*[60], in gnotobiotic primates go some way to resolving this dilemma. They have shown that human TF can induce specific DTH reactivity in naive recipients, not exposed to the antigens in question either naturally or by skin testing. Hopefully these findings will be confirmed in other systems, such as the mouse model which is more amenable to detailed analysis.

Positive results were obtained with a large range of antigens which, although encouraging in one sense, make comparisons between findings difficult. What is now required is a reproducible animal model with the potential for analysis in different laboratories. Until such time as this occurs it is unlikely that the sceptics will accept TF as a specific entity.

It was disappointing that little progress was made at the workshop towards identifying and characterizing the active component(s) in TF which continue to elude standard biochemical approaches. For this reason, the precise relationship between non-specific and specific activities remained unresolved.

MODE OF ACTION

The mechanism whereby TF transfers DTH reactivity in an apparently specific manner remains unsolved. This is largely related to the multiplicity of components in it coupled with the failure to identify a single fraction carrying specificity. From the theoretical point of view, TF could influence either the induction or effector phases or both of the DTH response. Its possible sites of action are shown schematically in Figure 3.1.

Induction of DTH requires the presence of macrophages and immunologically competent T cells. In a truly naive individual, such as the gnotobiotic primates used by Eichberg *et al.*[60], the number of antigen reactive T cells would be expected to be negligible. For TF to have an effect in this situation (see Figure 3.1), it would need to act as a gene derepressor capable of inducing uncommitted lymphocyte precursors to express antigen specific receptors. In other words, it might play a role in *lymphocyte differentiation*. The reports of partial reconstitution of dual deficiency states and thymic hypoplasia with TF[61] could be interpreted as indirect evidence in favour of this possibility as could its effect on E-rosette-forming cells[54]. Neither phenomenon is, however, antigen-specific and may be irrelevant to development of specific clones of T cells. Furthermore TF lacks colony stimulating activity on progenitor cells[13] when tested in the agar colony system of Metcalf[62]. Could TF act as the antigen specific receptor on T cells? Taken literally this implies that T cells exposed to TF would passively acquire antigen binding sites. There is no precedent for such a phenomenon. Furthermore, the receptors on T cells appear to be composed of idiotype components of immunoglobulin synthesized by the cells themselves[63]. For TF to influence receptor production it would need to act on precursor cells, i.e. once again as a differentiating agent.

Alternatively, TF could act at the stage of antigen presentation to T cells (see Figure 3.2). Normally this step in T-cell triggering requires macrophages, but if TF were to contain macrophage processed antigen fragments, i.e. *superantigen*, activation might occur more rapidly than usual particularly in presensitized individuals possessing memory T cells. The net result would be apparently specific transfer of DTH. The need to add additional antigen for TF to work *in vitro* or *in vivo* speaks against this possibility, although data formally excluding the presence of contaminating antigen are rare. On the other hand, TF does appear to contain the second component of the macrophage T-cell interaction, namely *Ia antigens*. When antigen is added, it will couple to the Ia molecules to form a complex which can stimulate T cells to proliferate and release lymphokines. In an *in vitro* system where macrophages may be limiting, this could result in an enhanced T-cell response. The fact that Ia antigens carry multiple specificities explains the non-specificity of augmentation observed in the lymphocyte transformation assay. It is, however, less easy to see how their presence can account for apparent specificity of transfer of DTH skin reactivity and the MMI response since the naive host already carries a full complement of Ia specificities. If the Ia component is assumed to be coupled with antigen fragments giving rise to another form of superantigen, TF should be effective on its own. Furthermore, its alleged capacity to transfer reactivity across species barriers would appear at first sight to minimize the potential importance of Ia component, but in this context it should be recalled that a significant degree of homology exists between histocompatibility antigens in different species.

The comments to date relate to possible ways in which TF or its components might exert a specific effect during induction of the DTH response. It could, however, influence the effector phase as well. The presence in the

Table 3.6 Effect of transfer factor in patients with chronic mucocutaneous candidiasis (CMC)

Clinical features	*Immunological abnormalities**	*Source of TF*	*No. of patients*	*Conversion of†*		*Other relevant therapy*	*Clinical outcome‡*	*References*
				DTH skin tests	In vitro *tests*			
Persistent vaginal candidiasis	DTH, MMI negative, LT positive with candida	Candida + (3–4 units)	3	3/3	2/3	Mycostatin and fungilin	3/3 no recurrence 6–12 months after TF	92
CMC without endocrinopathy	DTH skin test negative with candida	Candida +	6	5/6	Not done	Amphotericin B and 5-fluorocytosine	6/6 remission maintained by TF	93
	DTH skin tests and *in vitro* tests negative with candida	Candida +	4	1/1 remainder not tested	3/4	Amphotericin B	3/4 remission maintained by TF for 2–3 years. Partial remission in 4th case	92
CMC with endocrinopathy	DTH skin tests and *in vitro* tests negative with candida	Candida +	4	1/1 remainder not tested	2/4	Amphotericin B	4/4 improved with respect to mucous membranes, 1/4 showed improvement of nails, 1 subsequently died of Ca. stomach, follow-up 2–4 years	92
	DTH skin tests and MMI test negative, LT positive with candida	Candida + vs. candida –	1	1/1	1/1	Amphotericin B	1/1 remission maintained with *Candida* + TF but not *Candida* – TF	65
CMC	DTH skin tests and *in vitro* tests with candida	Candida + Candida +	6 5	6/6 5/5	Not done Not done	Nil Amphotericin B	0/6 improved 5/5 remission maintained by TF	66
CMC§	Candida specific tests negative abnormal neutrophil function	Candida +	1	1/1	1/1 (T cell and neutrophil function)	Mycostatin and iron	1/1 improvement	94
	Candida specific tests negative abnormal neutrophil chemotaxis	Candida +	1	1/1 (transient)	1/1	Nil	0/1	95
CMC¶ (unclassified)	No details given	Pooled TF_Z	22	No details given		No details	17/22 showed at least transitory improvement	13

* Relevant findings only given. In general patients reported had a selective T-cell deficiency to candida antigens. In patients with more severe candidiasis all DTH tests were negative, but in those with mild disease (vaginal) LT was usually positive

† Conversion of DTH tests correlated with clinical improvement

‡ The major effect of TF was to prevent recurrence in patients treated with adequate chemotherapy to reduce antigen load. It was ineffective given on its own

§ The patient had an additional defect in neutrophil function which was corrected by TF possibly due to its chemotactic activity

¶ Represent summary figures cited in International Workshop (1976). TF is prepared from pooled leukocytes from healthy blood donors

Table 3.7 Summary of clinical uses of TF

Diagnosis	*Source of TF*	*No. of patients*	*Conversion of*		*Other relevant therapy*	*Clinical outcome*	*References*
			DTH skin tests	In vitro *tests*			
Immunodeficiency states group							
Thymic dysplasia	Normal donors	4	0/4	0/4	Nil	0/4 3 died	96
	Normal donors	1	1/1	0/1	Nil	1/1 decreased frequency of infections for 3 years	97
Severe combined immunodeficiency	Normal donors	5	3/5	3/5	Thymus graft	3/5 reconstitution of T-cell function	61
	Normal donors	1	1/1	1/1	Thymus graft	1/1 T-cell function normal 5 months after transplantation; maintained on gammaglobulin	67
	Normal donors	1	1/1	not done	Thymus graft	DTH skin tests improved, but patient died of lymphoma	98
Variable immunodeficiency	Normal donors	1	1/1	1/1	Nil	1/1	38
Variable immunodeficiency with warts and autoimmune haemolytic anaemia	Normal donors	1	1/1	1/1 both transient	Intermittent prednisone, splenectomy	0/1 no effect on warts or episodes of haemolysis	92
Wiskott–Aldrich syndrome	Normal donors	12	7/12	6/8	Nil	6/10	99
	Normal donors	4	2/4	not done	Nil	2/4	100
	Normal donors	3	no details given		Nil	2/3 transitory benefit	13
	Normal donors	2	not done	1/2	Nil	2/2 decrease in incidence of infection and severity of eczema over period of 3 years	92
Ataxia telangiectasia	Normal donors	5	2/5	not done	Nil	3/5 partial	100
	Normal donors	2	no details given		Nil	1/2 transitory benefit	13
	Normal donors	1	not done	0/1	Nil	0/1 died of lymphoma 18 months after TF commenced	92
Humoral immunodeficiency group							
Primary acquired hypogammaglobulinaemia	Normal donors	1	Serum IgG levels rose		Gammaglobulin replacement	1/1 decreased frequency of injections of gammaglobulin required	39

crude extract of polynucleotides analogous to poly AU, and of components with both cGMP stimulatory and chemotactic activity supports this possibility. Although these activities are necessarily non-specific they do not exclude the coexistence of a specific component. Furthermore, possession of *adjuvant-like properties* may well contribute to the efficacy of TF as an immunopotentiating agent (see Figure 3.3).

CLINICAL USAGE

TF was first employed as an immunopotentiating agent in 1970 when Levin *et al.*[3] gave it to a patient with Wiskott–Aldrich syndrome. Since then it has been used to treat a wide variety of conditions in which cell-mediated immune responses have been compromised. These can be broadly divided into four groups:

1. Primary immunodeficiency states characterized by impaired T-cell activities;
2. Patients with recurrent or acute disseminated infections due to viruses, fungi or intracellular bacteria particularly in patients with compromised immune systems;
3. Patients with malignant disease;
4. Patients with disease with a suspected infectious aetiology.

When used clinically TF is usually expressed in units, one unit being the equivalent either of 5×10^8 lymphocytes (most commonly used) or 10^9 leukocytes.

Preparation

The conventional method of production of TF for clinical usage has been to prepare it by disruption of cells in the presence of DNase followed by extensive dialysis against large volumes of distilled water[64]. Volunteers from laboratory staff, students or relatives of the patient act as sources of cells. This method of collection of leukocytes for production of TF is obviously time-consuming and usually provides only a limited supply of material. Use of the cell separator has gone some way towards solving the problem of supply. A good run will yield up to 10^{10} mononuclear cells (20 units of TF). Access to such apparatus is not, however, always possible. Several groups including our own[6,12] have therefore established links with blood transfusion centres since healthy blood donors provide a continuous and ideal source of cells. In most centres, donors have all been carefully screened and each of their donations is checked routinely for the presence of hepatitis B antigen. Furthermore, it has been our experience that donors agree readily to DTH skin testing; TF from their cells can therefore be defined with respect to antigen specificity. In this way a bank of TFs can be accumulated for use in acute as well as chronic clinical situations.

Preparation of TF by dialysis has likewise proved a problem. The process is time-consuming and the risk of contamination significant. As mentioned in the section on physicochemical properties, it is now possible to use Amicon Ultrafiltration Diaflo cells instead of dialysis sacs for treatment of the crude leukocyte extract. Filtration is rapid and results in only a two-fold increase in dialysate so that volumes for lyophilization are easier to handle. The chance of contamination is minimal since the cell can be sterilized by autoclaving. Furthermore, the biochemical profile of TF prepared by filtration through PM 10 or PM 30 (our choice) is very similar to that of TF prepared in the classical manner (Figure 3.2). Further details are given in earlier reviews[6, 64].

The final point which should be stressed is that TF for both clinical and experimental use must be pyrogen tested. It is still surprising how often no specific mention of this is made in articles describing the results of its administration *in vivo* or its use *in vitro*.

Review of clinical experience

The results of clinical usage of TF have already been the subject of several extensive reviews[4–6]. The cases summarized in Tables 3.6–3.9 comprise a representative sample which is intended to allow a critical analysis of its efficacy and to establish guidelines for its subsequent use. Information given includes the nature and severity of the immune defect, i.e. whether selective or non-selective, the criteria for studying progress, and the degree of success achieved.

Primary immunodeficiency states

The most consistent successes reported have been in patients with chronic mucocutaneous candidiasis (CMC) where a selective defect in T-cell immunity has been demonstrable (Table 3.6). The characteristic laboratory findings include negative DTH skin tests and MIF production to candida antigens coupled with a variable LT response. After administration of TF, clinical improvement is usually accompanied by conversion of *in vitro* and *in vivo* DTH tests although the former, at least in our hands, tend to fluctuate significantly. The favourable response is not surprising if one accepts the existence in TF of an antigen specific component. In this context, the report of a patient by Littman *et al.*[65] is particularly interesting. They showed that TF prepared from candida positive but not from candida negative donors could prolong the clinical remissions induced by amphotericin B therapy. Three additional points have emerged from the study of patients with candidiasis. First, it is essential to give TF in conjunction with optimal drug

Table 3.8 Summary of clinical usage of TF

Disease	Source of TF	No. of patients	Conversion of: DTH skin tests	Conversion of: In vitro tests	Other relevant therapy	Clinical outcome	References
Recurrent or persistent infections group							
Hepatitis B antigen positive chronic active hepatitis	Donors recovered from hepatitis B infection	1	not done	1/1	Nil	0/1	101
		3	not done	1/1	Nil	? 2/3 improvement in T-cell and liver function. Patients remained HBAg positive	102
Coccidioidomycosis	Donors with strong DTH reactive to cocci	49	32/44	27/32 (LT) 24/28 (MMI)	Amphotericin B surgical drainage	12/44, clearly associated with TF 19/44, improvement not clearly associated with TF	67
Lepromatous leprosy	Donors with +ve DTH reactions to lepromin	5	1/5	1/5	Dapsone	4/5 showed reduction in bacteriological index; reversal reaction in 4/5	103
	Ditto	4	3/4	not done	Sulphones	Reversal reaction in 3/4	88
Progressive primary tuberculosis	Donors with +ve Mantoux reactions	1	1/1	1/1	Anti-tuberculosis drugs	1/1 after failure to respond to chemotherapy, dramatic improvement associated with TF	104
SSPE	Donors with +ve DTH reactions to measles	1	not done	not done	Nil	1/1 transient improvement	105
	Ditto	2	not done	1/2	Isoprinosine	0/2	92
	Normal donors	14	no details given		Nil	0/14	13
Herpes type 2 (genital)	Donors with previous history of herpes infection	4	not done	4/4 +ve LT before therapy	Topical	0/4 no convincing evidence of response	92
Urinary tract infection	Normal donors	20	20/20	not done	Nil	No details given	106
Malignancy group							
Malignant melanoma (disseminated)	Donors immunized against tumours	10	not done	not done	Surgery	4/10 duration?	107
	Melanoma in remission or relatives	10	not done	3/6	Surgery, chemotherapy and BCG	2/10 3 years later; remainder died	70
	Relatives and patients with other pigmented skin lesions	9	not done	5/9	No details given	1/9	90

Table 3.8—*continued*

Nasopharyngeal carcinoma	Donors recovered from infectious mononucleosis	2	1/1	not done	No details given	2/2 remission	125
	Ditto	1	1/1	1/1	Chemotherapy and radiotherapy	0/1	108
Carcinoma of breast (inoperable)	Normal donors	5	3/5	not done	Surgery	1/5 partial regression for 6 months	84
Osteogenic sarcoma	Cohabiting relatives with cytotoxic cells	13	not done	13/13	Surgery radiotherapy	Depends on extent of disease. 3 patients with small tumour disease free 13–19 months later	9
Hodgkin's diseases (stage IV)	HD in long-term remission	6	6/6	6/6	Nil	No details given	109
	Normal donors	8	6/8	8/8	Chemotherapy and/or radiotherapy 3 months before	No details given	92
Miscellaneous group of advanced malignancy	Cohabitants	35	13/35	no details given	Previous conventional therapy which had failed	13/35 transient for 2 weeks to 12 months	110
Miscellaneous diseases with suspected infectious aetiology group							
Multiple sclerosis	Normal donors	5	not done	5/5	Nil	0/5	73
	Normal donors	6	not done	1/2	Nil	2/6 possible arrest in progression of disease over 1-year period	92
	Normal (mumps +ve) donors	1	not done	not done	Nil	1/1 progressive disease apparently arrested. Leading active life	75
Sarcoidosis	Normal donors	7	2/7 (5/7 local only)	not done	Nil	No details given	110
	Normal donors	8	6/8	6/8	Nil	No details given	112
Rheumatoid arthritis	Normal donors	3	3/3	3/3	Steroids and azathioprine	3/3	78
Crohn's disease	Normal donors	13	3/12	13/13	Nil	No details given	113
	Normal donors	7	7/7	7/7	Azathioprine or ACTH	7/7	79

treatment. This is particularly important not only for minimizing antigen load, but because some patients will respond clinically and show DTH conversion following chemotherapy alone[66]. Secondly, TF is likely to be more successful when given to patients early in the disease. Once chronic nail changes have occurred, little improvement will occur unless surgery is used. Thirdly, TF appears to be less effective in those patients with associated endocrinopathies for reasons which are not clear.

Unfortunately there are almost no other diseases like CMC which have a well-defined selective T-cell deficiency and involve a micro-organism responsive to chemotherapy. Coccidioidomycosis might at first sight seem to fall into this category, but marked variability in response to TF and chemotherapy suggests that its pathogenesis is multifactorial and more complex than that of CMC[67]. Indeed preliminary reports of the TF trial in this disease sound disappointing. SSPE is likewise a poor model for analysis. Not only is the evidence for a selective defect to measles virus questionable, but the antigen load is not amenable to reduction by chemotherapy. The failure of TF to elicit significant improvement is therefore not surprising (Table 3.8).

The results of TF therapy in non-selective primary deficiencies in cell-mediated immunity have been variable (Table 3.7). Well-documented success has been reported in the Wiskott–Aldrich syndrome with respect to reduction in eczema and frequency of infections, but it is now apparent that TF does not influence the subsequent development of lymphoma (Blaese, personal communication). Clinical improvement appears to correlate with a lack of Fc receptors on patients' monocytes[4] and conversion in DTH reactivity *in vivo* and *in vitro*. Little or no success has been achieved in other deficiency states with one exception which is worthy of comment. Several investigators, for example Ammann[61] and Rachelefsky *et al.*[68], have reported permanent reconstitution with a combination of TF and thymus grafting in patients with severe combined immunodeficiency states. This is of interest with respect to the mode of action of TF (see section on mode of action), but may well be superseded as a primary form of therapy, at least in those cases with adenosine deaminase deficiency by irradiated red cells[69].

Acute disseminated or recurrent infections

The success of TF in treatment of chronic mucocutaneous candidiasis and Wiskott–Aldrich syndrome has led to its use in patients with either recurrent infections or acute disseminated infections which are severe and/or secondary to compromised host defences (Tables 3.8 and 3.9). The effects of TF in these situations can be broadly divided into three categories: (i) clinical benefit with conversion of DTH tests, (ii) no clinical benefit with conversion of DTH tests, and (iii) no clinical benefit or conversion of DTH tests. At first sight it is tempting to conclude that the positive responses simply represent chance

Table 3.9 Clinical experience with TF in compromised hosts with opportunistic infections

Infection	*No. of patients*	*Underlying disease*	*Source of TF**	*Other relevant therapy*	*Clinical response†*
Herpes zoster (disseminated)	6	Lymphoproliferative disorders	Donors herpes zoster positive	All receiving cytotoxic drugs. 2/6 given hyperimmune vaccinial globulin	5/6 complete recovery from infection. 1/6 died from underlying disease
Herpes simplex (disseminated)	5	4/5 lymphoproliferative disorders 1/5 carcinoma of bladder	Donors herpes simplex positive	4/5 receiving cytotoxic drugs	1/5 showed good response with clearing of lesions; 4/5 died with persistent infection
Perineal warts (recurrent)	1	Stage IV Hodgkin's disease in remission	Pool from 10 normal donors	Topical, no cytotoxic drugs for 18 months	1/1 with increasing disease-free intervals after removal of warts
Aspergillosis	1	Acute childhood leukaemia	Pool from 20 normal donors	On maintenance chemotherapy	1/1 with full recovery from infection. Died from leukaemia 9 months later
Listeriosis‡ (brain abscess)	1	Renal transplant recipient	Pool from 20 normal donors	On prednisone and azathioprine: removal of graft; ampicillin	1/1 full recovery from infection; since then has been retransplanted and is well 4 years later. No evidence for development of anti-HLA antibodies
Measles	2	Acute childhood leukaemia	Donor's measles positive	On cytotoxic drugs, 1 child in relapse	2/2 full recovery from infection. Both in remission 1–2 years later
Herpes simplex	1	Atopic eczema	Donor's herpes simplex positive	Topical	1/1 deteriorating with compromised T-cell function until TF given. Followed by complete recovery

* Donors chosen because of recent infection and/or high antibody titres. Potency of TF confirmed by stimulation of cells *in vitro*
† In all patients T-cell function was impaired. 3/3 patients with herpes simplex who died had no rise in E-rosettes after TF. 4/4 patients with other infections who showed a good clinical response did show a rise in E-rosettes
‡ Stewart *et al.*, 1974[126]

effects in an uncontrolled and heterogeneous group of disorders. Although almost all studies were indeed uncontrolled, certain lessons can be learnt about the use of TF from these reports. First, TF cannot be expected to help in the presence of a high antigen load (e.g. hepatitis B antigenaemia, SSPE, warts). Secondly, it is essential to use TF in conjunction with conventional therapy even though this may prevent precise analysis of the contribution made by TF. Thirdly, TF should be restricted to patients with infections due to micro-organisms (e.g. viruses, fungi, intracellular bacteria) requiring cell-mediated immune mechanisms for their control. Fourthly, it is difficult to compare results by different investigators in the absence of standard tests for potency and treatment schedules. Since *in vitro* assays for TF are now available, it is not unreasonable to expect that future reports should contain comments on potency.

Specific reference needs to be made to the use of TF in compromised hosts. Although it will never be possible to carry out controlled trials in this situation, a sufficient number of encouraging reports (Tables 3.8 and 3.9) now exists to justify a course of TF particularly where conventional therapy either is unavailable (e.g. drug-resistant tuberculosis) or is likely to be inadequate (e.g. immunosuppressed leukaemic or renal transplant with opportunistic infection). Furthermore, high dose TF is less likely to be accompanied by significant side-effects than other immunopotentiating agents such as levamisole and BCG. Ideally a 'specific' TF should be administered, but when lacking it may be necessary to rely on the general potentiating effects of pooled TF from 10–20 donors. Specific DTH testing is not feasible in this situation. A rise in E-rosette-forming cells does, however, seem to correlate with clinical response. From our experience, the only consistently disappointing results have been obtained with disseminated herpes simplex infections. In this situation it is reasonable to try different agents, particularly interferon or an interferon inducer when available.

Malignant disease

The selective action of TF in stimulating the cell-mediated arm of the immune response has led to its use as an immunotherapeutic agent in a wide range of malignant tumours including melanoma[70], nasopharyngeal carcinoma[71], Hodgkin's disease[72] and osteogenic sarcoma[9]. In theory TF has the advantage over other immunopotentiators (e.g. BCG) of exerting specific antitumour effects, but at present it is difficult if not impossible to evaluate the efficacy of TF in malignancy (Table 3.9). Most studies have been uncontrolled and their interpretation bedevilled by the small number of patients treated, the use of patients with advanced disease, the short duration of follow-up, the dual problem of specificity of TF and antitumour cytotoxicity mechanisms, and the presence of inhibitory phenomena such as suppressor cells and blocking factors. Osteogenic sarcomas may perhaps prove to be the exception to the rule. Evidence is available supporting the existence of specific cytotoxic T cells both in patients and in cohabiting relatives[40,41]. Leukocytes from the latter have provided a source of 'specific' TF which has been shown to stimulate production of cytotoxic T cells in tumour-bearing recipients. The results of a controlled trial of tumour specific TF from this source are eagerly awaited, although preliminary reports are encouraging[9]. Until such time as this information is available the value of TF as a specific immunotherapeutic agent in the treatment of malignant disease must remain anecdotal. The same guidelines described for treatment of infectious diseases apply to its usage here. TF is unlikely to work in the presence of a significant antigen (tumour) load and must therefore be administered in conjunction with optimal forms of conventional therapy, preferably early in the disease or in disease-free intervals. In this context, it should be noted that most of the studies summarized in Table 3.9 concern patients with advanced disease. The disappointing results of therapy are therefore hardly surprising.

The possibility that TF can act, like BCG and *Corynebacterium parvum*, in a non-specific manner should not be ignored particularly in view of its low toxicity. Comparisons of the efficacy of these agents could therefore be worthwhile. In the meantime, a case can be made for using TF not so much for its possible antitumour effect but rather to minimize opportunistic infections arising secondary to suppression of host defences by chemotherapy. This is applicable in childhood leukaemia, for example, where patients in good remission may still die from intercurrent infections (see Table 3.8).

Diseases with a suspected infectious aetiology

TF has been given to patients with a miscellaneous group of diseases in which an infectious agent is suspected to be playing an aetiological role. This group includes multiple sclerosis, juvenile and adult rheumatoid arthritis, sarcoidosis, and Crohn's disease (Table 3.9). To date no clearcut evidence of clinical improvement has been reported in patients with MS[73,74] although benefit has been claimed in isolated cases[75]. In view of the recent revival of interest in a possible viral aetiology coupled with the findings of cytopathic activity in blood of cohabiting relatives[76], our group has initiated a controlled trial with TF prepared from relatives' leukocytes. Particular attention is being paid to cases of early MS with minimal disability and with a presumed low antigen (? viral) load. The effect of TF versus placebo is being assessed by means of the sensitive electrophysiological technique of evoked response potentials[77].

Encouraging results have been claimed in juvenile rheumatoid arthritis[78] and Crohn's disease[79] but a definitive answer awaits adequate follow-up and treatment of sufficient numbers of patients. In the absence of a defined immune defect and aetiological agent, it is unlikely that these studies will shed much light on the nature or mode action of TF.

Clinical trials

The variation in diseases treated and results obtained in any particular disease highlight the need for properly controlled trials of TF. The problem, however, has been to find a suitable disease from the scientific and ethical points of view. This difficulty is further complicated by the controversy surrounding the nature and mode of action of TF. If one assumes that TF contains a specific component, then the ideal disease should be characterized by a selective defect in cell-mediated immunity to a defined antigen which is derived from a replicating agent (microbe or cell) amenable to treatment with conventional therapy and responses to which can be monitored *in vitro* and *in vivo*. The most suitable candidate would appear to be chronic mucocutaneous candidiasis, but even this is a disease where more than one defect is possible (Table 3.6) and it is rare. Nonetheless a trial is underway at NIH, the results of which should prove most interesting. The use of specific TF in osteogenic sarcoma may prove to be an alternative if T-cell mediated cytotoxicity is considered to be an acceptable alternative to the DTH response within the field of cell-mediated immune reactions.

Despite the difficulties in selecting an ideal group of patients, a number of trials with TF have been reported in the literature in the past 2 years. The key features are summarized in Table 3.10. With the exception of the study in malnourished children[80], no significant improvements were observed. The duration of the trials in three out of five instances was, however, 3 months or less. Furthermore the types of disease selected did not permit either reduction in antigen load or fully meaningful laboratory assessment of TF. In the absence of a defined causative agent, conversion of tests to marker antigens, although confirming the potency of TF in one study[81] is not an optimal way of monitoring its efficacy. It is to be hoped that other trials (e.g. those in leprosy and coccidiodomycosis) will be continued for longer periods of time and will include more comprehensive laboratory data.

Guidelines and recommendations for clinical usage

The variable results reported in the previous section coupled with the paucity of laboratory information available in many studies, emphasizes the importance of establishing guidelines for selection and treatment of patients with TF.

The need for comprehensive evaluation of recipients before and after therapy has already been stressed. Particular emphasis should be placed on defining (i) the selectivity or otherwise of the defect, (ii) its nature, i.e. whether cellular or mediated by serum factors, (iii) the existence of adequate numbers

Table 3.10 Summary of published controlled trials with transfer factor

Reference	Walker *et al.* (1975)[113]	José *et al.* (1976)[80]	Stevens *et al.* (1975)[114]	Behan *et al.* (1976)[74]	Maini *et al.* (1976)[81]
Disease/condition	Malnutrition	Malnutrition	Warts	MS	Rheumatoid arthritis
No. patients given TF	16	40	13	14	3
No. patients given placebo	16	35	17	15	3
Source of TF	Normal adults	Parents of patients	Normal adult whose warts had regressed spontaneously	Normal adults and relatives of patients	Normal adults
Total dose given (in cell equivalents)	10^9	$2 \times 5 \times 10^8$	$10^7 + 2 \times 10^8$	3 injections of TF from 1 pint of blood	3 injections of TF from 5,2,2 pints of blood, followed by 3 injections of saline
Parameters followed	Weight, haematocrit, reticulocytes, serum protein, albumin, globulin, DTH skin tests	Weight, number of chest, bowel, middle ear and skin infections	Condition of warts	Clinical condition, urinalysis, full blood counts, haematological examination, CSF analysis	Clinical condition, DTH skin tests, LT and LMI to marker antigen
Time of study	4 weeks	12 months	7 weeks	3 months	18 months
Difference between groups	No significant difference	Significantly fewer bowel infections in TF group	No significant difference	No significant difference	No significant difference

of target cells, viz. immunocompetent T cells, (iv) the extent of the antigen load (micro-organisms or tumour cell mass) and, (v) the general health of the patient including nutritional status.

The optimal usage of TF can be well exemplified by reference to management of patients with chronic mucocutaneous candidiasis. Treatment should be divided into two stages. Stage one consists of minimizing antigen (fungal) load by conventional and adequate chemotherapy (e.g. with amphotericin B), correction if necessary of iron deficiency[32] which may be present due to gastric atrophy in patients with the *Candida* endocrine syndrome[83] and removal of necrotic tissue such as infected nails. TF should then be used as a stage two procedure to maintain remission. Monitoring of the patient during as well as before therapy is vital, preferably by *in vitro* procedures to minimize the chance of subliminal sensitization by repeated DTH skin testing. Clearly this approach is not feasible in every patient, but the principles described should be followed as far as possible for optimal therapeutic benefit to be obtained. The potency of every TF batch should be tested before use, if any meaningful results, either positive or negative are to be obtained. The classical way of checking potency was to inject it into naive healthy recipients and demonstrate conversion of DTH skin test reactivity. This is not always possible, but the development of *in vitro* assays for measuring TF activity, has provided an acceptable alternative.

The amount and frequency of administration of TF poses another, yet unresolved problem. Some investigators have given daily injections for several weeks, others weekly, bi-weekly or monthly. At present there are no definitive guidelines since some regimes are likely to be more refractory than others. It is, however, clear that the activity of TF, although long-lived in normal individuals, may be transient in compromised hosts. TF should therefore be administered repeatedly depending on the clinical and immunological response of the recipients. Two examples from our own experience are worth citing in this context. First, in patients with chronic mucocutaneous candidiasis, good responses *in vivo* and *in vitro* have been achieved by giving one unit of TF weekly or bi-weekly for a month followed by monthly injections of one unit. Secondly, in acutely compromised hosts with disseminated infections, TF can be given in a dose of 1–2 units daily for up to a week. Monitoring with specific tests is often impracticable in this group of patients, but as mentioned previously, a rise in number of E-rosette-forming T cells does provide at least some guide to therapeutic response.

Complications

TF has now been administered to a large number of patients with a variety of diseases. To date remarkably few side-effects, immediate or delayed, have been reported. Indeed TF has an enviable record for a relatively new therapeutic agent. Patients occasionally complain of pain and erythema at the site of injection which may be associated with transient fever. From our experience with over 50 patients, these problems are rare and do not require any specific treatment. Furthermore, there is no evidence for development of significant biochemical or haematological abnormalities[84]. This is presumably related at least in part to the non-immunogenicity of TF. The relatively low toxicity of TF should always be borne in mind when selecting an immunopotentiating agent such as levamisole[85] particularly for use in non-malignant disease.

Isolated reports exist alleging the occurrence of more severe complications. Three are worthy of mention. The first involves a patient with Wiskott–Aldrich syndrome who developed haemolytic anaemia following a course of TF[86]. The patient did, however, have a weakly positive Coombs test before commencement of treatment and the severe episode of haemolysis was apparently triggered by a coxsackie B_5 infection. Although TF may have contributed by restoring autoaggressive T-cell function, haemolytic anaemia is a well-known occurrence in untreated cases of the Wiskott–Aldrich syndrome. The second complication likewise relates to this syndrome, viz. development of lymphoma after prolonged treatment with TF. As mentioned previously, TF reduces the incidence of severe infections. Since the result is to prolong life in patients with a high natural incidence of lymphomas, it is hardly appropriate to suggest that TF was a causative factor in their development. The third report described a case of severe combined immunodeficiency in whom a fatal illness occurred characterized by polyclonal gammopathy, leukocytosis and anti-i antibodies within 3 weeks of commencement of TF[87]. The precise cause of the relapse was, however, obscured by the severity of the underlying disease coupled with the administration of gammaglobulin and plasma as well as TF. Isolated reports of this kind should not therefore preclude the use of TF in diseases where no alternative modes of therapy are readily available.

Several theoretical complications deserve mention. The first relates to transmission of infectious agents such as hepatitis B or oncogenic viruses. Although recipients are often immunologically incompetent, no definite cases of virus transmission have been reported. Screening of donors for HBs antigen and the use of dialysis or ultrafiltration in its production presumably account for this. Secondly, enhancement of depressed T-cell function by TF could in theory lead to a severe host response which might in turn result in widespread tissue damage at the same time as eliminating any infectious agent present. That this complication can occur is shown by the appearance of reversal reactions in patients with leprosy given TF[88] and by development of inflammation around visible tumour deposits[89,90]. Presumably signs of this kind are indicative of a beneficial effect of TF, and their absence in patients with other diseases with presumed infectious activity such as multiple sclerosis or SSPE may therefore be a poor prognostic sign. Thirdly, TF donors might be sensitized (e.g. by pregnancy) to the histocompatibility antigens of the recipient which could lead to initiation of an autoimmune response, but apart from the two cases mentioned here, no evidence for autostimulation has appeared. Furthermore, the existence of suppressor T cells with regulatory activity in normal hosts[91] implies that TF may be as likely to stimulate self-surveillance mechanisms as autoaggressive T-cell activity. A more significant problem might arise in transplant recipients given TF for opportunistic infections. Theoretically graft rejection, if not already accepted as part of the therapeutic approach, could be accelerated, or alternatively retransplantation could become more difficult if new sensitivities to alloantigens were produced. It is, however, encouraging that the infected renal transplants given TF by our group (Table 3.9) did not develop evidence of sensitization to new HLA-A, B or D antigens. Fourthly, TF might transfer other unwanted specificities for example to drugs or contact irritants. To date no cases have been reported, which is presumably related to careful screening of the leukocyte donors. The final potential complication of TF relates particularly to its use in tumour-bearing subjects. The existence of isolated reports of effects on IgG antibody production by TF[38,39] raises the possibility of augmentation of blocking factor levels but this has yet to be confirmed.

In conclusion, the advantages of TF in selected cases seem to outweigh any potential disadvantages, particularly where no better alternative modes of therapy are available, but awareness of the possible complications is a valid part of its clinical usage.

CONCLUSIONS

Transfer factor was originally described 23 years ago and has been in regular clinical use for 8 years. It is therefore a relatively 'old' entity in the rapidly advancing field of modern immunology. Despite this, controversy continues to surround the nature of its active components and its precise mode of action. Although there is now general agreement that TF can exert a non-specific potentiating effect *in vitro* and *in vivo*, the existence of a component with definite immunological specificity still awaits confirmation. The treatment of more patients even with other diseases is unlikely to provide the answer. What is required to settle the issue is a good experimental model which utilizes well-defined antigens and which can be readily reproduced in many laboratories, and conforms to the requirements originally laid down by Lawrence. Perhaps further developments in basic immunology will be necessary before this goal can be achieved. In the meantime, it is, at least in our opinion, reasonable to continue using TF clinically in the treatment of certain disorders including chronic mucocutaneous candidiasis and recurrent or acute disseminated infections of 'T-cell type', particularly in compromised hosts. Furthermore, evaluation of TF with its potential advantage of specificity compared with other more toxic non-specific immunopotentiating agents in antitumour prophylaxis is probably worthwhile. Until such time as the basic properties of TF are better defined, it will be difficult to carry out a definitive controlled trial.

ACKNOWLEDGEMENT

The studies reported from our laboratory were carried out in collaboration with Ms C. van der Brink and Mrs J. Edwards. We are grateful to Ms D. Bartimote for typing text and tables. The project was supported by a grant from the Clive and Vera Ramaciotti Foundation of New South Wales.

References

1. Lawrence, H. S. (1954). The transfer of generalized cutaneous hypersensitivity of the delayed tuberculin type in man by means of the constituents of disrupted leucocytes. *J. Clin. Invest.*, **33**, 951
2. Lawrence, H. S. (1955). The transfer in humans of delayed skin sensitivity to streptococcal M substance and to tuberculin with disrupted leucocytes. *J. Clin. Invest.*, **34**, 219
3. Levin, A. S., Spitler, L. E., Stites, D. P. and Fudenberg, H. H. (1970). Wiskott–Aldrich syndrome, a genetically determined cellular immunologic deficiency: clinical and laboratory responses to therapy with transfer factor. *Proc. Nat. Acad. Sci. USA*, **67**, 821
4. Levin, A. S., Spitler, L. E. and Fudenberg, H. H. (1973). Transfer factor therapy in immune deficiency states. *Annu. Rev. Med.*, **24**, 175
5. Lawrence, H. S. (1974). Transfer factor in cellular immunity. *The Harvey Lectures*, **Series 68**, 239
6. Basten, A., Croft, S., Kenny, D. F. and Nelson, D. S. (1975). Uses of transfer factor. *Vox Sang.*, **28**, 257
7. Pizza, G., Viza, D., Boucheix, C. and Corrado, F. (1976). Studies with *in vitro* produced transfer factor. In: *Transfer Factor: Basic Properties and Clinical Applications* (M. S. Ascher, A. A. Gottlieb and C. H. Kirkpatrick, eds.), p. 173 (New York: Academic Press)
8. Wyborn, J., Levin, A. S., Spitler, L. E. and Fudenberg, H. H. (1973). Rosette-forming cells, immunologic deficiency diseases and transfer factor. *N. Engl. J. Med.*, **288**, 710
9. Levin, A. S., Byers, V. S., Fudenberg, H. H., Wybran, J., Hackett, A. J., Johnston, J. O. and Spitler, L. E. (1975). Osteogenic sarcoma. Immunologic parameters before and during immunotherapy with tumour specific transfer factor. *J. Clin. Invest.*, **55**, 487
10. Vadas, M. A., Miller, J. F. A. P., McKenzie, I. F. C., Chism, S. E., Shan, F.-W., Boyse, E. Z., Gamble, J. R. and Whitelaw, A. M. (1976). Ly and Ia antigen phenotypes of T cells involved in delayed-type hypersensitivity and in suppression. *J. Exp. Med.*, **144**, 10
11. Spitler, L. E., Levin, A. S. and Fudenberg, H. H. (1974). Transfer factor. *Clin. Immunobiol.*, **2**, 153
12. Basten, A., Croft, S. and Edwards, J. (1976). Experimental studies of transfer factor. In: *Transfer Factor: Basic Properties and Clinical Applications* (M. S. Ascher, A. A. Gottlieb and C. H. Kirkpatrick, eds.), p. 75 (New York: Academic Press)
13. Grob, P. J., Reymond, J.-F., Häcki, M. A. and Frey-Wettstein, M. (1976). Some physico-chemical and biological properties of a transfer factor preparation and its clinical application. In: *Transfer Factor: Basic Properties and Clinical Applications* (M. S. Ascher, A. A. Gottlieb and C. H. Kirkpatrick, eds.), p. 247 (New York: Academic Press)

14. Baram, P., Yuan, L. and Mosko, M. M. (1966). Studies on the transfer of human delayed-type hypersensitivity. *J. Immunol.*, **97**, 407
15. Spitler, L. E. (1973). In: *Workshop on Basic Properties and Clinical Applications of Transfer Factor* (C. H. Kirkpatrick and D. Rifkind, eds.), p. 235, NIH, USA
16. Rifkind, D., Frey, J. A., Petersen, E. A. and Dinowitz, M. (1976). Delayed hypersensitivity to fungal antigens in mice. III. Characterization of the active component in immunogenic RNA extracts. *J. Infect. Dis.*, **133**, 533
17. O'Dorisio, M. S., Neidhart, J. A. and Lobuglio, A. F. (1976). Identification of hypoxanthine as the major component of chromatographically prepared transfer factor. In: *Transfer Factor: Basic Properties and Clinical Applications* (M. S. Ascher, A. A. Gottlieb and C. H. Kirkpatrick, eds.), p. 215 (New York: Academic Press)
18. Krohn, K. J. E., Uotilla, A., Grohn, P. and Vaisanen, J. (1975). Uracil in transfer factor. *Lancet*, **ii**, 1209
19. Gallin, J. I. and Kirkpatrick, C. H. (1974). Chemotactic activity in dialysable transfer factor. *Proc. Nat. Acad. Sci. USA*, **71**, 498
20. Sandler, J. A., Smith, T. K., Manganiello, V. C. and Kirkpatrick, C. H. (1975). Stimulation of monocyte cGMP by leukocyte dialysates. An antigen-independent property of transfer factor. *J. Clin. Invest.*, **56**, 1271
21. Burger, D. R., Vandenbark, A. A., Daves, D., Anderson, W. A., Vetto, R. M. and Finke, P. (1976c). Nicotinamide: suppression of lymphocyte transformation with a component identified in human transfer factor. *J. Immunol.*, **117**, 797
22. Erb, P., Feldmann, M. and Hogg, N. (1976). Role of macrophages in the generation of T helper cells. IV. Nature of genetically related factor derived from macrophages incubated with soluble antigen. *Eur. J. Immunol.*, **6**, 365
23. Burger, D. R., Vetto, R. M. and Malley, A. (1972). Transfer factor from guinea-pigs sensitive to dinitrochlorobenzene: absence of super antigen properties. *Science*, **175**, 1471
24. Zuckerman, K. S., Neidhart, J. A., Balcerzak, S. P. and Lobuglio, A. F. (1974). Immunologic specificity of transfer factor. *J. Clin. Invest.*, **54**, 997
25. Kirkpatrick, C. H., Robinson, L. B. and Smith, T. K. (1976). The identification and significance of hypoxanthine in dialysable transfer factor. *Cell Immunol.*, **24**, 230
26. Burger, D. R., Vandenbark, A. A., Daves, D., Anderson, W. A., Vetto, R. M. and Finke, P. (1976b). Human transfer factor: fractionation and biologic activity. *J. Immunol.*, **117**, 789
27. Andron, L. A. and Ascher, M. S. (1976). Chromatography of transfer factor and assay of fractions *in vitro*. In: *Transfer Factor: Basic Properties and Clinical Applications* (M. S. Ascher, A. A. Gottlieb and C. H. Kirkpatrick, eds.), p. 291 (New York: Academic Press)
28. Parish, C. R., Jackson, D. C. and McKenzie, I. F. C. (1976). Low-molecular weight Ia antigens in normal mouse serum. III. Isolation and partial chemical characterization. *Immunogenetics*, **3**, 455
29. Rapaport, F. T., Lawrence, H. S., Millar, J. W., Pappagianis, D. and Smith, C. E. (1960). Transfer of delayed hypersensitivity to coccidioidin in man. *J. Immunol.*, **84**, 358
30. Maurer, P. H. (1961). Immunological studies with ethylene oxide-treated human serum. *J. Exp. Med.*, **113**, 1029
31. Sills, R. D., Rom, J. and Berk, J. E. (1959). Altered skin reactivity induced by repeated histoplasmin skin tests. *J. Allergy*, **30**, 541
32. Jensen, K., Patnode, R. A., Townsley, H. C. and Cummings, M. M. (1962). Multiple passive transfer of the delayed type of hypersensitivity in humans. *Annu. Rev. Resp. Dis.*, **85**, 373
33. Paterson, P. Y., Semo, R., Blumenschein, G. and Swelstad, J. (1971). Mucocutaneous candidiasis, anergy and a plasma inhibitor of cellular immunity: reversal after amphotericin B therapy. *Clin. Exp. Immunol.*, **9**, 595
34. Newberry, W. M., Chandler, J. W., Chin, T. D. Y. and Kirkpatrick, C. H. (1968).

Immunology of the mycosis. I. Depressed lymphocyte transformation in chronic histoplasmosis. *J. Immunol.*, **100**, 436

35. Nelson, D. S., Waters, M. F. R., Pearson, J. M. H., Penrose, J. M. and Nelson, M. (1975). Inhibition of lymphocyte transformation in mixed leucocyte cultures by serum from patients with leprosy. *Clin. Exp. Immunol.*, **22**, 385
36. Basten, A. and Miller, J. F. A. P. (1974). Cellular interactions in the immune response. In: *Cell Communication* (R. P. Cox, ed.), p. 187 (New York: J. Wiley and Sons)
37. Parish, C. R. (1971). Immune response to chemically modified flagellin. II. Evidence for a fundamental relationship between humoral and cell-mediated immunity. *J. Exp. Med.*, **134**, 21
38. Arala-Chaves, M. P., Proenca, R. and de Sousa, M. (1974). Transfer factor therapy in a case of complex immunodeficiency. *Cell Immunol.*, **10**, 371
39. Zaldivar, N. M., Papageorgicu, P. S., Kafee, S. and Glade, P. R. (1975). The use of TF in a patient with agammaglobulinaemia. *Pediatr. Res.*, **9**, 541
40. Thor, D. E., Cottman, C. A., Bearden, J. D., Williams, T. E. and Flippen, J. H. (1976). Adjunctive transfer factor in osteogenic sarcoma. II. Methodology and results of the immunological studies. In: *Transfer Factor: Basic Properties and Clinical Applications* (M. S. Ascher, A. A. Gottlieb and C. H. Kirkpatrick, eds.), p. 563 (New York: Academic Press)
41. Byers, V. S., Levin, A. S., Hackett, A. J. and Fudenberg, H. H. (1975). Tumour-specific cell-mediated immunity in household contacts of cancer patients. *J. Clin. Invest.*, **55**, 500
42. Thor, D. E., Jureziz, R. E., Veach, S. R., Miller, E. and Dray, S. (1968). Cell migration inhibition factor released by antigen from human peripheral lymphocytes. *Nature (Lond.)*, **219**, 755
43. Marsman, A. J. W., van der Hart, M., Walig, C. and Eijsvoogel, V. P. (1972). Migration inhibition experiments with mixtures of human peripheral blood lymphocytes and guinea-pig peritoneal exudate cells. *Eur. J. Immunol.*, **2**, 546
44. Fleer, A., van der Hart, M., Blok-Schut, B. J. T. and Schellekens, P. T. A. (1976). Correlation of PPD and BCG-induced leukocyte migration inhibition, delayed cutaneous hypersensitivity, lymphocyte transformation *in vitro* and humoral antibodies to PPD in man. *Eur. J. Immunol.*, **6**, 163
45. Søborg, M. and Bendixen, G. (1967). Human lymphocyte migration as a parameter of hypersensitivity. *Acta Med. Scand.*, **181**, 247
46. Ascher, M. S., Schneider, W. J., Valentine, F. I. and Lawrence, H. S. (1974). *In vitro* properties of leukocyte dialysates containing transfer factor. *Proc. Nat. Acad. Sci. USA*, **71**, 1178
47. Hamblin, A. S., Maini, R. N. and Dumonde, D. C. (1976a). Human transfer factor *in vitro*. I. Augmentation of lymphocyte transformation to tuberculin PPD. *Clin. Exp. Immunol.*, **23**, 290
48. Ahern, T. and Sanderson, C. J. (1976). Stimulation of lymphocytes by antigen in microplate cultures; absence of an effect of transfer factor *in vitro*. *Clin. Exp. Immunol.*, **23**, 499
49. Mueller-Eckhardt, C. and Ritts, R. E. (1976). Inhibitory activity of medium-dialysed transfer factor on lymphocyte blastogenesis. *Blut*, **32**, 353
50. Cohen, L., Holzman, R. S., Valentine, F. T. and Lawrence, H. S. (1976). Requirement of precommitted cells as target for the augmentation of lymphocyte proliferation by leucocyte dialysates. *J. Exp. Med.*, **143**, 791
51. Littman, B. H., Hirschman, E. M. and David, J. R. (1977). Augmentation of [^{3}H]thymidine incorporation by human lymphocytes in the presence of antigen and fractions of dialysable transfer factor: A non-specific phenomenon. *Cell Immunol.*, **28**, 158
52. Hamblin, A. S., Dumonde, D. C. and Maini, R. N. (1976b). Human transfer factor *in vitro*. II. Augmentation of lymphocyte transformation to phytohaemagglutinin. *Clin. Exp. Immunol.*, **23**, 303

53. Holzman, R. S., Schreiber, E. and Lawrence, H. S. (1976). Production of sheep erythrocyte rosette-forming cells by lymphocytes cultured with leucocyte dialysates. In: *Transfer Factor: Basic Properties and Clinical Applications* (M. S. Ascher, A. A. Gottlieb and C. H. Kirkpatrick, eds.), p. 205 (New York: Academic Press)
54. Khan, A., Garrison, O., Thometz, D. and Hill, J. M. (1976a). Fractionation of transfer factor with high-pressure liquid chromatography and E-rosette-enhancing activity of various fractions. In: *Transfer Factor: Basic Properties and Clinical Applications* (M. S. Ascher, A. A. Gottlieb and C. H. Kirkpatrick, eds.), p. 335 (New York: Academic Press)
55. Triglia, R. and Spitler, L. E. (1976). Human 'Transfer Factor' activity in guinea-pigs: further studies. In: *Transfer Factor: Basic Properties and Clinical Applications* (M. S. Ascher, A. A. Gottlieb and C. H. Kirkpatrick, eds.), p. 695 (New York: Academic Press)
56. Steele, R. W., Heberling, R. L., Eichberg, J. W., Eller, J. J., Kalter, S. S. and Kniker, W. T. (1976). Prevention of herpes simplex virus type 1 fatal dissemination in primates with human transfer factor. In: *Transfer Factor: Basic Properties and Clinical Applications* (M. S. Ascher, A. A. Gottlieb and C. H. Kirkpatrick, eds.), p. 381 (New York: Academic Press)
57. Welch, T. M., Wilson, G. B. and Fudenberg, H. H. (1976a). Human transfer factor in guinea-pigs: partial purification of the active component. In: *Transfer Factor: Basic Properties and Clinical Applications* (M. S. Ascher, A. A. Gottlieb and C. H. Kirkpatrick, eds.), p. 399 (New York: Academic Press)
58. Welch, T. M., Triglia, R., Spitler, L. E. and Fudenberg, H. H. (1976b). Preliminary studies on human TF activity in guinea-pigs. Systemic transfer of cutaneous delayed type hypersensitivity to PPD and SK/SD. *Clin. Immunol. Immunopathol.*, **5**, 407
59. Dunnick, W. and Bach, F. H. (1976). Guinea-pig 'Transfer Factor' *in vitro*: physico-chemical properties and partial purification. In: *Transfer Factor: Basic Properties and Clinical Applications* (M. S. Ascher, A. A. Gottlieb and C. H. Kirkpatrick, eds.), p. 185 (New York: Academic Press)
60. Eichberg, J. W., Steele, R. W., Kalter, S. S., Kniker, W. T., Heberling, R. L., Eller, J. J. and Rodriguez, A. R. (1976). Cellular immunity in gnotobiotic primates induced by TF. *Cell. Immunol.*, **26**, 114
61. Ammann, A. J., Wara, D. W., Doyle, N. E. and Globus, M. S. (1975). Thymus transplantation in patients with thymic hypoplasia and abnormal immunoglobulin synthesis. *Transplantation*, **20**, 457
62. Metcalf, D. (1970). Studies on colony formation *in vitro* by mouse bone marrow cells. *J. Cell. Physiol.*, **76**, 89
63. Binz, H. and Wigzell, H. (1975). Shared idiotypic determinants on B and T lymphocytes reactive against the same antigenic determinants. *J. Exp. Med.*, **142**, 1218
64. Lawrence, H. S. and Al-Askari, S. (1971). The preparation and purification of transfer factor. In: In vitro *Methods in Cell-Mediated Immunity* (Bloom and Glade, eds.), p. 531 (New York: Academic Press)
65. Littman, B. H., Rocklin, R. E., Parkman, R. and David, J. R. (1976). Combination transfer factor–amphotericin B therapy in a case of chronic mucocutaneous candidiasis: A controlled study. In: *Transfer Factor: Basic Properties and Clinical Applications* (M. S. Ascher, A. A. Gottlieb and C. H. Kirkpatrick, eds.), p. 495 (New York: Academic Press)
66. Kirkpatrick, C. H. and Smith, T. K. (1976). The nature of TF and its clinical efficacy in the management of cutaneous disorders. *J. Invest. Dermatol.*, **67**, 425
67. Catanzaro, A. and Spitler, L. (1976). Clinical and immunological results of transfer therapy in coccidioidomycosis. In: *Transfer Factor: Basic Properties and Clinical Applications* (M. S. Ascher, A. A. Gottlieb and C. H. Kirkpatrick, eds.), p. 477 (New York: Academic Press)

68. Rachelefsky, G. S., Stiehm, E. R., Ammann, A. J., Cederbaum, S. D., Opelz, G. and Terasaki, P. I. (1975). T-cell reconstitution of thymus transplantation and transfer factor in severe combined immunodeficiency. *Pediatrics*, **55**, 114
69. Polmar, S. H., Stern, R. C., Schwartz, A. L., Wetzler, E. M., Chase, P. A. and Hirshhorn, R. (1976). Enzyme replacement therapy for adenosine deaminase deficiency and severe combined immunodeficiency. *N. Engl. J. Med.*, **295**, 1337
70. Spitler, L. E., Levin, A. S. and Wybran, J. (1976). Combined immunotherapy in malignant melanoma. Regression of metastatic lesions in two patients concordant in timing with systemic administration of transfer factor and BCG. *Cell Immunol.*, **21**, 1
71. Goldenberg, G. J. and Brandes, L. J. (1976). *In vivo* and *in vitro* studies of immunotherapy of nasopharyngeal carcinoma with transfer factor. *Cancer Res.*, **36**, 720
72. Khan, A., Hill, J. M., MacLellan, A., Loeb, E., Hill, N. O. and Thaxton, S. (1975). Improvement in delayed hypersensitivity in Hodgkin's disease with TF: lymphophoresis and cellular immune reactions of normal donors. *Cancer*, **36**, 86
73. Jersild, C., Platz, P., Thomsen, M., Dupont, B., Svejgaard, A., Ciongoli, A. K., Fog, T. and Grob, P. (1976). TF treatment of patients with MS. I. Preliminary report of changes in immunological parameters. *Scand. J. Immunol.*, **5**, 141
74. Behan, P. O., Melville, I. D., Durward, W. F., McGeorge, A. P. and Behan, W. M. H. (1976). TF therapy in multiple sclerosis. *Lancet*, **i**, 988
75. Sacks, N., Potgieter, H. J. and van Rensburg, A. J. (1976). The use of transfer factor in the treatment of multiple sclerosis. *S. Afr. Med. J.*, **50**, 1556
76. Koldovsky, V., Koldovsky, P., Henle, W., Ackerman, R. and Haase, G. (1975). Multiple-sclerosis-associated agent transmission to animals and some properties of the agent. *Infect. Immunity*, **12**, 1355
77. Halliday, A. M., McDonald, W. R. and Mushin, J. (1973). Visual evoked response in diagnosis of multiple sclerosis. *Br. Med. J.*, **4**, 661
78. Kass, E., Frøland, S. S., Natvig, J. B., Blichfeldt, P., Hoyeraal, H. M. and Munthe, E. (1974). A new principle of immunotherapy in rheumatoid arthritis: treatment with transfer factor. *Scand. J. Rheumatol.*, **3**, 113
79. Asquith, P., Mallas, E., Ross, I., Montgomery, R. D., Cooke, W. T. and Thompson, R. A. (1975). Proceedings: TF in the treatment of Crohn's disease. *Gut*, **16**, 832
80. José, D. G., Ford, G. W. and Welch, J. S. (1976). Therapy with parents' lymphocyte TF in children with infection and malnutrition. *Lancet*, **i**, 263
81. Maini, R. N., Scott, J. T., Hamblin, A., Roffe, L. and Dumonde, D. C. (1976). Is the clinical benefit from transfer factor in rheumatoid arthritis a placebo effect? In: *Transfer Factor: Basic Properties and Clinical Applications* (M. S. Ascher, A. A. Gottlieb and C. H. Kirkpatrick, eds.), p. 601 (New York: Academic Press)
82. Joynson, D. H. M., Jacobs, A., Walker, D. M. and Dolby, A. E. (1972). Defect in cell-mediated immunity in patients with iron-deficiency anaemia. *Lancet*, **ii**, 1058
83. Valdimarsson, H., Higgs, J. M., Wells, R. S., Yamamura, M., Hobbs, J. R. and Holt, P. J. L. (1973). Immune abnormalities associated with chronic mucocutaneous candidiasis. *Cell. Immunol.*, **6**, 348
84. Oettgen, H. F., Old, L. J., Farrow, J. H., Valentine, F. T., Lawrence, H. S. and Thomas, L. (1974). Effects of dialyzable transfer factor in patients with breast cancer. *Proc. Nat. Acad. Sci. USA*, **71**, 2319
85. Graber, H., Takacs, L. and Vedrödy, K. (1976). Agranulocytosis due to levamisole. *Lancet*, **ii**, 1248
86. Ballow, M., Dupont, B. and Good, R. A. (1973). Autoimmune hemolytic anaemia in Wiskott–Aldrich syndrome during treatment with transfer factor. *J. Pediatr.*, **83**, 772
87. Gelfand, E. W., Baumal, R., Huber, J., Crookston, M. C. and Shumak, K. H. (1973). Polyclonal gammopathy and lymphoproliferation after transfer factor in severe combined immunodeficiency disease. *N. Engl. J. Med.*, **289**, 1385

88. Bullock, W. E., Fields, J. P. and Brandriss, M. W. (1972). An evaluation of TF as immunotherapy for patients with lepromatous leprosy. *N. Engl. J. Med.*, **287**, 1053
89. Khan, A., Thaxton, S., Hill, J. M., Hill, N. O., Loeb, E. and MacLellan, A. (1976b). Clinical trials with transfer factor. In: *Transfer Factor: Basic Properties and Clinical Applications* (M. S. Ascher, A. A. Gottlieb and C. H. Kirkpatrick, eds.), p. 583 (New York: Academic Press)
90. Silva, J., Allen, J., Wheeler, R., Bull, F., Morley, G. and Plouffe, J. (1976). Transfer factor therapy in disseminated neoplasms. In: *Transfer Factor: Basic Properties and Clinical Applications* (M. S. Ascher, A. A. Gottlieb and C. H. Kirkpatrick, eds.), p. 573 (New York: Academic Press)
91. Taylor, R. B. and Basten, A. (1976). Suppressor cells in humoral immunity and tolerance. *Br. Med. Bull.*, **32**, 152
92. Basten, A., Croft, S. and van der Brink, C. (1977). Clinical usage of transfer factor: review of 3 years experience. (In preparation)
93. José, D. G. (1975). Treatment of chronic mucocutaneous candidiasis by lymphocyte transfer factor. *Aust. N.Z. J. Med.*, **5**, 318
94. Lawton, J. W. M., Costello, C., Barclay, G. R., Urbaniak, S. J., Darg, C., Raeburn, J. A., Uttley, W. S. and Kay, A. B. (1976). The effect of TF on neutrophil function in CMC. *Br. J. Haematol.*, **33**, 137
95. Kirkpatrick, C. H. and Gallin, J. I. (1975). Suppression of cellular immune responses following transfer factor: report of a case. *Cell. Immunol.*, **15**, 470
96. Pachman, L. M., Kirkpatrick, C. H., Kaufman, D. H. and Rothbert, R. M. (1974). The lack of effect of TF in thymic displasia with immunoglobulin synthesis. *J. Pediatr.*, **84**, 681
97. Ballow, M. and Good, R. A. (1975). Report of a patient with T-cell deficiency and normal B-cell function: A new immunodeficiency disease with response to transfer factor. *Cell. Immunol.*, **19**, 219
98. Stoop, J. W., Eijsvoogel, V. P., Zegers, B. J. M., Blok-Schut, B., van Bekkum, D. W. and Ballieux, R. E. (1976). Selective severe cellular immunodeficiency. Effect of thymus transplantation and TF administration. *Clin. Immunol. Immunopathol.*, **6**, 289
99. Spitler, L. E., Levin, A. S., Stites, D. P., Fudenberg, H. H., Pirofsky, B., August, C. S., Stiehm, E. R., Hitzig, W. H. and Gatti, R. A. (1972). The Wiskott–Aldrich syndrome. Results of transfer factor therapy. *J. Clin. Invest.*, **51**, 3216
100. Griscelli, C., Rivillard, J. P., Betvel, H., Herzog, G. and Touraine, J. L. (1973). Transfer factor therapy in immunodeficiencies. *Biomedicine*, **18**, 220
101. Tong, M. J., Nystrom, J. S., Redeker, A. G. and Marshall, G. J. (1976). Failure of TF therapy in chronic active type B hepatitis. *N. Engl. J. Med.*, **295**, 209
102. Jain, S., Thomas, H. C. and Sherlock, S. (1975). The effect of lymphocytic TF on hepatitis B surface antigen-positive chronic liver disease. *Gut*, **16**, 836
103. Hastings, R. C., Morales, M. J., Shannon, E. J. and Jacobson, R. R. (1976). Preliminary results on the safety and efficacy of transfer factor in leprosy. In: *Transfer Factor: Basic Properties and Clinical Applications* (M. S. Ascher, A. A. Gottlieb and C. H. Kirkpatrick, eds.), p. 465 (New York: Academic Press)
104. Whitcomb, M. E. and Rocklin, R. E. (1973). Transfer factor therapy in a patient with progressive primary tuberculosis. *Ann. Intern. Med.*, **79**, 161
105. Vandvik, B., Frøland, S. S., Høyeraal, H. M., Stein, R. and Degre, M. (1973). Immunological features in a case of subacute sclerosing panencephalitis treated with transfer factor. *Scand. J. Immunol.*, **2**, 367
106. Anttila, R., Grohn, P. and Krohn, K. (1976). TF and cell-mediated immunity in urinary tract infections in children. *Lancet*, **i**, 315
107. Morse, P. A., Dercas, G. D., Smith, G. V., Raju, S. and Haray, J. D. (1973). Transfer factor therapy of human cancer. *Clin. Res.*, **21**, 71

108. Ng, R. P., Alexopoulos, C. G., Moran, C. J. and Bellingham, A. J. (1975). Transfer factor in Hodgkin's disease. *Lancet*, **ii**, 901
109. Vetto, R. M., Burger, D. R., Notte, J. E., Vandenbark, A. A. and Baker, H. W. (1976). Transfer factor therapy in patients with cancer. *Cancer*, **37**, 90
110. Lawrence, H. S. and Zweiman, B. (1968). Transfer factor deficiency response—a mechanism of anergy in Boeck's sarcoid. *Trans. Assoc. Am. Physicians*, **81**, 240
111. Horsmanheimo, M. and Virolainen, M. (1976). Transfer of tuberculin sensitivity of TF in sarcoidosis. *Cell. Immunol. Immunopathol.*, **6**, 231
112. Ng, R. P. and Vicary, F. R. (1976). Cell-mediated immunity and transfer factor in Crohn's disease. *Br. Med. J.*, **2**, 87
113. Walker, A. M., Garcia, R., Pate, P., Mata, L. J. and David, J. R. (1975). TF in the immune deficiency of protein-calorie malnutrition: a controlled study of 32 cases. *Cell. Immunol.*, **15**, 372
114. Stevens, D. A., Ferrington, R. A., Merigan, T. C. and Marinkovich, V. A. (1975). Randomized trial of transfer factor treatment of human warts. *Clin. Exp. Immunol.*, **21**, 520
115. Baram, P. and Condoulis, W. (1976). Fractionation of rhesus monkey dialyzable KLH-transfer factor and the *in vitro* assay of specific biologic activity using the indirect MIF assay. In: *Transfer Factor: Basic Properties and Clinical Applications* (M. S. Ascher, A. A. Gottlieb and C. H. Kirkpatrick, eds.), p. 301 (New York: Academic Press)
116. Huard, T. and Baram, P. (1976). 'Nonspecific' effects of human dialyzable transfer factor. In: *Transfer Factor: Basic Properties and Clinical Applications* (M. S. Ascher, A. A. Gottlieb and C. H. Kirkpatrick, eds.), p. 359 (New York: Academic Press)
117. Steele, R. W., Eichberg, J. W., Heberling, R. L., Eller, J. J., Kalter, S. S. and Kniker, W. T. (1976). Transfer of cellular reactivity to 3 non-human primate species with human and baboon transfer factor. In: *Transfer Factor: Basic Properties and Clinical Applications* (M. S. Ascher, A. A. Gottlieb and C. H. Kirkpatrick, eds.), p. 371 (New York: Academic Press)
118. Petersen, E. A., Frey, J. A., Dinowitz, M. and Rifkind, D. (1976). Transfer of delayed hypersensitivity to mice with human immune cell extracts. In: *Transfer Factor: Basic Properties and Clinical Applications* (M. S. Ascher, A. A. Gottlieb and C. H. Kirkpatrick, eds.), p. 387 (New York: Academic Press)
119. Vandenbark, A. A., Burger, D. R. and Vetto, M. R. (1976). Human transfer factor: trials with an assay in guinea-pigs. In: *Transfer Factor: Basic Properties and Clinical Applications* (M. S. Ascher, A. A. Gottlieb and C. H. Kirkpatrick, eds.), p. 425 (New York: Academic Press)
120. Jeter, W. S., Paquet, A. Jr., Ferebee, R. N., Olson, G. B. and Roinestad, F. (1976). In: *Transfer Factor: Basic Properties and Clinical Applications* (M. S. Ascher, A. A. Gottlieb and C. H. Kirkpatrick, eds.), p. 431 (New York: Academic Press)
121. Trepo, C. G. and Prince, A. M. (1976). Attempted immunotherapy with dialyzable transfer factor in hepatitis B carrier chimpanzees: induction of delayed hypersensitivity to hepatitis B surface antigen (HBsAg). In: *Transfer Factor: Basic Properties and Clinical Applications* (M. S. Ascher, A. A. Gottlieb and C. H. Kirkpatrick, eds.), p. 449 (New York: Academic Press)
122. Basten, A., Croft, S. and Edwards, J. (1976). Experimental studies of transfer factor. In: *Transfer Factor: Basic Properties and Clinical Applications* (M. S. Ascher, A. A. Gottlieb and C. H. Kirkpatrick, eds.), p. 75 (New York: Academic Press)
123. Read, S. E., Espinoza, L. R. and Zabriskie, J. B. (1976). *In vitro* assay for transfer factor using direct migration inhibition. In: *Transfer Factor: Basic Properties and Clinical Applications* (M. S. Ascher, A. A. Gottlieb and C. H. Kirkpatrick, eds.), p. 129 (New York: Academic Press)
124. Clinton, B. A. and Magoc, T. J. (1976). *Leishmania enriettii* infections in guinea-pigs and transfer factor obtained from convalescent yet immune animals. In: *Transfer Factor:*

Basic Properties and Clinical Applications (M. S. Ascher, A. A. Gottlieb and C. H. Kirkpatrick, eds.), p. 709 (New York: Academic Press)
125. Goldenberg, G. J. and Brandes, L. J. (1972). Immunotherapy of nasopharyngeal carcinoma with transfer factor from donors with previous infectious mononucleosis. *Clin. Res.*, **20**, 947
126. Stewart, G. J., Basten, A. and Tiller, D. J. (1974). Cerebral infection with *Listeria monocytogenes* in renal transplant patients. *Austr. N.Z. J. Med.*, **4**, 431
127. Burger, D. R., Vandenbark, A. A., Finke, P., Nolte, J. E. and Vetto, R. M. (1976a). Human transfer factor: effects on lymphocyte transformation. *J. Immunol.*, **117**, 782

4
Manipulation of States of Altered Immunity

RICHARD HONG
University of Wisconsin, Center for Health Sciences, Madison, Wisconsin, USA

INTRODUCTION

In recent years, an impressive amount of information involving the cellular and molecular processes of immune processes has accumulated. This greater understanding has permitted a number of novel approaches to restore, augment or modulate states of altered immunity. In Table 4.1 I have listed the approaches which will be discussed. Although the chapter is primarily concerned with deficiency states, it is of interest to consider two other situations of general importance first.

Soluble immune response suppressor (SIRS)

When one considers the great power and destructive capability of the immune system as exemplified by rejection of transplanted organs, graft-versus-host reactions, systemic lupus erythematosus, etc., one can appreciate that immune mechanisms must be modulated to maintain good health. A major controlling influence of the immune system is generated by a population of thymocytes known as T suppressor cells (reviewed by Gershon[1]). Rich and Pierce[2] showed that supernatants obtained from splenocytes stimulated by a mitogen, concanavalin A, showed suppressive capability. Based on this observation, Krakauer *et al.*[3] were able to suppress the autoimmune phenomenon observed in the naturally occurring animal model of lupus erythematosus, the NZB/W mice. Particularly impressive in this study was the demonstration that 93% of the treated population was still alive at the end of 1 year as compared to only 7% of the control group. Animals were injected early in infancy prior to the appearance of overt disease so at present the full therapeutic capability of this manoeuvre is incompletely defined.

Another mechanism of restoring suppressor activity is described below in the section on cultured thymic epithelium.

Table 4.1 Immunological engineering

I. Soluble immune response suppressors (SIRS)
II. Passive antibody administration
III. Newer strategies in immunodeficiency
   A. Fetal tissues
      1. Liver
      2. Thymus
   B. Thymic hormone
   C. Transfer factor
   D. Erythrocyte infusions in adenosine deaminase (ADA) deficiency
   E. Cultured thymic epithelium
      1. Combined immunodeficiency diseases
      2. Other

Passive antibody administration

The use of antibody to antigens of the Rh blood group to eliminate the antigen and prevent sensitization of Rh negative mothers following pregnancy was an ingenious application of the fundamental principle of the immunologic reaction viz., the specific binding of antigens by an immunoglobulin. The principle involved is simply that the Rh positive erythrocytes which leak into the maternal circulation at the time of delivery (probably during placental separation) are coated with antibody which promotes clearance by splenic phagocytes[4]. Except in the area of infectious agents and their products, antibodies have not been otherwise widely employed to control the distribution of harmful agents within the body. Recently, experience with an antibody to digitalis has been reported by Butler *et al.*[5,6]. Administration of intact sheep antidigoxin antibodies removes digoxin from the extravascular space. The protein-bound glycoside is pharmacologically inactive and it has been suggested that immunological control of pharmacokinetics can be employed in situations of life threatening digoxin intoxication. Intact antibody molecules are retained, however, and the digoxin is released in a free and active form. Furthermore, administration of heterologous antiserum can cause anaphylaxis or serum sickness. To circumvent these problems, Butler *et al.*[6] have employed Fab fragments of sheep antibody. Fab–digoxin complexes are continuously excreted in the urine so that the bound, inactive digoxin is eliminated from the body. Furthermore, Fab fragments are less immunogenic and antisheep antibodies were not produced in recipient animals.

IMMUNODEFICIENCY STATES

Fetal liver and fetal liver–thymus combination

The rationale for the use of fetal liver rests upon the early demonstration that such infusions were effective in the correction of thymectomized irradiated animals[7]. In fact, the infusions were as effective as bone marrow. However, the early use of fetal liver in human immunodeficiency syndromes led to very disappointing results (reviewed in ref. 8). This negative experience was in all probability due to the use of frozen cells or cells which were non-viable due to the length of time which elapsed between the time of organ removal and transplantation. A resurgence in interest followed the successful report by Keightley *et al.*[9]. The successful fetal liver transplants recorded to date are summarized in Table 4.2. It is of interest to note that the most significant B-cell reconstitution observed was seen in the two patients who were deficient for adenosine deaminase. In the patients who are adenosine deaminase positive, there is a significant change in the T-cell function and improvement in the clinical course. Significant B-cell reconstitution has not been observed however.

It is apparent that in fetal liver transplantation a small graft of immunocompetent cells has been given to the patient. So far the fatal complications of overwhelming graft-versus-host reaction (GVHR) seen with immunocompetent cell transfusions obtained from unmatched random donors has not been observed. A subacute or chronic graft-versus-host reaction has been seen (Rothberg, cited in ref. 8). In Keightley's case, the fatal immune complex nephritis may have represented an unusual manifestation of chronic GVHR[9].

It is of interest to note that fetal liver which is a putative source of stem (hence both B and T) cells acts in this transplant situation much more similar to fetal thymus. The aggressor reaction, i.e. GVHR is a T-cell reaction and the reconstitution as has been noted primarily involves the T cells.

It is important to emphasize that the immunological reconstitution observed with fetal liver requires many months and that should this form of therapy be selected, protection of the child from overwhelming infections will be required for prolonged periods, probably several months, before significant protective capability of the transplant can be observed.

O'Reilly *et al.*[10] combined fetal liver and fetal thymus transplantation in the treatment of two severe combined immunodeficiency (SCID) patients. In one instance, the thymus and the liver were obtained from different donors. With the demonstration of chimerism, chronic *Mycobacterium avium* infection was finally brought under control and granulomas were detected. Presently the patient showed *in vitro* responsivity to mitogens and modest increases of immunoglobulin levels. In the other patient, two fetal liver transplants were unassociated with significant laboratory evidence of improvement. Thereafter, an irradiated thymus from an 18-week-old donor

Table 4.2 Fetal liver transplantation

Case	*Diagnosis*	*Transplant*	*GVHR*	*T-cell reconstitution*	*B-cell reconstitution*	*Chimerism*	*Clinical status*
1. Keightley *et al.* 1975	SCID (ADA−)	2.5×10^8 cells i.p. from 4.2 cm, 8.5 wk. fetus at 3 months of age	± (7–10 weeks)	+[1]	+[5]	+	1. Did well for 12 months 2. Died of nephrotic syndrome secondary to immune complex nephritis 15 months after transplantation
2. Ackeret *et al.* 1976	SCID (ADA−)	1.23×10^9 cells (liver and thymus) IV from 12 wk. fetus at 7½ months of age	?	+[2]	+[2] ?	?	1. Immunologically normal to 18 months 2. Died suddenly after viral infection
3. Whisnant *et al.* 1975; Buckley*	SCID (ADA+)	3.8×10^8 cells i.p. from 9 wk. fetus at 11 months of age	+ (7–10 weeks)	↑ total E-rosettes	0	0	1. No change 2. Died 10 months after transplantation of chronic pulmonary disease
4. Whisnant *et al.* 1975; Buckley*	SCID (ADA+)	8×10^7 cells i.p. from 8 wk. fetus at 13 months of age	+ (7–10 weeks)	+[3]	+[6]	+	1. Clearing of oral candidiasis 2. Doing well 12 months after transplantation
5. Rothberg,* 1975	SCID (ADA+)	3.7×10^6 cells i.p. from 1.7 cm, 4–5 wk. fetus at 5 months of age	+ (3 weeks to present)	+[4]	0	?	1. Normal height and weight 2. Doing well 13 months after transplantation 3. Fluctuating skin rash, alopecia, and eosinophilia

[1] ↑ lymphocyte count, ↑ total E-rosettes, normal *in vitro* response to mitogens, allogeneic cells, and *Candida*
[2] Normal B- and T-cell function at 18 months of age
[3] ↑ total E-rosettes, normal *in vitro* responses to PHA and PWM, positive skin test
[4] ↑ total E-rosettes, normal *in vitro* responses to allogeneic cells and *Candida*, significantly increased response to PHA and PWM
[5] B lymphocytes present, serum IgG, IgM, and IgA, poor antibody response to ØX-174 and *Salmonella typhimurium*
[6] Small amount of IgM, no IgA and IgA
* Personal communication
From: Horowitz, S. D. and Hong, R. (1977). *The Pathogenesis and Treatment of Immunodeficiency* (Basel: S. Karger) (with permission)

was transplanted followed a month later by another fetal liver transplant. Normal *in vitro* response to mitogens and modest increase of IgG and IgM levels were noted.

Fetal thymus

As with fetal liver, the early attempts with fetal thymus also met with failure, probably for the same reasons. The definition of the DiGeorge syndrome as a disorder primarily involving the thymus gland spurred new interests in the use of fetal thymus transplantation and successful implantation was accomplished in 1968[11,12]. The rapidity of the response and the subsequent demonstration that some cases of DiGeorge syndrome showed spontaneous improvement have made the mechanisms of reconstitution in these situations difficult to explain. It is quite likely that a hormonal mechanism was involved. In fact, Steele *et al.*[13] demonstrated transient T-cell restoration following implantation of the thymus in a Millipore® chamber. In that same year, a fetal thymus transplant was given to a young man with chronic mucocutaneous candidiasis and transient improvement was observed[14]. A few years later, however, the patient suffered two bouts of *Pneumocystis carinii* pneumonia. Although he recovered, he gradually developed pulmonary fibrosis which resulted in death about 3 years after the original transplant.

The first impressive benefit in SCID was recorded by Ammann *et al.* in 1973[15]. A significant aspect of this experience was the use of transfer factor (TF) shortly before the transplant. Proliferating lymphoid cells of donor origin were demonstrated in the child with the acquisition of *in vitro* responses to phytohaemagglutinin and allogeneic cells. The T-cell reconstitution was limited, however, and cutaneous reactivity was never observed. Nevertheless, at 4 years of age, 95% of the circulating lymphocytes in the child were still of donor origin. However, *in vitro* responsivity had declined at this time and the child subsequently died of chronic pulmonary disease (Ammann, personal communication). Two other patients with SCID who received thymus transplantation after transfer factor have also shown marked clinical improvement subsequent to the transplant. One patient is still alive 2 years after the transplant with positive cutaneous reactivity and increased numbers of E-rosettes; the patient has chronic encephalopathy, however[16]. A third patient demonstrates virtually no change in the lymphocyte studies with the exception of an increase in the number of E-rosettes and concomitant decrease in the number of surface immunoglobulin-bearing cells. This child is maintained on gammaglobulin therapy and has been completely asymptomatic for 2 years following the transplant[17].

It appears that in fetal thymus transplantation, some T-cell replacement occurs. The children have demonstrated long periods of wellbeing subsequent to transplant but the eventual outcome is as yet unknown. Whether transfer factor is in fact necessary to improve the efficiency of the take or works in some other fashion, is at present unknown.

Thymic hormone

A number of groups have studied humoral factors obtained by extraction of thymus glands. There are numerous products obtained from these separations and chemical characterization has begun[18–21]. Clinical use of a crude preparation derived from calf thymuses (fraction 5) has been reported and large clinical trials are presently in progress[22]. An impressive response in a case demonstrating deficiency of the T cells and present but non-functional immunoglobulins was reported by Wara *et al.*[23]. Decrease in IgA, normalization of IgG levels and increase in T-cell rosettes and phytohaemagglutinin response was observed. There was a marked decrease in the number of infections and chronic diarrhoea abated. Use of thymosin in SCID and other forms of immunodeficiency has not produced very gratifying results (Table 4.3). It seems likely that as better definition and delineation of the thymic factors is accomplished, more consistent benefit will be seen (reviewed in ref. 8).

Transfer factor (TF)

Transfer factor is a low molecular weight dialysable material originally described by Lawrence[24]. It is a material of amazing biological potential and has the capability of transferring cutaneous reactivity to skin-test negative individuals. The material is obtained by disrupting leukocytes, usually by repeated cycles of freezing and thawing. When such material is injected into a non-reactive but immunologically normal individual, the acquired cutaneous reactivity usually involves only antigens to which the donor is highly sensitive although recent reports describing the acquisition of reactivity to antigens other than those to which the donor was sensitive indicate a certain degree of non-specificity to the transfer reaction. Transfer factor obtained from a primary recipient will also confer upon a secondary non-reacting recipient the newly acquired sensitivity; thus, the leukocytes of the recipient actually acquire a transferable substance.

In approximately half of the patients with SCID, cutaneous reactivity and containment of infectious processes have been reported. Nevertheless, long-term clinical benefit and significant prolongation of life have not been attained by the use of TF in SCID. In Wiskott–Aldrich syndrome (WAS), more striking results have been reported. Diminished bleeding tendency, clearing of eczema, and reduction of splenomegaly have been observed in approximately 50% of patients treated. A predictor of beneficial response from transfer factor appears to be the presence of monocytes demonstrating decreased IgG receptors[25].

Perhaps the most striking benefit of TF has been observed in chronic mucocutaneous candidiasis. Prior therapy with antifungal agents is usually necessary to obtain the clinical benefit. There is no reliable predictor as to which patients will demonstrate improvement. However, when observed, the clinical improvement is most dramatic[26].

The mechanism of action of transfer factor is unknown. However, recent work by Kirkpatrick and Smith[27] indicates that the active moiety in transfer factor preparations is a small polypeptide. It can be shown that minimal substitutions in a polypeptide of only six amino acids can generate a tremendous number of variations (500 000) accounting for a large repertoire of different antigen specificities. If it is recalled that the antibody combining site of immunoglobulins is very small, it is not surprising that a similar small stretch of amino acids in TF can account for numerous reactivities.

The use of transfer factor in immunodeficiency may be associated with the development of malignancy. Gelfand *et al.*[28] observed a polyclonal gammopathy and lymphoproliferative disorder in a child with SCID treated with TF. Similar experiences have also been seen by us. No definite proof of causation is available and it is well known that patients with immunodeficiency are prone to lymphomas and leukaemias. However, these observations plus a recent report of five patients with WAS treated with transfer factor who acquired malignancies soon after onset of therapy are enough to excite concern[29].

Erythrocyte infusions

The first biochemical defect associated with immunodeficiency was reported in 1972[30]. Adenosine deaminase (ADA), an enzyme important in the metabolism of adenosine to inosine was found to be absent in two patients with SCID. Exhaustive investigation of a large series quickly uncovered 13 cases of ADA deficiency associated with immunodeficiency[31]. The enzyme defect apparently results in the build-up of toxic levels of cyclic nucleotides with a resultant attrition of lymphoid elements.

Polmar *et al.*[32] showed that proliferative responses of ADA deficient lymphocytes to mitogens could be increased by the addition of ADA to the culture media. Encouraged by this observation, they gave small transfusions of frozen, irradiated blood. The ADA present in erythrocytes was sufficient to increase lymphocyte counts and proliferative responses. Normal weight gain and appearance of a thymic shadow was reported.

The description of a biochemical defect marks the beginning of the molecular definition of immunodeficiency. One can anticipate that a whole series of related biochemical lesions will soon be described. The availability of other novel forms of enzyme replacement[33,34] will provide unique approaches to therapy.

Cultured thymic epithelium (CTE)

Jacobs and Huseby[35] showed that ovarian tumours maintained in tissue culture would be accepted across histocompatibility barriers. Subsequently, Opelz and Terasaki[36] demonstrated that leukocytes maintained in culture

Table 4.3 Results of thymosin treatment

Reference	*Age*	*Sex*	*Duration of therapy*	In vitro *total-E-rosette assay with thymosin*	In vivo *effect of thymosin*
SCID					
1. August*	1 year	F	2½ months	+	1. No increase in T-cell markers or function 2. Clearing of *Pneumocystis* pneumonia
2. Goldman*	10 months	M	18 days	−	1. No change 2. Thymosin stopped because of skin reaction 3. Developed hepatitis post-therapy
3. Goldman*	11 months	M	1 month	−	1. No change
4. Seeger*	7 months	M	3 weeks	−	1. No change
5. Griscelli*	4 months	M	4 weeks	+†	1. No change
Cellular immunodeficiency with immunoglobulin					
6. August*	11 years	M	2 days	+	1. Positive skin tests to mumps and SK/SD 2. Treatment terminated due to hives at injection site
7. Goldman*	6 years	M	5 weeks	±	1. Possible decrease in total E-rosettes 2. Possible increase lymphocyte blastogenesis 3. Disappearance of IgG-K gammopathy
8. Hill*	8 months	M	1 month	+	1. Increased total E-rosettes 2. Clearing of *Pneumocystis* pneumonia 3. Child died with evidence of hepatitis at autopsy
9. Reid (ADA−)*	2½ years	M	2 months	+	1. Clinical improvement 2. Increased total E-rosettes 3. + *Candida*, tetanus, and diphtheria skin test 4. Lymphopenia persists
10. Wara *et al.* 1975	6 years	F	>21 months	+	1. Normal IgG (no Ab following immunization), no change in IgM and IgA 2. Increased total E-rosettes and PHA response; no MLC reactivity 3. Positive mumps and *Candida* skin tests 4. Decreased infections and diarrhoea; weight gain

Table 4.3—*continued*

T-cell deficiency					
11. Griscelli (partial DiGeorge)*	3 months	M	>3 months	+	1. Clinical improvement; decreased infections 2. Increased total E-rosettes; *in vitro* response to PHA, ConA, PWM 3. Positive PHA skin test
12. Ammann and Wara (NP def.) (personal communication)‡	5 years	F	8 months	+	1. No change in immunoglobulins 2. Increased total E-rosettes, PHA and MLC response 3. No positive skin tests 4. Clinical improvement 5. Thymosin stopped due to sensitization
Ataxia telangiectasia					
13. Waldman*	9 years	F	10 months	+	1. Increased total E-rosettes 2. Increased lymphocytes
14. Waldman*	6 years	F	5 months	+	1. Increased total E-rosettes 2. Increased MLC reactivity 3. Increased response to PWM and ConA 4. Positive tetanus skin test
15. Waldman*	7 years	F	5 months	+	1. Increased total E-rosettes
16. Ammann and Wara (personal communication)‡	4 years	M	3 months	+	1. Skin test conversion 2. Increased total E-rosettes 3. No change in PHA or MLC response 4. No change in clinical status
Wiskott–Aldrich syndrome					
17. Ammann and Wara (personal communication)‡	11 years	M	11 months	+	1. Increased total E-rosettes 2. Normal PHA response; increased MLC reactivity 3. Eczema improved 4. Decreased herpes stomatitis 5. Decreased bacterial infections

* Cited in ref. 22
† Response with haemolysed RBC also
+ = positive, − = negative, ± = equivocal
‡ From Horowitz, S. D. and Hong, R. (1977). *The Pathogenesis and Treatment of Immunodeficiency* (Basel: S. Karger) (with permission)

for at least 12 days lost their ability to stimulate allogeneic responder cells in the mixed leukocyte culture reaction. Since this test can be equated to the initial sensitization which occurs in the early phase of an allograft rejection reaction, it can be inferred that a loss of sensitizing capability results from the culture. Of even greater relevance to replacement therapy for immunodeficiency, however, was the demonstration of functional integrity by Lafferty *et al.*[37] who were able to completely restore thyroidectomized recipients with thyroid grafts previously maintained for short periods in culture.

Encouraged by these observations Schulte-Wissermann *et al.*[38] studied cultured thymic epithelium as a possible modality of therapy. When cultured thymic epithelium was transplanted into immunologically normal recipients, lymphoid repopulation occurred even across xenogeneic barriers. Cultured thymic epithelium was employed in a case of SCID in February 1976. Within a month, signs of reconstitution were observed. Diarrhoea stopped and a normal pattern of weight gain was resumed. The proliferative responses to mitogens and allogeneic cells increased although they remained at subnormal levels. Delayed cutaneous reactivity was acquired.

Amazingly, a B-cell response was observed as well as T-cell benefit. At present, immunoglobulin levels are normal and functional antibody has been detected. We are especially gratified to find that antibodies to newly acquired infections have been detected. Exhaustive testing in this case and other transplants, both in man and mouse, have demonstrated that the functioning lymphocyte population is of recipient origin. Therefore, the donor epithelium has differentiated the stem cells of the host. The unexpected but impressive effect of the thymic transplant upon the B cells demonstrates that the B-cell system in man can be profoundly dependent upon the thymus[39]. Cultured thymic epithelium offers an exciting new approach to immunotherapy, and additionally provides impetus for a similar approach to transplantation of other organs. The major change which occurs during culture is the loss of cells which are highly stimulatory in the initial sensitization of allograft rejection. These cells have been termed passenger leukocytes[40] and are, most likely, B lymphocytes and macrophages[41]. It seems quite certain that transplantation of other organs in man may become possible using culture techniques.

Cultured thymic epithelium can be used *in vitro* to differentiate bone marrow cells or peripheral blood leukocytes. Horowitz *et al.*[42] showed a suppressor deficiency in 14/14 patients with lupus erythematosus. When lymphocytes from seven of those patients were incubated with cultured thymic epithelium (CTE), suppressor reactivity returned. Encouraged by these results, we have recently transplanted CTE to a child with non-responsive autoimmune haemolytic anaemia associated with suppressor deficiency. She has now regained *in vitro* suppressor activity and maintains a normal haemoglobin with minimal steroid therapy.

CONCLUSIONS

In an era of space travel and electronic wizardry man has begun to engineer his own bodily functions. The ingenuity displayed is awesome and frightening. Hopefully, as these new approaches create new problems we can engineer our intellects to meet the challenge.

References

1. Gershon, R. K. (1974). T-cell control of antibody production. *Contemp. Top. Immunobiol.*, **3**, 1
2. Rich, R. R. and Pierce, C. W. (1974). Biological expressions of lymphocyte activation. III. Suppression of plaque-forming cell responses *in vitro* by supernatant fluids from concanavalin A-activated spleen cell cultures. *J. Immunol.*, **112**, 1360
3. Krakauer, R. S., Strober, W., Rippeon, D. L. and Waldman, T. A. (1977). Prevention of autoimmunity in experimental lupus erythematosus by soluble immune response suppressor. *Science*, **196**, 56
4. Clark, C. A. (1969). Prevention of rhesus iso-immunization. *Sem. Hematol.*, **6**, 201
5. Butler, V. P., Jr. (1977). Digoxin: immunologic approaches to measurement and reversal of toxicity. *N. Engl. J. Med.*, **283**, 1150
6. Butler, V. P., Jr. (1977). Effects of sheep-digoxin-specific antibodies and their Fab fragments on digoxin pharmacokinetics in dogs. *J. Clin. Invest.*, **59**, 345
7. Uphoff, D. E. (1958). Preclusion of secondary phase of irradiation syndrome by inoculation of fetal hematopoietic tissue following lethal total body irradiation. *J. Nat. Cancer Inst.*, **20**, 625
8. Horowitz, S. D. and Hong, R. (1977). *The Pathogenesis and Treatment of Immunodeficiency.* (Basel: S. Karger)
9. Keightley, R. G., Lawton, A. R., Cooper, M. D. and Yunis, E. J. (1975). Successful fetal liver transplantation in a child with severe combined immunodeficiency. *Lancet*, **ii**, 850
10. O'Reilly, R. and Good, R. A. (1976). Fetal liver and fetal thymus transplants. Presented at the *3rd Workshop of the International Co-operative Group for Bone Marrow Transplantation in Man*, August 19–21, Tarrytown, New York
11. Cleveland, W. W., Fogel, B. J., Brown, W. T. and Kay, H. E. M. (1968). Foetal thymic transplant case of DiGeorge's syndrome. *Lancet*, **ii**, 1211
12. August, C. S., Rosen, F. S., Filler, R. M., Janeway, C. A., Markowski, A. and Kay, H. E. M. (1968). Implantation of a foetal thymus restoring immunological competence in a patient with thymic aplasia (DiGeorge syndrome). *Lancet*, **ii**, 1210
13. Steele, R. W., Limas, C., Thurman, G. B., Schulein, M., Bauer, H. and Bellanti, J. A. (1972). Familial thymic aplasia. Attempted reconstitution with fetal thymus in a millipore diffusion chamber. *N. Engl. J. Med.*, **287**, 787
14. Levy, R. L., Huang, S. W., Bach, M. L., Bach, F. H., Hong, R., Ammann, A. J., Bortin, M. and Kay, H. E. M. (1972). Thymic transplantation in a case of chronic mucocutaneous candidiasis. *Lancet*, **ii**, 898
15. Ammann, A. J., Wara, D. W., Salmon, S. and Perkins, H. (1973). Thymus transplantation. Permanent reconstitution of cellular immunity in a patient with sex-linked combined immunodeficiency. *N. Engl. J. Med.*, **1**, 298
16. Rachelefsky, G. S., Stiehm, E. R., Ammann, A. J., Cederbaum, S. D., Opelz, G. and Terasaki, P. I. (1975). T-cell reconstitution by thymus transplantation and transfer factor in severe combined immunodeficiency disease. *Pediatrics*, **55**, 114
17. Shearer, W. T., Wedner, H. J., Strominger, D. B., Tissane, J. and Hong, R. (1977). Successful transplantation of the thymus in Nezelof's syndrome. *Pediatrics* (In press)

18. Basch, R. S. and Goldstein, G. (1974). Induction of and cell differentiation *in vitro* by thymin, a purified polypeptide hormone of the thymus. *Proc. Nat. Acad. Sci. USA*, **71**, 1474
19. Bach, J. F., Bach, M. A., Charrier, J., Dardenne, M., Fournier, C., Papiernik, M. and Pleau, J. M. (1975). The circulating thymic factor (TF). Biochemistry, biological activities and clinical applications. A summary. In: *Biological Activity of Thymic Hormones* (D. W. van Bekkum, ed.) (Rotterdam: Kooyer Scientific Publications)
20. Goldstein, A. L., Asanuma, Y. and White, A. (1970). The thymus as an endocrine gland: properties of thymosin, a new thymus hormone. *Recent Prog. Horm. Res.*, **26**, 505
21. Trainin, N. and Small, M. (1970). Studies on some physicochemical properties of a thymus humoral factor conferring immunocompetence on lymphoid cells. *J. Exp. Med.*, **132**, 885
22. Goldstein, A. L., Cohen, G. H., Rossio, J. L., Thurman, G. B. and Ulrich, H. T. (1976). Use of thymosin in the treatment of primary immunodeficiency diseases and cancer. *Med. Clin. N. Am.*, **60**, 591
23. Wara, D. W., Goldstein, A. L., Doyle, N. E. and Ammann, A. J. (1975). Thymosin activity in patients with cellular immunodeficiency. *N. Engl. J. Med.*, **292**, 70
24. Lawrence, H. S. (1969). Transfer factor. *Adv. Immunol.*, **11**, 195
25. Spitler, L. E., Levin, A. S., Stites, D. P., Fudenberg, H. H., Pirofsky, B., August, C. S., Stiehm, E. R., Hitzig, W. H. and Gatti, R. A. (1972). The Wiskott–Aldrich syndrome. Results of transfer factor therapy. *J. Clin. Invest.*, **51**, 3216
26. Kirkpatrick, C. H., Rich, R. R. and Bennett, J. E. (1971). Chronic mucocutaneous candidiasis: model building in cellular immunity. *Ann. Intern. Med.*, **74**, 955
27. Kirkpatrick, C. W. and Smith, T. K. (1977). Specific and non-specific activities in dialyzable transfer factor. *Proc. 11th Leukocyte Conference* (In press)
28. Gelfand, E. W., Baumal, R., Huber, J., Crookston, M. C. and Shumak, K. H. (1973). Polyclonal gammopathy and lymphoproliferation after transfer factor in severe combined immunodeficiency disease. *N. Engl. J. Med.*, **289**, 1385
29. Sellars, W. A. and South, M. A. (1975). Wiskott–Aldrich syndrome with 18-year survival. Treatment with transfer factor. *Am. J. Dis. Child.*, **129**, 622
30. Giblett, E. R., Anderson, J. E., Cohen, F., Pollara, B. and Meuwissen, H. J. (1972). Adenosine deaminase deficiency in two patients with severely impaired cellular immunity. *Lancet*, **ii**, 1067
31. Meuwissen, H. J., Pickering, R. J., Pollara, B. and Porter, I. H. (eds.) (1975). *Combined Immunodeficiency Disease and Adenosine Deaminase Deficiency. A Molecular Defect.* (New York: Academic Press)
32. Polmar, S. H., Stern, R. C., Schwartz, A. L., Wetzler, E. M., Chase, P. A. and Hirschorn, R. (1976). Enzyme replacement therapy for adenosine deaminase deficiency and severe combined immunodeficiency. *N. Engl. J. Med.*, **291**, 989
33. Brady, R. O., Pentchev, P. G., Gal, A. E., Hibbert, S. R. and Dekaban, A. S. (1974). Replacement therapy for inherited enzyme deficiency. Use of purified glucocerebrosidase in Gaucher's disease. *N. Engl. J. Med.*, **291**, 989
34. Ihler, G. M., Glew, R. H. and Schnure, F. W. (1973). Enzyme loading of erythrocytes. *Proc. Nat. Acad. Sci. USA*, **70**, 2663
35. Jacobs, B. B. and Huseby, R. A. (1967). Growth of tumors in allogeneic hosts following organ culture explantation. *Transplantation*, **5**, 420
36. Opelz, G. and Terasaki, P. I. (1974). Lymphocyte antigenicity loss with retention of responsiveness. *Science*, **184**, 464
37. Lafferty, K. J., Cooley, M. A., Woolnough, J. and Walken, K. R. (1975). Thyroid allograft immunogenicity is reduced after a period in organ culture. *Science*, **188**, 259
38. Schulte-Wissermann, H., Manning, D. and Hong, R. (1977). Transplantation of cultured thymic epithelium. I. Morphological and technical considerations (In preparation)
39. Hong, R., Santosham, M., Schulte-Wissermann, H., Horowitz, S., Hsu, S. H. and Winkelstein, J. A. (1976). Reconstitution of B and T lymphocyte function in severe

combined immunodeficiency disease after transplantation with thymic epithelium. *Lancet*, **ii**, 1270

40. Stuart, F. P., Bastien, Holter, A., Fitch, F. W. and Elkins, W. L. (1971). Role of passenger leucocytes in the rejection of renal allografts. *Transplant. Proc.*, **3**, 461
41. Talmadge, D. W., Dart, G., Radovich, J. and Lafferty, K. J. (1976). Activation of transplant immunity: effect of donor leukocytes on thyroid allograft rejection. *Science*, **191**, 385
42. Horowitz, S. D., Borcherding, W., Moorthy, A. V., Chesney, R., Schulte-Wissermann, H. and Hong, R. (1977). Induction of suppressor T cells in systemic lupus erythematosus by thymosin and cultured thymic epithelium. *Science*, **197**, 999

5
Immune Response in Cancer Patients

R. MARK VETTO

Department of Surgery, US Veterans' Hospital, and the University of Oregon Health Sciences Center, Portland, Oregon 97207, USA

Clinicians who care for patients afflicted with cancer frequently observe wide variations in the behaviour of the tumour. This has led to various speculations, including the notion that immune influence, if not control, may be responsible for these variations in behaviour. Supporting data for this belief includes (1) the discovery of tumour-specific antigens; (2) the documentation of spontaneous regression of tumours, even though infrequent; (3) the development of animal models in which effective antitumour immunization has been accomplished; and (4) the similarity of what is thought to be tumour immunity response to cell-mediated and humoral reactions occurring during tissue transplantation rejection and during bacterial infections. The study of tumour immunity has suggested possible ways in which responses might be manipulated, or engineered, to achieve an influence over the progress of the tumour. Although a vast amount of work has been done in this area by a host of investigators working in both the pre- and post-transplant eras, our present knowledge is primitive and often empirical. Nevertheless, progress has been made in assessing the immune status of cancer patients and changes in status which occur during the clinical course.

In order to assess immune responses to neoplasms, and to rationally utilize these responses as a basis for therapy, an analysis of the tumour immunity data base must be undertaken. An arbitrary scheme for analysis is as follows:

I. Immune response to tumours.
  1. Immunogenicity of tumour antigens.
  2. Defined response systems.
    (a) Cell-mediated mechanisms.
    (b) Humoral mechanisms.

II. The influence of tumours on the immune response.
  1. Immunocompetence as an indicator of prognosis.
  2. Suppression of immune response.
III. Use of immunological engineering to alter immune response to tumour.
  1. Repair and replacement of inadequate immune mechanisms.
  2. Use of non-specific immunostimulators.
  3. Specific active immunotherapy.
  4. Specific adoptive immunotherapy.
IV. Immune instructional methods to establish or augment specific immunity.
  1. Lymphocyte transfer factor (TF).
  2. Immune RNA (I-RNA).
V. Use of specific antibodies in tumour therapy.
  1. Cytotoxic antibodies.
  2. Antibody carriers for tumouricidal agents.

THE IMMUNE RESPONSE TO TUMOURS

Immunogenicity of tumour antigens

Tumours, which are either induced with carcinogens, or arise spontaneously, express a variety of neoantigens on their cell surfaces. These have been demonstrated by tumour rejection responses in syngeneic animals which have been immunized in a number of ways, including partial surgical excision of existing tumour or administration of irradiated tumour cells. In the case of animals with large progressive tumours, smaller tumour challenges at a different site may be rejected, demonstrating that a concomitant relationship exists with each tumour site and that it may be largely dependent on the size of tumour challenge in terms of cell numbers[1,2]. Stimulation of these responses may be heightened by injection of an adjuvant such as Bacillus Calmette-Guerin (BCG)[3,4].

The degree of specific immunogenicity produced by various tumour neoantigens is found to vary greatly and may even be absent. For instance, rat hepatic and mammary tumours produced by 2-acetoamino-fluorene (AAF) do not express distinct neoantigens capable of inducing tumour rejections[5]. Another possibly important observation is that the degree of immunogenicity induced by 3-methycholanthrene (MCA) sarcomas is related to the inducing dose of the carcinogen. Thus low doses of carcinogen produce tumours of low immunogenicity[6]. Furthermore, spontaneously arising tumours are less frequently immunogenic than carcinogen-produced tumours. Also the level of immunity following spontaneously arising tumours is usually less than that seen following carcinogen-induced tumours, where protection against tumour challenge may be frequently established[7].

Baldwin has observed that carcinogen-induced and spontaneously arising rat tumours also express a variety of non-specific embryonic antigens. These embryonic antigens are usually not capable of inciting a tumour rejection response, but such a response when observed, is restricted to individually distinct neoantigens.

Failure to induce tumour rejection response

The failure of specific neoantigens to consistently induce tumour rejection responses has given rise to several possible explanations.

(a) The 'sneaking through' hypothesis[8] suggests that an emerging tumour is not associated with sufficient immunogenicity until the cell number reaches a point beyond host control. After this critical time immunity is induced and is measurable by cytotoxic reactivity[9].

(b) Modification of neoantigen expression and characteristics may render tumour cells poor targets for tumour rejection mechanisms. For example, in carcinogen-induced tumours (amino-azo dye-induced rat hepatomas) tumour rejection antigens are stable integral components of the cell surface, whereas embryonic antigens are labile components[10]. Antibody against tumour-specific antigen therefore has been found to remain cell-bound for longer periods compared to antibodies against embryonic antigens which are rapidly lost from the cell surface during incubation[11].

(c) Changes in cell-mediated immunity or humoral factors may occur. These are largely reflections of changes in cell population, as measured, for example, by T-cell rosettes and numbers of suppressor and null cells. Humoral factors include excess antigens[12], antigen–antibody complexes[13], 'masking' antibody[14], and low molecular weight blocking factors[15].

(d) Host immunodeficiencies may precede the induction of tumour, such as is seen in the athymic nude mouse or in the clinical immunodeficiencies such as Swiss type agammaglobulinaemia and Wiskott–Aldrich syndrome. Immunodeficiency may also be present in malnutrition states.

Correlation between in vivo *and* in vitro *evidence of immunity*

Important discrepancies exist between evidence of immunity in the tumour host and the *in vitro* assessment of such immunity. An example is seen in induced tumours which exhibit lymphoid immunity to tumour-specific and embryonic neoantigens, but after tumour excision response to embryonic antigen can no longer be demonstrated[16]. Further, serum from tumour-immune animals produces complement-dependent and cell-dependent cytotoxicity *in vitro* but is without effect in controlling transplanted tumours in syngeneic animals.

Much recent attention has been focused on exact ways in which antigen exposure and the resulting immune state occur *in vivo* and what the effects are on control of the tumour by immune states produced in different ways. Soluble tumour antigens are immunogenic whether prepared by the commonly used 3 M KCl extract method or by other methods. Under highly restricted conditions tumour antigen administrations have been noted to afford some degree of protection against tumour challenge[17,18]. In some instances, however, tumour antigens have either abrogated or interfered with tumour rejection. Rats made immune to an MCA-induced sarcoma were not capable of tumour rejection after treatment with large amounts of soluble tumour antigen administered intraperitoneally[19]. In another example, rats pretreated with DAB-induced hepatoma membranes containing tumour antigen were unable to reject the tumour after subsequent induction of immunity[20]. Other studies have shown that preimmunization with either crude membrane preparations or 3 M KCl extracts of MCA-induced sarcoma renders the animal incapable of producing a tumour rejection response when subsequently immunized with irradiated tumour cells. These observations have given rise to the view that exposure to acellular antigens prior to induction of immunity produces a population of suppressor cells which interfere with lymphocyte cytotoxicity[21].

Immune inhibitory agents

Herberman has attempted to analyse factors which influence *in vitro* cellular responses by working with a series of virus-induced tumours. A number of factors were identified which inhibited immune responses to tumour antigens. One such factor was inhibition of cellular immunity by suppressor cells. It was observed that depression of phytohaemagglutinin (PHA) responses occurred in mice bearing murine sarcoma virus (MSV)-induced tumours, and that the depressed response persisted as the tumour progressed. But PHA responses are restored by removal of cells after passage on rayon adherence columns[22,23]. The activity of suppressor cells is restricted to mitogen-induced responses, since no effect is exerted on the activity of cytotoxic effector cells[24].

Another suppressive factor is the tumour cell itself or products of the tumour. Addition of cells from a viral-induced tumour (C58NT)D to normal thymocytes caused a marked inhibition of mixed lymphocyte culture (MLC) response to allogeneic normal cells. Other viral-induced tumours were found to have similar properties. In general, this was also true for tumour

Table 5.1 Response of normal lymphocytes to blocking serum*

Serum source	*Tumour patient cells*		*Normal cells*	
	PHA	*PWM*	*PHA*	*PWM*
Tumour patient serum†	14 000	10 000	21 000	16 000
Normal serum	58 000	38 000	85 000	46 000

* Counts per minute of tritiated thymidine incorporation
† Adenocarcinoma of sigmoid colon with hepatic metastases. (After Vetto, R. M., Burger, D. R. and Lilley, D. P. (1974). *Arch. Surg.*, **108**, 558)

cell sonicates. There is evidence that tumour cell suppression of lymphoid responses in these systems is due to the KR virus isolated from the tumour cells, since KRV itself produces suppression which can be eliminated by incubation with anti-KRV serum[25].

In addition to the inhibitory effects of suppressor cells and viruses in tumour cells, serum factors which are either specific or non-specific may interfere with *in vitro* immune response and perhaps also with *in vivo* responses. Specific antitumour serum[26], or non-specific factors in tumour-bearing animals such as immunoregulatory globulin (IRA)[27] or serum blocking factor (SBF)[28,29] produce suppression. Blocking of phytohaemagglutinin response by SBF obtained from a tumour patient is shown in Table 5.1.

Methods for increasing tumour antigen immunogenicity

Augmentation of immunogenicity of tumour antigens has been accomplished by treating tumour cells with *Vibrio cholerae* neuraminidase (VCN). This finding has been supported by several observations including: (1) fetal tissue incubated in VCN induces a greater degree of sensitization than fetal tissue treated with heat inactivated VCN[30]; (2) small ordinarily non-immunogenic numbers of lymphocytes when treated with VCN produce accelerated skin-graft rejection in allogeneic recipients[31]; (3) cyclophosphamide-prepared mice do not become tolerant to VCN-treated bone marrow cells[32];

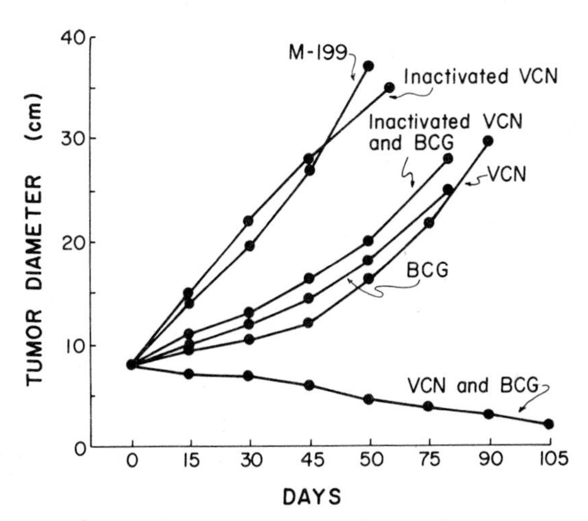

Figure 5.1 Response of a spontaneous mammary adenocarcinoma to repeated intratumour injection of *Vibrio cholerae* neuraminidase (VCN) and/or *Mycobacterium bovis* (BCG). The results with inactivated VCN were similar to injections with M-199 culture medium. VCN alone, BCG alone and inactivated VCN with BCG produced intermediate results in tumour size control. VCN in combination with BCG prevented tumour growth. (After Simmons, R. L. and Rios, A. (1975). In: *Host Defense Against Cancer and its Potentiation*, p. 227 (Tokyo: University Park Press)

(4) VCN-treated human lymphocytes are several-fold more stimulating in a one-way mitomycin-C mixed lymphocyte culture[33]. VCN acts on cell surfaces to release sialic acid residues[34–36] which reduce the negative charge on the cell surface, increase cell deformability and susceptibility of the cell to phagocytosis[37,38]. Thus the tumour cell alterations may render antigens more available to the immunoreactive cells of the host. The use of VCN and BCG in a spontaneous mouse mammary adenocarcinoma is shown in Figure 5.1.

There are a variety of other methods by which tumours may be modified to express immunogenicity. This general area has been reviewed by Prager and Baechtel[39]. One example of tumour cell modification is iodoacetamide treatment of murine ascites lymphoma cells, which permits immunization of syngeneic hosts with some degree of protection against transplanted tumours. Another example is glutaraldehyde modified tumour cells which produce primarily a cellular response and offer protection against tumour transplant[40,41]. It is interesting that glutaraldehyde modified spleen cells from the tumour host also offer protection against tumour transplant.

Defined response systems

Immunity is presently thought of as consisting of a cellular arm, mediated by thymic-derived lymphocytes and a humoral arm derived from bursal equivalent cells. In clinical settings there has been a tendency to further fragment such responses in terms of what is thought to be most important in a given circumstance, such as the predominant role of cellular responses in transplanted organ rejection. It does not seem reasonable, however, that a well-developed humoral mechanism acts as an innocent, relatively non-participating bystander in a response as complex and important as immunity. Perhaps more reasonable is the possibility that other systems exist which are as yet unidentified and which occupy a position as important and necessary as cellular and humoral immunity to produce the intricate machinations of immune response. Possible examples of this are 'natural immunity', Klein's observation of highly specific natural killing[42] and Kumar's strontium-sensitive marrow rejection factor[43]. Certain cell systems such as suppressor or null cells, augmentor cells or macrophages, all of which are now regarded as participators, may eventually be shown to comprise major systems of immunity and may lend themselves to manipulation or engineering. For the present, however, immune responses may be most conveniently considered as cellular and humoral.

Cell-mediated mechanisms

The presence of macrophages in tumours—It has been pointed out by Alexander[44] that a tumour is composed of malignant cells supported by a stroma and vascular system made of normal cells, and that in addition there are present varying amounts of inflammatory cells including lymphocytes, neutrophils and macrophages. The presence of macrophages has been particularly intriguing for investigators since as these cells process antigens, they seem necessary for the conversion of memory lymphocytes to a cytotoxic state in response to antigen and can themselves be generally and specifically tumouricidal[45]. Large numbers of macrophages, whose presence is established by specific means such as binding by antimacrophage sera, are found in experimental animal tumours[46] and in human tumours[47]. In chemically-induced rat sarcomas macrophage content ranged from 3 to 58% of the total cell population of the tumour. In a variety of human tumours the macrophage content ranged from 0 to 30%. In malignant breast tumours it was noted that those which had metastasized contained few macrophages, whereas localized tumours had higher numbers of macrophages. There is as yet no information regarding the relation between host survival and macrophage content of the tumour[48].

In the case of melanomas, all metastatic tumours had a low macrophage content whereas all primary tumours without metastases, or locally recurrent tumours without metastases contained 9 to 30% macrophages.

The mechanism by which macrophages enter tumours is thought to be partly dependent on the presence of T lymphocytes and to be similar to the way that monocytes enter sites of inflammation in a delayed hypersensitivity response. Macrophage response to rat sarcoma is diminished as the result of T-lymphocyte depletion. Macrophage entrance into tumour may be a partially T-cell dependent specific host reaction against tumour antigens, since immunogenicity of the tumour in terms of protective sensitization is related to the macrophage content. Furthermore, transplanted rat sarcomas with large numbers of macrophages are less likely to metastasize unless transplanted into T-cell deficient rats[48] (Table 5.2).

Table 5.2 Relationship between macrophage content and incidence of distant metastases within 1 year of removal of transplanted chemically induced sarcomas from syngeneic recipients

Tumour	*Macrophage content %*		*Incidence % of metastasis**	*Immunogenicity†*
	Mean	*Range*		
MC-3	8	2–12	100	$<10^3$
HSH	12	10–15	100	10^4
ASBP-1	22	18–26	52	10^5
MC-1 (M)	38	26–42	25	10^6
HSN	40	34–44	32	5×10^6
HSBPA	54	42–63	11	5×10^7

* Following amputation of tumour-bearing limb 14 days after tumour cell inoculation
† Number of cells required to induce i.m. tumour in rats immunized by tumour excision
(After Gauci, C. L. and Alexander, P. (1975). *Cancer Lett.*, **1**, 29)

Stimulation of macrophages—Macrophage mobilization in the clinical treatment of malignant tumours has been investigated with the use of agents such as Bacillus Calmette Guerin (BCG) and *Corynebacterium parvum*. In experimental animal systems activation of macrophages by the above agents and other immunopotentiators such as *Toxoplasma gondii*, *Mycobacterium bovis* and synthetic reticuloendothelial stimulants such as polyriboinosinic acid, polyribocytodylic acid, polyacrylic acid–maleic anhydride, and pyran, a copolymer of maleic anhydride–divinyl ether, produced an 'arming' effect on macrophages which induces specific or non-specific cytotoxicity against tumour cells[49–57]. There is also some suggestion that macrophages function as effector cells in resistance to tumours as demonstrated by massive proliferation of histiocytes in the lymph drainage area of transplanted non-metastasizing hamster lymphomas[58]. Moreover, activated macrophages administered intravenously 48 h after intravenous innoculation of B-16 melanoma cells reduced the number of pulmonary metastases[59].

In vivo *lymphocyte sensitization*—An example of immune engineering is shown by the series of experiments aimed at inducing lymphocyte sensitization *in vitro* by presentation of tumour antigen. This approach is attractive for a number of reasons which include its obvious possible application to tumour immunotherapy, the observation that cell-mediated lysis (CML) manifested by lymphocytes sensitized *in vitro* is seven- to ten-fold greater than that obtained by *in vivo* sensitization[60], that weak immunogens can

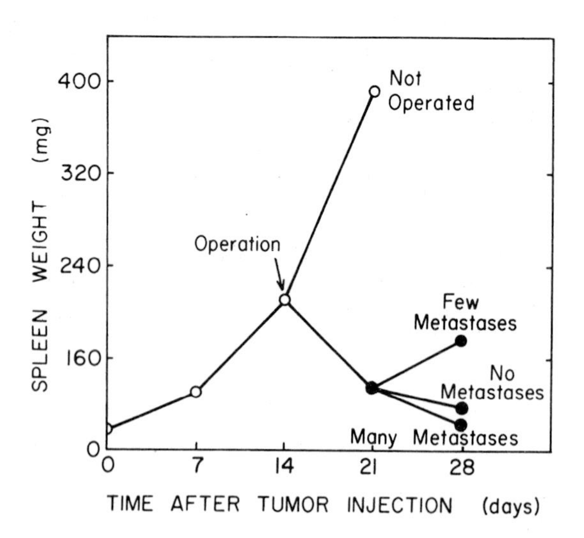

Figure 5.2 Spleen weight increases due to accumulation of suppressor cells after establishment of tumour by foot-pad injection of 5×10^5 3LL cells. If the tumour is removed at day 14, an enhancement-free period results during which further spleen size changes are dependent upon existing metastases. The post-tumour excision period is used for testing specifically sensitized T lymphocytes. (After Treves, A. J., Cohen, I. R. and Feldman, M., *Isr. J. Med. Sci.* In press)

evoke CML *in vitro*, whereas this does not occur *in vivo*, that lymphocytes can be sensitized *in vitro* against autoantigens[61], and that lymphocytes sensitized *in vitro* can, after inoculation, recruit effector cells *in vivo*[62]. The method used for sensitization consisted of culturing T lymphocytes on

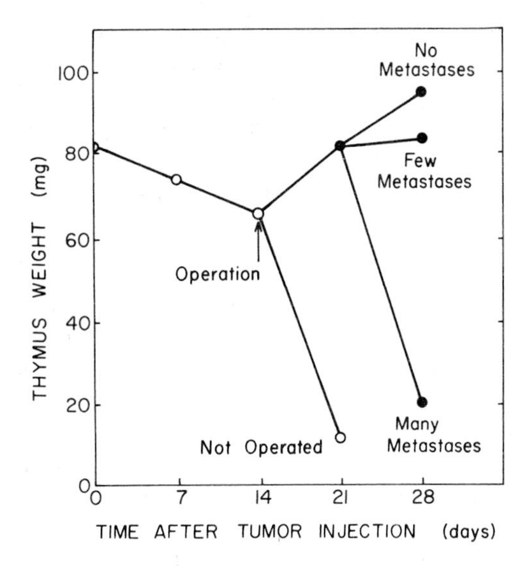

Figure 5.3 Thymus size decreases after establishment of 3LL tumour. If the primary tumour is excised the thymus increases in size and further changes are related to appearance of metastases. (After Treves, A. J., Cohen, I. R. and Feldman, M., *Isr. J. Med. Sci.* In press)

foreign monolayers for 5 days, in order to produce blastoid cells capable of specifically lysing target cells syngeneic to the sensitizing monolayer[63]. In this particular model the tumour was the 3LL Lewis lung carcinoma in C57BL mice[64]. During the period of uncontrolled tumour growth splenomegaly resulted from an accumulation of lymphocytes which have been subsequently shown to enhance tumour growth by suppression of the host's immune response[65]. Control of enhancement could be attained by resection of the primary tumour (Figure 5.2), and this enhancement-free interval was used to test with sensitized T lymphocytes in order to prevent eventual pulmonary metastases from the 3LL tumour. T lymphocytes administered 1 day after surgical removal of the tumour resulted in protection of 50% of the animals from lethal metastases. The specificity of this protection was demonstrated by the fact that lymphocytes sensitized against fibroblasts offered no protection[66]. Concurrent thymic suppression occurs with progressing tumour but is prevented by control of the tumour (Figure 5.3).

Of additional interest is the finding that antigen-fed syngeneic macrophages are capable of specifically sensitizing T lymphocytes. Furthermore, the *in vitro* CML resulting from macrophage-sensitized lymphocytes is significantly greater than that observed from lymphocytes sensitized by tumour monolayers[67]. In addition, tumour growth is inhibited when tumour cells are injected subcutaneously with sensitized lymphocytes.

An apparently purely cellular response against tumour can be produced. An autochthonous MCA-induced rat sarcoma system, in which immunity was induced by a vascular ligation-and-release technique[68], exhibited tumour destruction due to lymphoid cells from the host[69]. No humoral antibody directed against the tumour could be detected by cytotoxicity testing, immunofluorescence or immune adherence techniques[70]. Participation in tumour destruction by T lymphocytes and also macrophages was shown by time lapse phase-contrast cinemamicrography.

Lymphocytes in tumours—Recently more attention has been given toward defining the significance of lymphocytes which infiltrate the tumour since their presence has frequently been taken to indicate a favourable response. In Burkitt's lymphoma, which is an Epstein–Barr virus-associated tumour and which is composed primarily of B-cell lymphoblasts, infiltrating T cells occupied 4–38% of the tumour cell population[71]; T cells were observed to kill EB virus cell lines[72].

In infectious mononucleosis (IM), which may in some instances be a precursor to neoplastic disease[73], the atypical cells during the acute phase of the disease were shown to be both T and B cells[74,75]. Since only B cells can be infected by the EB virus, it was thought that T cells represent an immune response against EBV-infected B cells[76]. Blood lymphocytes were assayed, and after removal of lymphocytes with complement receptors for cytotoxicity against EBV positive and negative lymphoblasts, it was found that the remaining lymphocytes were cytotoxic against EBV positive cell lines only[77,78].

Nasopharyngeal carcinomas are highly infiltrated with lymphocytes. The epithelial cells of the tumour are shown to carry the EB virus genome[79,80]. Lymphocytes isolated from these tumours are cytotoxic against EB virus cell lines and remain so after complement receptor carrying cells are removed[81].

Lymphocytes isolated from a human osteosarcoma metastasis could not be stimulated in culture against osteosarcoma tumour cells although peripheral blood lymphocytes underwent blastogenesis under these conditions. These lymphocytes did, however, respond to PHA stimulation[82].

Thus, from the limited number of functional studies carried out it is becoming evident that the nature of infiltrating lymphoid cells may vary in different systems. Their presence in tumours, which is capable of being assayed by various anatomical and functional means, usually indicates an immune response which is often cytotoxic. The place of this response in influencing the outcome of the clinical course is not yet clear.

Other cellular responses—A narrowly defined population of marrow-dependent cells (M cells) has been described which mediate genetic resistance to Friend virus (FV) erythroleukaemia[43]. M-cell resistance differs from T- and B-cell functions in several ways, including that thymic influence is not required for maturation, that M-cell function is not suppressed by acute lethal whole body radiation and steroid administration, that M-cell function is selectively abrogated by administration of radioactive strontium and also by silica particles and cyclophosphamide, and that function is regulated by immune response genes not linked to the H-2 complex[83]. Strontium-89 treatment is especially useful in this model since T and B cell and macrophage functions remain intact.

Interference with cellular responses—A radioisotope foot-pad assay demonstrated that E_4 tumour homogenate derived from mice produces immunosuppression as measured by a decreased delayed hypersensitivity response[84]. This followed the observation that immune responses to tumour cells increased during early phases of tumour induction, became suppressed as the tumour enlarged, and was restored after the tumour was excised[85]. The data suggest that cell-mediated immune response is suppressed by a tumour-derived substance that interacts with a serum component, probably to produce an antigen–antibody complex as shown in other systems[86–88]. This experiment illustrates the difficulty in considering humoral and cellular responses separately.

Interference with cell-mediated responses is thought to be at least partially due to blocking serum factors composed of antibody or antigens, or related immune complexes. The mode by which interference or blocking results is not known, but these factors are on the surface of lymphocytes and presumably either render them incapable of functioning as effector cells if they are sensitized, or possibly block sensitization to the tumour[89,90].

Other blocking factors have also been described which are of smaller size (1000–2000 M.W.), are composed of peptide chains, are probably lymphocyte products and migrate in the alpha-2 band in electrophoresis[15,27]. These have been previously referred to.

Humoral mechanisms

Antibodies—Cells against which antibodies are directed may undergo destructive lysis by one of two ways; the lysis may be complement-mediated in the presence of antibody, or lysis may be entirely antibody-dependent, complement-independent but carried on with the aid of helper cells. In either case the fatal lesion is a defect in the cell wall which permits escape of potassium and ingress of water into the hypertonic milieu[91]. In the case of complement-induced lysis it is thought that the lesion is produced by the insertion of terminal protein complement components into the lipid matrix of the target cell membrane. This insertion results in a rigid hollow channel that exposes the interior of the cell[92].

In experimental animal or *in vitro* systems the effectiveness of complement-mediated lysis varies greatly depending upon the type of tumour or other conditions of the experiment. Reasons for variability include density of distribution of antigenic determinants, deficiency in complement binding sites and differences in cell repair mechanisms[93,94]. Complement-mediated cytolysis is most efficiently triggered in association with a single IgM molecule. Lysis also takes place with two or more IgG-class molecules, but this requires a situation where cell surface antigenic groups form a closely spaced repeated pattern[95].

Antibody-dependent cell-mediated cytolysis is effected by IgG-class antibodies which require an intact Fc portion of the molecule[96]. The helper or effector cell may be one of several types and in fact need not be obtained from the immune animal. Thus it is the antibody molecule which confers specificity on the reaction.

A variety of distinctive cells have been effective in this cytolytic reaction, including neutrophils, platelets, macrophages, fetal liver cells and null (without B or T antigenic markers) lymphocytes. All these cells, however, are capable of binding the IgG molecule Fc terminal and thus have Fc receptors[97]. All cells, however, which possess the Fc receptor are not cytotoxic effectors. Cell–cell interaction associated with antibody-dependent lysis is represented in Figure 5.4.

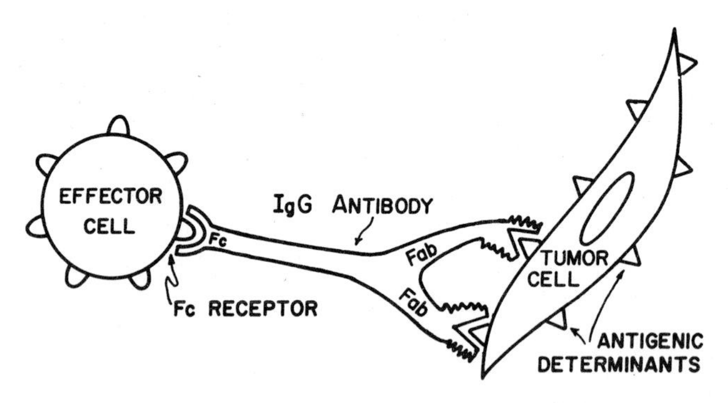

Figure 5.4 Schematic representation of antibody-dependent cell-mediated cytolysis (ADCC). Specific tumour cell binding occurs at the variable sites of the IgG molecule. Several types of cells, including hepatic fetal cells, platelets and null cells may serve as effectors

Anti-antibodies—The network theory of immune regulation proposed by Jerne[98] indicates that the immune response is a finely balanced company of humoral and cell-mediated reactions which at times, under conditions of immunogenic challenge or acquired immune deficiency results in a negative feedback reaction which is intended to control the immune response and restore the organism to its original balance. While such a hypothesis, in view of the deluge of immunological information that has recently been developed, seems to be an oversimplification of actual events, it is useful, at least for the present, to think of immune responses along the lines that Jerne has suggested. Indeed, there is much evidence that tends to support the network theory. One such example of support is the production of anti-antibodies directed against tumour antibodies[99–101].

Antitumour antibodies react with a number of tumour antigen types. Included are those which are directed against the surface membrane of the tumour cell and exhibit specificity[102], and those directed against intracytoplasmic tumour antigens and which show a greater degree of cross-reactivity. In human melanoma these two antigen types are present during the early phases of primary tumour growth, but if metastases and widespread dissemination result, antimembrane antibody disappears from the serum whereas anticytoplasmic antibody persists[103]. One of the explanations for this change is that specific anti-antibodies against membrane antibodies have been raised.

Antigammaglobulin antibodies have been recognized for a number of years in relation to several medical disorders such as rheumatoid arthritis, systemic lupus erythematosus and various autoimmune conditions[104–106]. Anti-antibodies are specifically directed against different areas of the

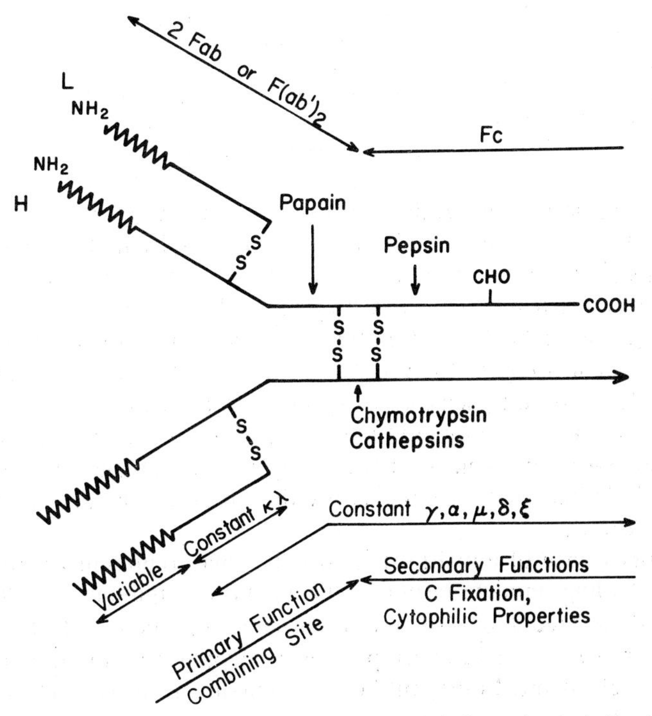

Figure 5.5 Schematic representation of IgG immunoglobulin molecule indicating regions where enzymatic degradation may produce antigenic fragments

immunoglobulin molecule depending upon what regions have been exposed to act as an antigen. Some of the regions which may result from physiological or laboratory molecule cleavage are shown in Figure 5.5.

Anti-idiotypic antibodies are directed against tumour membrane specific antibodies[107] and react at the variable region site of the tumour-specific antibody[108,109]. *Anti-cytoplasmic antibodies* have been shown to combine with $F(ab)_2$ fragments at the hinge site of the IgG molecule[110–114]. *Anti-Fc antibodies* (rheumatoid factor-like) have been identified in the sera of melanoma patients and are specifically directed against the Fc fraction of IgM or IgG. Anti-Fc antibodies increase as the tumour progresses and are both 19 S and 7 S. The target antibody against which anti-Fc is directed is not yet identified but appears to differ from anti-$F(ab)_2$ specificities[115,116]. The anti-antibodies studied in melanoma are summarized in Table 5.3.

Table 5.3 Anti-antibodies in melanoma

Type	*Class*	*Antigenic site*
1. Anti-idiotype* (Antimembrane)	IgG	Variable Region (Fab)
2. Anticytoplasmic†	IgG	Hinge Region $F(ab')_2$
3. Rheumatoid factor	IgM (19 S) IgG (7 S)	Fc

* Individually specific
† Group specific

The production of anti-antibodies may result partially from the exposure of new antigenic sites after splitting of the IgG molecule by enzymes such as cathepsins which are released from tumour cells. This reaction occurs *in vitro* only when host cells are present in the substrate suggesting that tumour infiltrating host cells are ultimately necessary for formation of anti-antibody. Some support for this concept is lent by the observation that similar IgG splitting by leukocytes is observed in abscess fluid[117].

The role of anti-antibodies in tumour regulation is presently the subject of speculation. Anti-idiotypic antibodies may regulate cellular immune mechanisms[118,119] but what factors enhance their production and for what purpose is unknown.

The appearance of anti-$F(ab)_2$ antibodies may represent an attempt to support a failing immune response during chronic immune stimulation, as shown by elevated levels of anticytoplasmic antibodies which occur as tumours progress. This has been previously suggested as an explanation for elevated levels of anti-$F(ab)_2$ antibodies occurring in chronic Gram-positive infections[120].

Further evidence for a beneficial effect of anti-$F(ab)_2$ antibodies may be inferred from the high levels occurring in patients with localized or stable tumours who also exhibit a low level of anticytoplasmic antibodies. Conversely, the opposite is true in patients in whom tumours are widespread or progressing[121].

Both beneficial and harmful effects of anti-tumour antibodies may be explained in terms of disordered regulation and control as implied by Jerne's network theory[98].

THE INFLUENCE OF TUMOURS ON THE RESPONSE

Immunocompetence as an indicator of prognosis

There has been much recent interest, especially in clinical settings, in the effect which a tumour exerts upon the ability of the host to respond immunologically in an effective manner. Thus, the initial immunocompetency of the host, measured in a variety of manners, at the time when the tumour is first discovered, has been correlated with the ultimate prognosis for the patient. For instance in patients undergoing definitive surgery for cancer, 90% of those who had complete resection of their tumour and remained disease-free for six months were capable of being sensitized to dinitrochlorobenzene (DNCB) prior to beginning therapy. Those patients who had non-resectable tumour, or in whom tumour recurred within 6 months were mostly not able to respond to DNCB prior to therapy. Additional follow-up has demonstrated correlation with definitive surgery, DNCB reactivity and long-term recurrence-free intervals and survival times[122–124] (Figure 5.6).

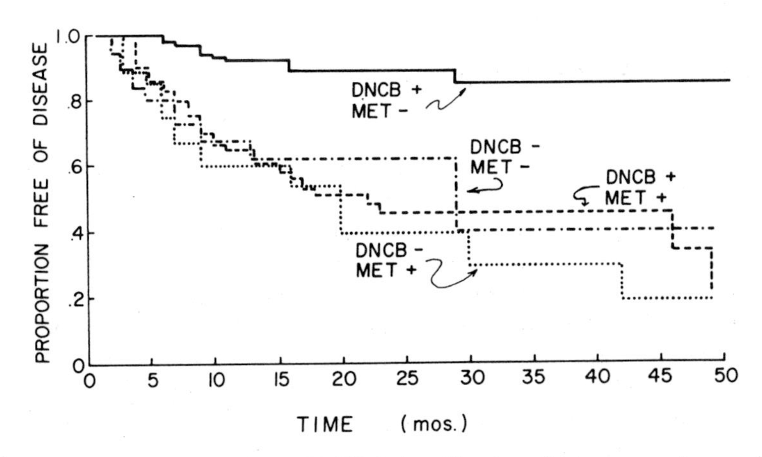

Figure 5.6 Tumour patients who are DNCB (+) and in whom the tumour can be completely resected and who have no metastases have a much lower tumour recurrence rate than similar patients who are DNCB (−). If complete resection is not possible or metastases are present DNCB response does not seem to influence tumour progress. (After Pinsky, C. M., El Domeiri, A., Caron, A. S. *et al.* (1974). *Cancer Res.*, **47**, 37)

DNCB is a skin-sensitizing hapten which is useful for inducing and measuring *de novo* delayed hypersensitivity.

At the present time methods for correlation with prognosis have proceeded far beyond the monitoring of non-specific delayed cutaneous hypersensitivity (DCH) reactions. A large variety of immune tests have been employed and are currently being studied. For example, PHA blastogenesis of lymphocytes in cancer patients has been correlated with a generally favourable prognosis[24]. Extensive attempts to correlate the outcome of various human malignancies with specific moieties such as migration inhibition factor (MIF), lymphocyte cytotoxin and macrophage chemotactic factor have been described[125]. A list of some of the determinations presently being used is shown in Table 5.4.

Table 5.4 Tests for immune response in malignancy

In vivo	*In vitro*
Primary DCH (DNCB or KLH)	Lymphocyte function:
Recall DCH (measles, mumps, SK-SD, PPD)	Blastogenesis (PHA, Con-A, PWM, Specific Ag)
T-Lymphocyte levels (E-rosettes)	Mediator production (LIF)
B-Lymphocyte levels (EAC-rosettes)	Direct cytoxicity
Monocyte levels	ADCC
Primary Ab response (precipitin, agglutinin reactions)	Monocyte–macrophage function:
Serum Ig levels	Cytotoxicity
Local inflammation (croton oil)	Chemotaxis
RES particle clearance	Phagocytosis
PHA dermal response	Complement function:
	C^3 Screen

Suppression of immune response

Chemotherapeutic agents

An important variable affecting testing of immune response of the patient to his tumour is the type of chemotherapy the patient is receiving. Certain drugs are very immunosuppressive, while other drugs are non-immunosuppressive or only slightly so[126]. Some of the more immunosuppressive drugs include the thiopurines, folic acid antagonists, alkylating agents, adriamycin, the nitrosureas and corticosteroids. Less immunosuppressive drugs include imidazole carboxamide, bleomycin, vincristine, 5-fluorouracil and cytosine arabinoside. Continuous daily therapy with chemotherapeutic agents results in immunosuppression, while cycled courses every few weeks are less immunosuppressive[127], but even cycled therapy is suppressive if maintained for long periods, especially to B-cell function[128]. This may resemble modulation of immune response seen when small amounts of chemotherapy are given which spare T-cell function while suppressing B-cell function and antibody production[129] (Table 5.5).

Tumour viruses

Oncogenic viruses, including Friend, Gross, Maloney and Rauscher leukaemia viruses cause impaired immune responses in mice to most non-viral antigens[130–135]. The inductive phase of the response is most sensitive to virus-induced suppression and IgG production is more susceptible to suppression than IgM production. In Friend virus tumours the suppression takes place, not at the antibody-producing B-lymphocyte level, but at the bone marrow stem precursor level[136]. There is some evidence that cell-mediated response to antigen or plant mitogens is also suppressed[137–139].

Although oncogenic viruses are immunosuppressive, virus-free spleen cells and cell extracts from mice with non-viral induced plasmacytoma and mastocytoma have also been shown to be immunosuppressive in terms of antibody production[140,141]. This is demonstrated *in vitro* against tumour host spleen cells and may be due to suppressor lymphocytes or suppressive factors liberated by the donor spleen cells or contained within them. Furthermore, cell-free mastocytoma extracts yield a dialysable ninhydrin-positive factor of approximately 1000–5000 molecular weight which is immunosuppressive. This may be the same material which was described by others in human malignancy as immunoregulatory alpha globulin (IRA)[27] or serum blocking factor (SBF)[15].

In at least one murine tumour system (Rowson–Parr virus—RPV) the immunodepressive effect on B-cell function can be ameliorated both *in vitro* and *in vivo* by addition of a relatively small number of normal syngeneic macrophages, suggesting that in this particular system the ultimate reason for the appearance of immunosuppression is a macrophage defect. In other tumour systems, however, such as the Friend virus (FLV) this is not entirely the case, and the reason for immunosuppression appears due to several factors including perhaps macrophage defect[142].

Table 5.5 Relation of chemotherapy to immune response

Strongly immunosuppressive drugs:
6-MP, MTX, Cytox, Pred, Adria, BCNU
Less immunosuppressive drugs:
DTIC, BLEO, VCR, 5-FU, ARA-C
Chemotherapy administration schedule:
(a) Continuous Rx strongly immunosuppressive
(b) Intermittent Rx less immunosuppressive
(c) Long duration intermittent Rx strongly immunosuppressive
Possible response modulation during treatment:
Unchanged or augmented DCH
Suppression of Ab

Repair of tumour-induced immune suppression by supplying normal immunocompetent cells is partly supported by the finding of bone marrow stem cell changes in animals treated with oncogenic viruses[143].

It has been suggested that E series prostaglandins (PGE_2) may play a role in allowing syngeneic tumours to escape immunological control, since PGE_2 is immunosuppressive *in vitro*. This effect may be reversed with prostaglandin inhibitors such as indomethacin and aspirin[144,145].

THE USE OF IMMUNOLOGICAL ENGINEERING TO ALTER THE IMMUNE RESPONSE TO TUMOURS

The repair and replacement of inadequate immune mechanisms

Lymphocyte transfer

The concept of transferring immunity with lymphoid cell dates from the observation of Landsteiner and Chase[146] who, in 1942, using guinea-pigs, demonstrated that cutaneous delayed hypersensitivity could be transferred from immune donors to non-immune recipients using lymphoid cells. A similar immune transfer using a lymphocyte extract was later demonstrated by Lawrence, transferring tuberculin sensitivity in man[147]. In a more recent clinical study lymphocytes obtained from the thoracic duct of an HL-A identical non-twin sibling were given to seven patients with a variety of cancers. A state of chimerism was detected in three of these patients who could be karyotyped because of opposite sex of the donor, and four patients exhibited mild signs of graft-versus-host reaction. Three of the seven patients exhibited a clinical effect on the tumour manifested by complete regression in one case and partial regression or control in two cases. In the remaining four patients no beneficial clinical effect was observed. In two of the karyotyped patients donated lymphocytes were not observed in the recipient beyond a week. In one patient who showed no clinical response to treatment 60% chimerism was present at 5 weeks. An additional observation was that skin reaction to recall antigens was restored in five of the patients[148,149].

Immunocompetent cell transplant, even with identical HL-A lymphocytes, is subject to a number of limitations. For instance, the donor may not be immune, serum blocking factors may be present which preclude cell–cell interaction, or the size of the tumour burden may simply be too large.

Humoral factors

A humoral recognition factor (HRF) has been described[150] which is an alpha-2 macroglobulin found in the plasma of normal subjects and which is thought necessary for proper macrophage function against tumours. This factor is depleted after surgery[151,152], has been found to inhibit the growth of primary and metastatic tumours[153], and (HRF) can be raised in the blood by employing reticuloendothelial stimulants (RES) such as BCG[154,155]. One of the new RES substances studied is the beta-1,3-glucopyranose polysaccharide, glucan, which is prepared from the inner part of the outer membrane of the yeast *Saccharomyces cerevisiae*[156,157]. This material may have advantages over other RES substances such as BCG, *Corynebacterium parvum* and levamisole, because it is a defined chemical compound which can be quantitated accurately, does not depend on viability for effect and is, on the basis of early testing, non-toxic.

Lymphocyte activation

Immune T lymphocytes which have bound antigen may be mistaken as the antigen source or tumour by macrophages which may phagocytize the T lymphocytes[158,159]. In order to avoid this autochthonous T lymphocytes have been activated with the non-antigenic mitogen phytohaemagglutinin and then administered to patients with cancer. In five patients with widespread cancer, 10^9 autochthonous activated T lymphocytes were administered daily on a 5-day monthly schedule. In three of these patients regression of pulmonary nodules occurred[160]. It is of considerable interest that while the pulmonary nodules regressed in these patients, in two patients concurrent progression of hepatic metastases was noted. One explanation is that an insufficient number of T lymphocytes was given; a more reasonable explanation, perhaps, is that the anatomical site of the tumour is important, and that local metabolic factors may modulate immune effectiveness. Although experiments of this type are interesting and perhaps give some insight into antitumour cell kinetics, the amount of persisting tumour makes it unlikely that approaches such as these will be successful[161].

The therapeutic use of non-specific immune stimulators

The use of non-specific immunostimulants has attracted considerable interest since it represents a way in which immune response of a tumour host may be manipulated. The interest has been heightened by clinical reports that some human tumour systems are favourably affected by treatment with these agents[162–164]. A considerable amount of research with non-specific immunostimulants in animal tumour systems has been done and has recently been reviewed[165]. The agents most commonly used include Bacillus Calmette-Guerin (BCG), other mycobacteria, *Corynebacterium parvum*, levamisole, glucan[156], the synthetic polynucleotide poly AU and various non-viable bacterial components and extracts. The clinical use of these agents has been disappointing, but this may be because they have necessarily been used in an empiric, non-discriminative manner, in salvage type situations. Furthermore, the precise mode of action of these agents and what sort of a substrate is necessary in the host for them to be effective is unknown. It seems that these agents are most effective when applied into the tumour, and that direct contact with the cell may be necessary[166]. They are most effective in more antigenic tumour systems[167] and therefore a well-developed existing immune response of the host to the tumour may be necessary for their effectiveness. They are most effective in the treatment of small accessible tumours[168] and have been reported to stimulate growth in large tumours[169]. The histological response to these agents is that of chronic inflammation and granuloma formation, although this varies greatly and a favourable anti-tumour response may occur without marked visible cellular changes[170]. The immunostimulants which are antitumour effective possess some specific quality which is not known since other agents such as turpentine, *Vaccinia* virus and oxazalone are capable of eliciting chronic inflammatory responses but have no antitumour activity[171].

The most commonly used immunostimulant in clinical studies is Bacillus Calmette-Guerin (BCG). BCG has been used as an adjuvant to therapy and administered by scarification in a variety of human tumours including melanomas, colorectal carcinoma and breast cancer. There seemed to be a modest advantage to BCG therapy in terms of survival when compared to historical control patients[172]. Other studies have indicated that early favourable results with the use of BCG in melanoma do not appear to be holding up after prolonged follow-up of the patient[173]. A recent review of the use of BCG in a variety of therapeutic combinations concludes that some encouragement remains for this agent, but that greatly beneficial effects in treatment of clinical cancer have not yet occurred[174].

Non-viable mycobacteria cell wall skeletons (CWS) have been shown to be as effective as BCG in the treatment of the line-10 hepatoma in guinea-pigs[175]. Similar material has produced prolonged survival in Stage IV lung cancers over a 15-month observation period[176]. The activity of CWS resides in the trehalose mycolate fraction termed P3[177].

The use of *Corynebacterium parvum* as an adjuvant to chemotherapy has produced longer survival in patients with disseminated breast and lung cancer. The mechanism by which *C. parvum* is effective is probably similar to BCG[178].

Levamisole is a phenylimidazole thiazole derivative that has been used as an antihelminthic for several years. Recently it was described as possessing immunotropic properties and shown to restore deficient immune responses in deficient hosts[179–181]. Levamisole does not suppress growth of primary experimental tumours, but after tumour reduction it prolongs the remission period and lengthens the time of survival. The ability to inhibit metastasis formation has been described[182,183]. Clinical studies in resected lung cancer have indicated that in short follow-up periods the incidence of tumour recurrence is diminished[184]. However, objective measurement of immune effects from levamisole and also *C. parvum* are difficult to establish[185].

The use of tumour vaccines (specific active immunotherapy) in cancer treatment

The animal or patient with a tumour may be non-immune or weakly immune to his tumour. Lack of adequate immune response of the host may be due to a number of reasons, including anergy, serum blocking factors, and depletion of immunocompetent cells due to the size of the tumour. One additional reason, however, is that sufficient exposure of the host to cell surface antigens has not occurred. This may be the result of tumour cell surface masking by antibody, immune complexes, or tumour protective substance such as acid residues. In this circumstance tumour antigen either in the form of cells or extracts administered to the host in an immunoreactive site may elicit greater degrees of humoral and cell-mediated responses in the host.

Neuraminidase-treated tumour cells

The immunogenicity of leukaemia and lymphosarcoma tumour cells in mice was significantly increased after treatment of the tumour cells with *Vibrio cholerae* neuraminidase. Neuraminidase cleaves the terminal N-acetyl-neuraminic acid residue from the tumour cell surface which results in alterations of physical and biological properties of the cells without affecting their viability[186,187]. Patients with acute myelocytic leukaemia have shown an increased remission rate when neuraminidase-treated allogeneic myeloblasts were administered in addition to chemotherapy (Figure 5.7).

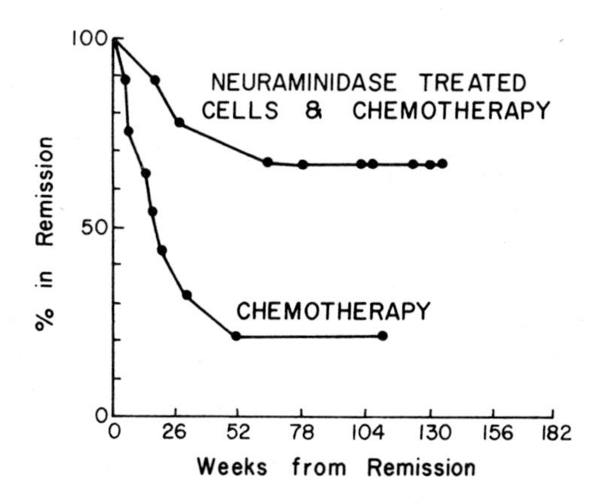

Figure 5.7 Duration of remission in randomly selected patients with acute myelocytic leukaemia given neuraminidase treated leukaemic cells and chemotherapy compared to a group treated with chemotherapy alone. Chemotherapy consisted of cytosine arabinoside and adriamycin. (After Bekesi, J. G., Roboz, J. P. and Holland, J. F. (1976). In: *International Conference on Immunotherapy of Cancer*, **277**, 313. New York Academy of Sciences)

Other work has shown regression of chemically reduced tumours in animals treated by neuraminidase altered autochthonous cells[188].

Tumour vaccine combined with other therapy

Several investigators have used adjuvant immunotherapy with autologous tumour vaccine combined with immunostimulators such as BCG and levamisole[189–192]. Tumour vaccine in Freund's adjuvant followed by BCG was used in 19 patients with Stage II bronchogenic carcinoma who had all visible tumours removed at surgery. Mean survival time was 25.7 months with three patients alive and disease-free at 32, 42 and 44 months. Mean survival in the control group was 8.1 months. Immune studies carried out revealed increased response of lymphocytes to PHA stimulation and in five patients tested, conversion to specific immunity as indicated by migration inhibition[193].

Attempts to characterize immune changes occurring after various therapies in carcinoma of the lung have shown the following: after high dose methotrexate and citrovorum factor rescue patients exhibited no change in dermal response to antigens but there was a reduction in blocking factor activity. Patients immunized with allogeneic tumour antigens exhibited conversion and enhancement of dermal responses and a tendency to develop serum blocking factors. Patients treated with combination immunochemotherapy exhibited increases and persistence in dermal responses and reduction of serum blocking factor production[194].

Specific adoptive immunotherapy

Adoptive immunotherapy is produced by infusing lymphocytes sensitized against tumour antigen in order to impart a specific immune reaction against the tumour. The duration of response is partly dependent upon the length of lymphocyte survival, and therefore, autochthonous cells seems preferable to HL-A incompatible allogeneic lymphocytes. The lymphocytes can be sensitized to tumour antigens *in vitro* by incubation with tumour antigens[195,196]. In human tumours there is an added variable since the lymphocytes are not entirely naive. In this circumstance induction of cytotoxicity is accelerated[197,198]. A parallel may be drawn with induction of cell-mediated immunity with transfer factor which is best accomplished in antigen-primed but non-immune animals[199,200].

Clinical studies in adoptive immunotherapy have been carried on with the use of adjuvants such as BCG and with chemotherapy. In general, the benefit of such therapy is not clearly established although changes in immunity often result, such as response to recall antigens, induction of migration inhibition to antigen and induction of *in vitro* cytotoxicity against the tumour[201–203].

IMMUNE INSTRUCTION METHODS OF THERAPY

Immune instruction implies that an agent is administered to a suitable subject which produces specific immunity in the recipient to an antigen, presumably by inducing recognition in immunocompetent cells. The two substances presently used for immune instruction are transfer factor (TF) and immune RNA (I-RNA).

Transfer factor

Transfer factor is a low molecular weight polypeptide which is extracted from immune leukocytes by vacuum dialysis. The molecule, which is heat-stable, is not degraded by enzymes such as RNase and DNase, but loses its activity when incubated with pronase. TF transfers the cell-mediated immunity of the donor to a recipient. It does not transfer humoral immune responses and is itself non-immunogenic[161,204]. Transfer of cell-mediated immunity is confirmed by dermal response to specific antigen and by leukocyte adherence inhibition.

Discovery of the existence of transfer factor[205,206] and its subsequent study both in the laboratory and clinically, has been carried out by a number of investigators[207–211]. It has been shown to be effective in transferring sensitivity, and presumably immunity, across species barriers[212]. Work is in progress to raise specific xenogeneic transfer factor for clinical use[213]. Efforts to define the active moiety in TF has disclosed that the leukocyte dialysate may be separated into numerous fractions by utilizing column chromatography, isoelectric focusing and high-pressure reverse phase chromatography[214]. The active fraction has been isolated[215] and study of the remaining fractions shows that a cellular immunodepressant which is

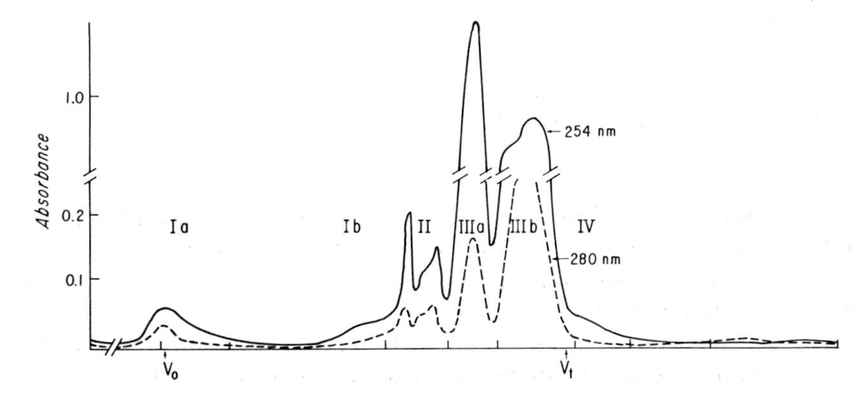

Figure 5.8 Sephadex G-25 exclusion chromatography of human TF. Fraction IIIa contains dermal transfer activity. Fraction IIIb contains antigen-independent dermal activity and may be augmentive. Fraction IV suppresses lymphocyte transformation

nicotinamide resides in at least one of the subfractions[216] (Figure 5.8). The molecular structure of TF appears to consist of a polypeptide chain linked to a chromophore[217]. Transfer factor has recently been reviewed in Conference[218].

Clinical studies

The use of transfer factor in cancer therapy has been studied by a number of investigators. The largest clinical study reported describes 35 patients with a variety of far-advanced tumours who were treated with TF[161]. One-third of these patients exhibited some favourable response and in six patients the index lesion regressed more than 50%. In three patients the tumour disappeared completely. The effect, however, persisted for only 1–12 months with an average of 3.6 months, and thus in this situation was not considered to be of great benefit to the patient, with one or two possible exceptions. During the period of tumour remission the patients developed positive dermal responses to allotype specific tumour antigen. The induced immunity was specific, since dermal responses to other tumour antigens did not occur. Recurrence of tumour was associated with loss of dermal response (Table 5.6). In addition, blocking factors often appeared in the serum as shown by suppression of blastoid lymphoid response to phytohaemagglutinin and by isolation of blocking factor by discontinuous electrophoresis.

Table 5.6 Delayed cutaneous hypersensitivity (DCH) responses to tumour antigens during transfer factor therapy

Patient groups	*No. of patients tested*	*No. of DCH responses*
Patients not responding clinically	8	0
Patients exhibiting serum blocking	5	0
Patients exhibiting a favourable clinical response (regression of tumour)	7	7
Patients with progression of tumour, after previously experiencing a favourable clinical response and +DCH	7	0

Of the remaining patients one-third clearly did not respond to TF therapy. Of these most exhibited serum blocking factors prior to beginning therapy. The remaining patients, although not blocked, exhibited depressed lymphoblastoid response (Table 5.7).

TF has been used in osteosarcoma to prevent metastases in patients either with or without remaining tumour after surgery. Donors for TF were tested for immunity by assaying lymphocyte cytotoxicity against tumour cells in culture. Specific immune response in the patient is also determined by cytotoxic assay[219].

Table 5.7 Pre-existence of serum blocking in 11 tumour patients not responding to TF immunotherapy

Patients	*Lymphocyte transformation (PHA)**		*Serum† blocking*
	Autologous serum	*Control serum*	
1	5 400	95 000	+
2	11 000	34 000	+
3	3 800	16 000	+
4	900	27 000	+
5	14 000	39 000	+
6	35 000	102 000	+
7	1 200	31 000	+
8	22 000	24 500	−
9	41 000	38 500	−
10	62 000	42 000	−
11	27 000	29 000	−

* CPM of [^{3}H]thymidine uptake in cultures supplemented with either autologous or control serum
† + serum blocking was significant ($p < 0.05$)

Assessment of immunity in patients and donors

Of paramount importance is the ability to detect and measure immunity in the patient and the donor of biological material. Immunity encompasses a wide variety of responses and cannot really be measured as a single entity. Of more importance is the dissection of immune response and ability to measure its component parts in order that specific deficiencies may be identified and treated. Cell-mediated responses and presumably immunity may be measured by skin testing with specific antigen, although in tumour systems there is often the question of the validity of the antigen. More recently migration inhibition factor, which is a lymphokine, has been used to test specific immunity. Still more recently Halliday reported the phenomenon where leukocytes from an immune individual were inhibited from adhering to a wettable surface such as glass after the cells had been incubated with antigen[220]. This observation has been developed into the leukocyte adherence inhibition (LAI) test for specific immunity. The test has been shown to correlate well with dermal response to antigen in melanoma, squamous cell carcinoma and neuroblastoma and exhibits specificity for the antigen tested[221]. The results in testing by dermal response and LAI in 234 subjects are shown in Figures 5.9 and 5.10.

The leukocyte adherence inhibition test

The test has been modified in order to make it clinically applicable and is performed in our laboratory as follows:[222]

Leukocyte preparation:
1. Collect 5 ml heparinized blood
2. Add 1 ml 3% dextran

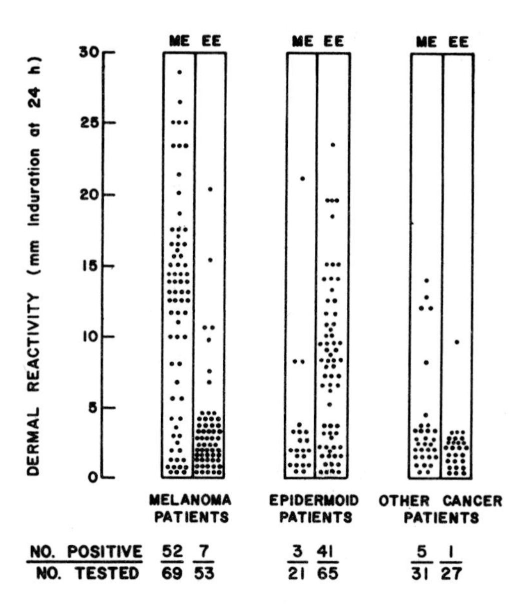

Figure 5.9 Delayed cutaneous hypersensitivity (DCH) results in cancer patients tested with 3 M KCl extracted melanoma (ME) and epidermoid carcinoma (EE) antigens. A high degree of specificity of DCH response is seen in each patient group

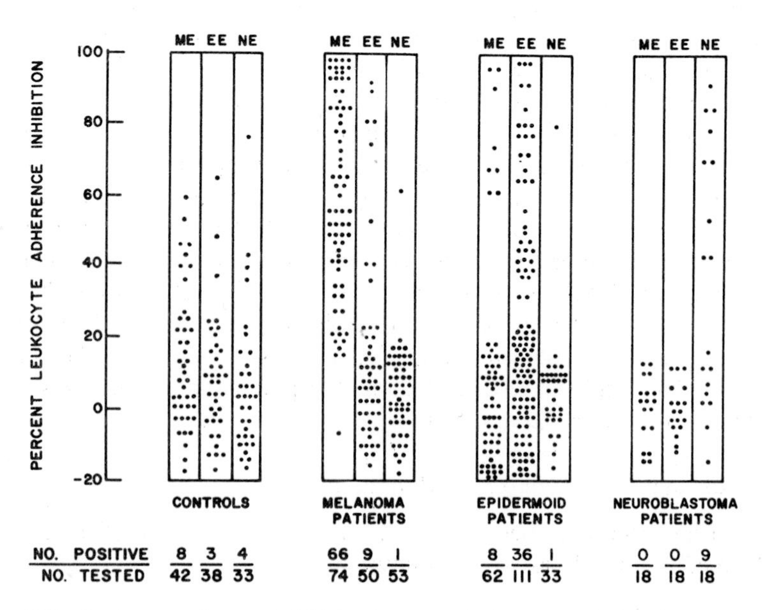

Figure 5.10 Leukocyte adherence inhibition (LAI) results in patients with melanoma, epidermoid carcinoma and neuroblastoma tested against 3 M KCl antigen extracts of these tumours (ME, EE, NE). A high degree of (+) LAI response is seen in each patient group

3. Incubate in plastic syringes for 30 min at 37 °C
4. Collect leukocyte layer
5. Add NH_4Cl for 10 min at 4 °C
6. Wash, count, dilute to 1–2 × 10^7/ml

Antigen preincubation:
1. Conduct incubation in non-wettable tubes
2. Add 0.60 ml media and 0.20 ml cells to control tubes
3. Add 0.15 ml media, 0.15 ml antigen, and 0.10 ml cells to 'test' tubes
4. Incubate at 37 °C for 30 min

Adherence incubation:
1. Transfer cell mixture to 10 ml conical glass centrifuge tubes
2. Count total cells in one control tube immediately
3. Incubate controls and 'test' tubes for 1–2 h at 37 °C

Cell quantitation and LAI calculations:
1. After incubation add 10 ml diluent to all tubes
2. Add red cell lysing agent (ZAP)
3. Count all tubes in Coulter Counter
4. $\text{LAI\%} = \dfrac{\text{Antigen induced non-adherent cells*}}{\text{Total adherent cells†}} \times 100$

The LAI test is particularly useful because it is an *in vitro* test for CMI and avoids the problems associated with skin testing with tumour antigen, especially in normal potential donors of biological immune material. Furthermore, the LAI test is easily performed and applied clinically.

Examples of the sequential use of the LAI test to determine CMI are as follows:

Patient A is a 60-year-old Caucasian male with level IV melanoma of the foot associated with groin metastases. He was treated with isolated hyperthermic perfusion of the involved extremity with L-phenylalanine mustard followed by wide resection of the primary lesion. At the same time ilio-inguinal lymphadenectomy was performed which subsequently revealed metastatic tumour in eight lymph nodes. LAI (Figure 5.11A) shows that CMI response was initially absent on two occasions. TF was added to the patient's therapy and CMI was established.

Patient B is a 4-year-old female child with Stage IV neuroblastoma who had been made tumour-free with a four-drug chemotherapy regimen. Serial LAI determinations (Figure 5.11B) show a waning CMI level although

---

* 'Test' – control
† Immediate control – control

the patient remained clinically well. At the 6-month point CMI is absent, but the definite diagnosis of recurrent tumour was not made until the ninth month. The patient was retreated with chemotherapy with return of CMI.

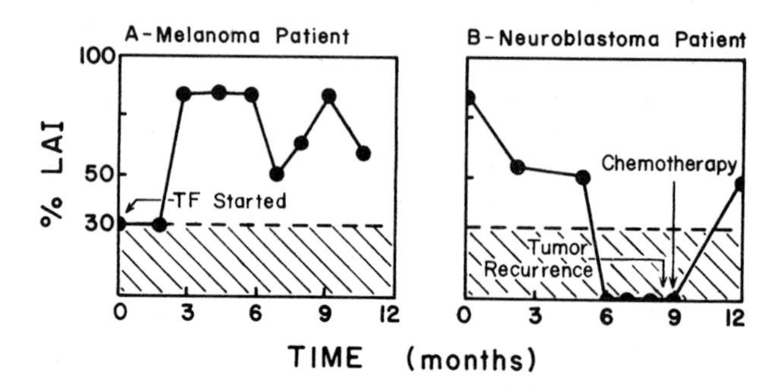

Figure 5.11 Sequential leukocyte adherence inhibition (LAI) testing in two patients with melanoma and neuroblastoma. Figure 5.11A shows establishment of (+) LAI response in melanoma following administration of transfer factor. Figure 5.11B shows loss of LAI response in neuroblastoma preceding discovery of tumour recurrence

Immune RNA

In 1962–4 Mannick and Egdahl first reported the mediation of immune responses to normal transplantation antigens with immune RNA (I-RNA)[223,224]. Immunity to skin allografts in rabbits was transferred by incubation of autologous spleen cells *in vitro* with RNA extracted from skin and lymph nodes of rabbits who had been specifically immunized. The autologous cells were later infused and accelerated skin graft rejection resulted. It was later found that I-RNA treated cells were cytotoxic to target cells *in vitro*[225,226]. After demonstration of tumour-specific antigenicity of most spontaneous virus tumours and carcinogen-induced animal tumours[227] a way was suggested for transfer of cellular tumour immunity. Subsequently growth retardation and occasional temporary regression of rat sarcoma was demonstrated after injection of RNA extracted from lymphocytes of sheep immunized against the rat sarcoma[228]. Other investigators using various animal models showed that the progress of tumours could be influenced by administering autologous or syngeneic lymphocytes which had been I-RNA instructed[229–231]. Finally I-RNA was administered directly with an RNase inhibitor and was found to confer resistance to a transplantable tumour[232,233].

Clinical trials using I-RNA have been carried out in two types of patients, those with grossly detectable metastatic disease, and those apparently free of tumour with a high expectancy of recurrence. The results are indeterminate but indicate that a small number of patients may have been helped[234].

At the present time it remains to be demonstrated, in spite of positive changes in cytotoxic indices, that I-RNA is clearly useful in the treatment of patients with cancer. There is no conclusive evidence that regression of established murine or human tumours occurs after I-RNA therapy. I-RNA, however, offers several possible advantages, at least for the present, over other methods of adoptive or instructional immunotherapy: (1) serum or plasma which may contain blocking factors need not be given; (2) sensitization to foreign leukocyte antigens is avoided; (3) possibility of graft-versus-host reaction is avoided; (4) I-RNA is not itself a strong antigen; (5) adjuvants are not required; (6) I-RNA may be more effective in conferring specific immunity than tumour antigens; and (7) I-RNA may be effective in spite of host anergy.

SPECIFIC ANTIBODIES FOR THE TREATMENT OF CANCER

Cytotoxic antibodies

Immune serum has been used successfully in the therapy of some infectious diseases. For this reason tumour immune serum obtained from 'cured' cancer patients or donors who have demonstrated antitumour antibodies has been used sporadically in the clinical care of cancer patients, but without consistent or sufficiently encouraging results. Some reasons proposed for lack of success is that specific antibodies may coat tumour cells, perhaps as antibody–antigen complexes, and thus enhance tumour growth[235,236], or specific antibodies may not be cytotoxic *in vivo*. Nevertheless, the use of specific antibodies in animal systems has been found to inhibit induction of experimental tumours[237,238], or even cause tumour regression[239]. Antibodies against an avian reticuloendotheliosis virus-induced tumour are specific for the tumour as shown by absorption against virus and tumour cells. The effect of specific antibodies on experimental tumours is partially dependent on host cellular response[240].

Antibody carriers for tumouricidal agents

A more recent and potentially quite useful approach is to employ specific antibodies as carriers of cytotoxic drugs or other agents such as toxins and isotopes. Antibodies have been used as carriers of radionuclides for detection of occult tumour as long as 30 years ago[241], but there is some evidence now that antitumour synergism exists between antibodies and a cytotoxic drug[242]. One of the problems with using immune globulin as a 'homing' device for a drug is that so much of the activity is distributed to the lungs, liver and spleen. This is not surprising since only a small amount of the globulin fraction consists of specific antitumour antibody. The method would be technically improved by isolation of specific antibody, perhaps by immunoabsorption as previously described for antilymphocyte antibody[243].

Globulin combined with chlorambucil has been used in a mouse lymphoma system resulting in improved survivals[244]. Thirteen patients with progressive metastatic melanoma were treated with antimelanoma globulin bound to chlorambucil against a control of imidazole carboximide-treated patients. Seven of the chlorambucil-antibody group experienced a favourable clinical response exhibiting a significant survival beyond 11 months in comparison to the test group[245]. Similar studies showing positive results have utilized antibody conjugated with such toxic substances as methotrexate[246], radioactive iodine[247], boron[248] and glucose oxidase[249].

SUMMARY AND CONCLUSIONS

Current concepts on tumour antigens and host responses to tumour antigens have been examined. There are numerous methods presently under study by which immune responses may be induced or otherwise affected by various biological engineering methods. Application of the host's immune response may someday become a most potent therapy against cancer. At present all clinical immunotherapy is investigative, the major role of such therapy at present being as an adjunct to conventional therapy. Under these conditions the contribution of immunity to tumour control is enormously difficult to evaluate. Reasons for this are that the definition of immunity itself is not entirely clear, and the significance of various *in vitro*, or for that matter *in vivo* tests, is not known. On the positive side, however, impressive advances in understanding immune response have occurred, and the increasing instances of favourable clinical reports in isolated cases or in small numbers of patients is a spur to the scientific and clinical investigative community. The future of the immune response as a cancer weapon should still be regarded with optimism.

ACKNOWLEDGEMENTS

The author wishes to thank his colleagues Denis R. Burger and Arthur A. Vandenbark for their review of the manuscript.

References

1. Chandradasa, K. D. (1973). The development and specific suppression of concomitant immunity in two syngeneic tumour-host systems. *Int. J. Cancer*, **11**, 748
2. Lausch, R. N. and Rapp, F. (1969). Concomitant immunity in hamsters bearing DMBA-induced tumor transplants. *Int. J. Cancer*, **4**, 226
3. Baldwin, R. W. and Pimm, M. V. (1973). BCG immunotherapy of a rat sarcoma. *Br. J. Cancer*, **28**, 281
4. Baldwin, R. W. and Price, M. R. (1976). Immunobiology of rat neoplasia. In: *International Conference on Immunobiology of Cancer*, **276**, 3 (New York Academy of Sciences)
5. Baldwin, R. W. and Embleton, M. J. (1969). Immunology of 2-acetylaminofluorene-induced rat mammary adenocarcinomas. *Int. J. Cancer*, **4**, 47
6. Prehn, R. T. (1975). Relationship of tumor immunogenicity to concentration of the oncogen. *J. Natl. Cancer Inst.*, **55**, 189
7. Baldwin, R. W. and Embleton, M. J. (1969). Immunology of spontaneously arising rat mammary adenocarcinomas. *Int. J. Cancer*, **4**, 430
8. Old, L. J. and Boyse, E. A. (1964). Immunology of experimental tumors. *Annu. Rev. Med.*, **15**, 167
9. Zöller, M., Price, M. R. and Baldwin, R. W. (1975). Cell-mediated cytotoxicity to chemically-induced rat tumours. *Int. J. Cancer*, **16**, 593
10. Baldwin, R. W. and Price, M. R. (1975). In: *Cancer: A Comprehensive Treatise* (F. F. Becker, ed.), **1**, 353 (New York: Plenum Press)
11. Currie, G. A. and Alexander, P. (1974). Spontaneous shedding of TSTA by viable sarcoma cells: its possible role in facilitating metastatic spread. *Br. J. Cancer*, **29**, 72
12. Vaage, J. (1974). Circulating tumor antigens versus immune serum factors in depressed concomitant immunity. *Cancer Res.*, **34**, 2979
13. Kaliss, N. (1958). Immunological enhancement of tumor homografts in mice: a review. *Cancer Res.*, **18**, 992
14. Hellstrom, K. E. and Möller, G. (1965). Immunological and immunogenetic aspects of tumor transplantation. *Progr. Allergy*, **9**, 158
15. Vetto, R. M., Burger, D. R., Vandenbark, A. A. and Nolte, J. (1975). The influence of serum blocking factors on cancer patients undergoing immunotherapy. *Am. J. Surg.*, **130**, 237
16. Zöller, M., Price, M. R. and Baldwin, R. W. (1976). Inhibition of cell-mediated cytotoxicity to chemically induced rat tumours by soluble tumour and embryo cell extracts. *Int. J. Cancer*, **17**, 129
17. Pellis, N. and Kahan, B. D. (1976). Specific tumor immunity induced with soluble materials: restricted range of antigen dose and of challenge tumor load for immunoprotection. *J. Immunol.*, **115**, 1717
18. Price, M. R., Preston, V. and Zöller, M. (1976). Evaluation of 51Cr release for detecting cell-mediated cytotoxic responses to solid chemically induced rat tumours. *Br. J. Cancer*, (In press)
19. McLaughlin, P. J., Pimm, M. V., Price, M. R. and Baldwin, R. W. (1976). *Int. J. Cancer* (In press)
20. Baldwin, R. W., Embleton, M. J. and Moore, M. (1973). Immunogenicity of rat hepatoma membrane fractions. *Br. J. Cancer*, **28**, 389
21. Embleton, M. J. Effect of BCG on cell-mediated cytotoxicity and serum blocking factor during growth of rat hepatoma. *Br. J. Cancer* (In press)
22. Kirchner, H., Chused, T. M., Herberman, R. B., Holden, H. T. and Lavrin, D. H. (1974). Evidence of suppressor cell activity in spleens of mice bearing primary tumors induced by Moloney sarcoma virus. *J. Exp. Med.*, **139**, 1473

23. Kirchner, H., Herberman, R. B., Glaser, M. and Lavrin, D. H. (1974). Suppression of *in vitro* lymphocyte stimulation in mice bearing primary Moloney sarcoma virus induced tumors. *Cell. Immunol.*, **13**, 32
24. Kirchner, H., Holden, H. T. and Herberman, R. B. (1975). Inhibition of proliferation of lymphoma cells and T lymphocytes by suppressor cells from spleens of tumor-bearing mice. *J. Immunol.*, **114**, 206
25. Herberman, R. B., Campbell, D. A. Jr., Oldham, R. K., Bonnard, G. D., Ting, C., Holden, H. T., Glaser, M., Djen, J. and Oehler, R. (1976). Immunogenicity of tumor antigens. In: *International Conference on Immunobiology of Cancer*, **276**, 26 (New York Academy of Sciences)
26. Ting, C. C. and Herberman, R. B. (1975). Specific afferent interference by antiserum of *in vivo* immunity. *Nature*, **257**, 801
27. Occhino, J. C., Glasgow, A. H., Cooperband, S., Mannick, J. A. and Schmid, K. (1973). Isolation of an immunosuppressive peptide fraction from human plasma. *J. Immunol.*, **110**, 685
28. Lilley, D. P., Burger, D. R. and Vetto, R. M. (1974). Tumor growth in the guinea-pig: alpha globulin changes associated with lymphocyte suppression. *J. Natl. Cancer Inst.*, **53**, 701
29. Vetto, R. M., Burger, D. R. and Lilley, D. P. (1974). Evaluation of immune status in tumor patients. *Arch. Surg.*, **108**, 558
30. Simmons, R. L., Lipschultz, M. L., Rios, A. *et al.* (1971). Failure of neurominidase to unmask histocompatibility antigens on trophoblast. *Nature New Biology*, **231**, 111
31. Simmons, R. L., Rios, A. and Ray, P. K. (1971). Immunogenicity and antigenicity of lymphoid cells treated with neurominidase. *Nature New Biology*, **231**, 179
32. Im, H. M. and Simmons, R. L. (1971). Modification of graft versus host disease by neurominidase treatment of donor cells. Decreased tolerogenicity of neurominidase treated cells. *Transplantation*, **12**, 472
33. Lundgren, G. and Simmons, P. O. (1971). Effect of neurominidase on the stimulatory capacity of cells in human mixed lymphocyte cultures. *Clin. Exp. Immunol.*, **9**, 915
34. Bagshawe, K. D. and Currie, G. A. (1968). Immunogenicity of L1210 Murine leukemia cells after treatment with neurominidase. *Nature (Lond.)*, **218**, 1254
35. Currie, G. A. and Bagshawe, K. D. (1968). The role of sialic acid in antigenic expression. Further studies of the Landschurz ascites tumor. *Br. J. Cancer*, **22**, 843
36. Bekesi, J. G., Arneault, G. Sr., Walter, L. *et al.* (1972). Immunogenicity of leukemia L1210 cells after neurominidase treatment. *J. Natl. Cancer Inst.*, **49**, 107
37. Weiss, L., Mayhew, E. and Ulrich, K. (1966). The effect of neurominidase on the phagocytic process in human monocytes. *Lab. Invest.*, **15**, 1304
38. Lee, A. (1968). Effect of neurominidase on the phagocytosis of heteralogous red cells by mouse peripheral macrophages. *Proc. Soc. Exp. Biol. Med.*, **128**, 891
39. Prager, M. D. and Bafechtel, F. S. (1973). Methods for modification of cancer cells to enhance their antigenicity. In: *Methods in Cancer Research* (H. Busch, ed.), **9**, 339 (New York: Academic Press)
40. Sanderson, C. J. and Frost, P. (1974). The induction of tumor immunity in mice using gluteraldehyde treated tumor cells. *Nature (Lond.)*, **248**, 690
41. Frost, P. and Sanderson, C. J. (1975). Tumor immunoprophylaxis in mice using gluteraldehyde treated syngeneic tumor cells. *Cancer Res.*, **35**, 2646
42. Klein, G. (1976). Discussion of natural immunity. In: *International Conference on Immunobiology of Cancer*, **276**, 39 (New York Academy of Sciences)
43. Kumar, V., Bennett, M. and Eckner, R. J. (1974). Mechanisms of genetic resistance to Friend virus leukemia in mice. *J. Exp. Med.*, **139**, 1093

44. Alexander, P., Eccles, S. A. and Gauci, C. L. L. (1976). The significance of macrophages in human and experimental tumors. In: *International Conference on Immunobiology of Cancer*, **276**, 124 (New York Academy of Sciences)
45. Levy, M. H. and Wheelock, E. F. (1974). The role of macrophages in defence against neoplastic disease. *Adv. Cancer Res.*, **18**, 131
46. Evans, R. (1972). Macrophages in syngeneic animal tumours. *Transplantation*, **14**, 468
47. Gauci, C. L. and Alexander, P. (1975). *Cancer Lett.*, **1**, 29
48. Eccles, S. A. and Alexander, P. (1974). Macrophage content of tumours in relation to metastatic spread and host immune reaction. *Nature (Lond.)*, **250**, 667
49. Hibbs, J. B., Lambert, L. H. and Remington, J. S. (1972). Possible role of macrophage mediated non-specific cytotoxicity in tumor resistance. *Nature New Biology*, **235**, 48
50. Evans, R. and Alexander, P. (1970). Co-operation of immune lymphoid cells with macrophages in tumour immunity. *Nature (Lond.)*, **228**, 620
51. Kaplan, A. M., Morahan, P. S. and Regelson, W. (1974). Induction of macrophage mediated tumor cell cytotoxicity by Pyran Co-polymer. *J. Natl. Cancer Inst.*, **52**, 1919
52. Keller, R. (1973). Cytostatic elimination of syngeneic rat tumor cells *in vitro* by non-specifically activated macrophages. *Journal*, **138**, 625
53. Hibbs, J. R., Lambert, L. H. and Remington, J. S. (1971). Resistance to Murine tumors conferred by chronic infection with intracellular protozoa Toxoplasma gondii and Besnoitia jellisoni. *J. Infect. Dis.*, **124**, 587
54. Parr, I., Wheller, E. and Alexander, P. (1973). Similarities of the antitumor actions of endotoxin lipid A and double stranded RNA. *Br. J. Cancer*, **27**, 370
55. Holterman, O. A., Klein, E. and Casale, G. P. (1973). Selection cytotoxicity of peritoneal leukocytes for neoplastic cells. *Cell. Immunol.*, **9**, 339
56. Ghaffar, A., Cullen, R. T., Dunbar, N. and Woodruff, M. F. A. (1974). Anti-tumor effect *in vitro* of lymphocytes and macrophages from mice treated with Corynebacterium parvum. *Br. J. Cancer*, **29**, 199
57. Cleveland, R. P., Meltzer, M. S. and Zbar, B. (1974). Tumor cytotoxicity *in vitro* by macrophages from mice infected with Mycobacterium bovis strain BCG. *J. Natl. Cancer Inst.*, **52**, 1887
58. Gershon, R. K., Carter, R. L. and Lane, N. J. (1967). Studies on homotransplantable lymphoma in hamsters. IV. Observations on macrophages in expression of tumor immunity. *Am. J. Pathol.*, **51**, 1111
59. Fidler, I. J. (1974). Inhibition of pulmonary metastasis by intravenous injection of specifically activated macrophages. *Cancer Res.*, **34**, 1074
60. Berke, G., Clark, W. R. and Feldman, M. (1971). *In vitro* induction of a heterograft reaction. Immunological parameters of the sensitization of rat lymphocytes against mouse cells *in vitro*. *Transplantation*, **12**, 237
61. Cohen, I. R., Globerson, A. and Feldman, M. (1971). Autosensitization *in vitro*. *J. Exp. Med.*, **133**, 834
62. Cohen, I. R. (1973). The recruitment of specific effector lymphocytes by antigen reactive lymphocytes in cell mediated autosensitization and autosensitization reactions. *Cell. Immunol.*, **8**, 209
63. Feldman, M., Cohen, I. R. and Wekerle, H. (1972). T-cell mediated immunity *in vitro*. An analysis of antigen recognition and target cell lysis. *Transplant. Rev.*, **12**, 57
64. Sugiura, K. and Stock, C. C. (1955). Studies in a tumor spectrum. III. The effect of phosphonomides on the growth of a variety of mouse and rat tumors. *Cancer Res.*, **34**, 1074
65. Treves, A. J., Carnaud, C., Trainin, N., Feldman, M. and Cohen, I. R. (1974). Enhancing T-lymphocytes from tumor-bearing mice: suppress host resistance to a syngeneic tumor. *Eur. J. Immunol.*, **4**, 722

66. Treves, A. J., Cohen, I. R. and Feldman, M. (1975). Immunotherapy of lethal metastases by lymphocytes sensitized against tumor cells *in vitro*. *J. Natl. Cancer Inst.*, **54**, 777
67. Treves, A. J., Schechter, B., Cohen, I. R. and Feldman, M. (1975). Sensitization of T-lymphocytes *in vitro* by syngeneic macrophages fed with tumor antigens. *J. Immunol.*, **116**, 1059
68. Takeda, K., Aizawa, N., Kikuchi, Y., Yamawaki, S. and Nakamura, K. (1966). Autoimmunity against methylcholanthrene-induced sarcomas of the rat in the autocthonous host. *GANN*, **57**, 221
69. Kikuchi, K., Ishii, Y., Ueno, H., Kanaya, T. and Kikuchi, Y. (1974). Analysis of tumor-specific cell-mediated immune reactions in the primary autocthonous host. *GANN Monograph on Cancer Research*, **16**, 99
70. Kikuchi, K., Kikuchi, Y., Phillips, M. E. and Southam, C. M. (1972). Tumor-specific, cell-mediated immune resistance to autocthonous tumors. *Cancer Res.*, **32**, 516
71. Gross, R. L., Steel, C. M., Levine, A. G., Singh, S. and Brubaker, G. (1975). *In vitro* immunological studies on East African cancer patients. III. Spontaneous rosette formation by cells from Burkitt lymphoma biopsies. *Int. J. Cancer*, **15**, 139
72. Jondal, M., Svedmyr, E., Klein, E. and Singh, S. (1975). Killer T cells in a Burkitt's lymphoma biopsy. *Nature (Lond.)*, **255**, 405
73. Stevens, D. A. (1972). Infectious mononucleosis and malignant lymphoproliferative diseases. *J. Am. Med. Assoc.*, **219**, 897
74. Sheldon, P. J., Hemsted, E. H., Papamichail, M. and Holborrow, E. J. (1973). Thymic origin of atypical lymphoid cells in infectious mononucleosis. *Lancet*, **i**, 2253
75. Vivolainen, M., Anderson, L. C., Lalla, M. and Von Essen, R. (1973). T-lymphocyte proliferation in mononucleosis. *Clin. Immunol. Immunopathol.*, **2**, 114
76. Jondal, M. and Klein, G. (1973). Surface markers on human B and T lymphocytes. II. Presence of Epstein-Barr virus receptors on B lymphocytes. *J. Exp. Med.*, **138**, 1365
77. Svedmyr, E. and Jondal, M. (1975). Cytotoxic effector cells specific for B-cell lines transformed by Epstein-Barr virus are present in patients with infectious mononucleosis. *Proc. Natl. Acad. Sci. USA*, **72**, 1622
78. Royston, I., Sullivan, J. L., Periman, P. O. and Perlin, E. Cell-mediated immunity to Epstein-Barr virus transformed lymphoblastoid cells in acute infectious mononucleosis. *N. Engl. J. Med.* (In press)
79. Klein, G., Giovanella, B. C., Lindahl, T., Fialkow, P., Singh, S. and Stehlin, J. S. (1974). Direct evidence for the presence of Epstein-Barr virus DNA and nuclear antigen in malignant epithelial cells from patients with poorly differentiated carcinoma of the nasopharynx. *Proc. Natl. Acad. Sci. USA*, **71**, 4737
80. Wolf, H., Zurhausen, H. and Becker, V. (1973). EB viral genomes in epithelial nasopharyngeal carcinoma cells. *Nature (Lond.)*, **244**, 245
81. Klein, E., Becker, S., Svedmyr, E., Jondal, M. and Vanky, F. (1976). Tumor infiltrating lymphocytes. In: *International Conference on Immunobiology of Cancer*, **276**, 207 (New York Academy of Sciences)
82. Vanky, F., Klein, E., Cornain, S., Bakacs, T., Stjernsward, J. and Nilsonne, U. Search for antitumor response in a bone tumor patient with a long clinical history. (In preparation)
83. Cudkowicz, G. and Bennett, M. (1971). Peculiar immunobiology of bone marrow allografts. I. Graft rejection by irradiated responder mice. *J. Exp. Med.*, **134**, 83
84. Paranjpe, M. S. and Boone, C. W. (1972). Delayed hypersensitivity to simian virus 40 tumor cells in Balb/c mice demonstrated by a radioisotope foot pad assay. *J. Natl. Cancer Inst.*, **48**, 563
85. Paranjpe, M. S. and Boone, C. W. (1974). Kinetics of the antitumor delayed hypersensitivity response in mice with progressively growing tumors: stimulation followed by specific suppression. *Int. J. Cancer*, **13**, 179

86. Nelson, K., Pollack, S. B. and Hellstrom, K. E. (1975). Specific antitumour responses by cultured immune spleen cells. I. *In vitro* culture method and initial characterization of factors which block immune cell-mediated cytotoxicity *in vitro*. *Int. J. Cancer*, **15**, 806
87. Thompson, D. M., Steele, P. K. and Alexander, P. (1973). The presence of tumor specific membrane antigen in the serum of rats with chemically induced sarcoma. *Br. J. Cancer*, **27**, 27
88. Baldwin, R. W., Bowen, J. G. and Price, M. R. (1973). Detection of circulation hepatoma D23 antigen and immune complexes in tumor-bearing serum. *Br. J. Cancer*, **28**, 16
89. Hellstrom, K. E. and Hellstrom, I. (1974). Lymphocyte-mediated cytotoxicity and blocking serum activity to tumor antigens. *Adv. Immunol.*, **18**, 209
90. Sjogren, H. O., Hellstrom, I., Bansal, L. C. and Hellstrom, K. E. (1971). Elution of 'blocking factors' from human tumor, capable of abrogating tumor-cell destruction by specifically immune lymphocytes. *Proc. Natl. Acad. Sci. USA*, **68**, 1372
91. Humphrey, J. H. and Dourmashkin, R. R. (1969). The lesions in cell membranes caused by complement. *Adv. Immunol.*, **11**, 75
92. Mayer, M. M. (1972). Mechanism of cytolysis by complement. *Proc. Natl. Acad. Sci. USA*, **69**, 2954
93. Henney, C. S. (1977). In: *Mechanisms of Tumor Immunity* (I. Green, S. Cohen and R. T. McCluskey, eds.), p. 55 (New York: John Wiley and Sons)
94. Segerling, M., Okanian, S. H. and Borsos, T. (1975). Chemotherapeutic drugs increase killing of tumor cells by antibody and complement. *Science*, **188**, 55
95. Borsos, T. and Rapp, H. J. (1965). Complement fixation on cell surfaces by 19S and 7S antibodies. *Science*, **150**, 505
96. MacLennan, I. C. M. (1972). Antibody in the induction and inhibition of lymphocyte cytotoxicity. *Transplant. Rev.*, **13**, 67
97. MacLennan, I. C. M. and Harding, B. (1974). Some characteristics of immunoglobulin involved in antibody dependent lymphocyte cytotoxicity. In: *Progress in Immunology* (L. Brent and J. Holborrow, eds.), **3**, 347 (New York)
98. Jerne, N. K. (1974). Towards a network theory of the immune system. *Am. Immunol. (Inst. Pasteur)*, **125C**, 373
99. Lewis, M. G., Ikonopisov, R. L., Nairn, R. C. *et al.* (1969). Tumour-specific antibodies in human malignant melanoma and their relationship to the extent of the disease. *Br. Med. J.*, **3**, 547
100. Morton, D. L., Eilber, F. R. and Malmgren, R. A. (1971). Immune factors in human cancer: malignant melanomas, skeletal and soft tissue sarcomas. *Prog. Exp. Tumor Res.*, **14**, 25
101. Boburtha, A. J., Chee, D. O., Laucius, J. F. *et al.* (1975). Clinical and immunological significance of human melanoma cytotoxic antibody. *Cancer Res.*, **35**, 189
102. Lewis, M. G. and Phillips, T. M. (1972). The specificity of surface membrane immunofluorescence in human malignant melanoma. *Int. J. Cancer*, **10**, 105
103. Lewis, M. G., Avis, P. J. G., Phillips, T. M. *et al.* (1973). Tumor-associated antigens in human malignant melanoma. *Yale J. Biol. Med.*, **46**, 661
104. Vaughn, J. H. (1972). In: *Arthritis and Allied Conditions* (J. L. Hollander and D. J. McCarthy, Jr., eds.), p. 153 (Philadelphia: Lee *b*nd Febiger)
105. Christian, C. L. (1975). In: *Laboratory Diagnostic Procedures in the Rheumatic Diseases* (A. J. Cohen, ed.), p. 95 (Boston: Little, Brown and Co.)
106. Cathcart, E. S. (1975). In: *Laboratory Diagnostic Procedures in the Rheumatic Diseases* (A. J. Cohen, ed.), p. 105 (Boston: Little, Brown and Co.)
107. Lewis, M. G., Phillips, T. M., Cook, K. B. *et al.* Possible explanation for loss of detectable antibody in patients with disseminated malignant melanoma. *Nature (Lond.)*, **232**, 52

108. Drew, R. L., Thompson, S. and Purdue, G. I. (1972). The immunogenicity of Proteus vulgaris OX 19 in the rabbit. *Pathol. Microbiol.*, **38**, 184
109. Oudin, J. (1966). The genetic control of immunoglobulin synthesis. *Proc. R. Soc. Ser. B.*, **166**, 207
110. Avrameas, S., Tadou, B. and Chuilon, S. (1969). Glutaraldehyde, cyanuric chloride and tetrazotized O-dianisidine as coupling reagents in the passive hemagglutination test. *Immunochemistry*, **6**, 67
111. Waller, M., Curry, S. and Richard, A. (1968). Serological specificity of IgG and IgM antiglobulin antibodies in anti-Gm(a) antisera. *Clin. Exp. Immunol.*, **3**, 631
112. Natvig, J. B. (1970). Human anti-gamma-globulin antibodies specific for gamma G heavy chain subclasses. *Immunology*, **19**, 125
113. Hartmann, D. and Lewis, M. G. (1974). Presence and possible role of anti-IgG antibodies in human malignancy. *Lancet*, **i**, 1318
114. Osterland, C. K., Harboe, M. and Kunkel, H. G. (1963). Anti-y-globulin factors in human sera revealed by enzymatic splitting of anti-Rh antibodies. *Vox Sang.*, **8**, 133
115. Singer, J. M. and Plotz, C. M. (1956). The latex fixation test. I. Application to the serologic diagnosis of rheumatoid arthritis. *Am. J. Med.*, **21**, 888
116. Winchester, R. I. and Agnello, V. (1970). 5th Pan American Congress of Rheumatology, p. 42 (Uruguay: Ponta del Este)
117. Fish, F., Witz, I. P. and Klein, G. (1975). The fate of immunoglobulin disappearing from the surface of coated tumour cells. *Clin. Exp. Immunol.*, **16**, 355
118. Cojenza, H. and Kohler, H. (1972). Specific suppression of the antibody response by antibodies to receptors. *Proc. Natl. Acad. Sci. USA*, **69**, 2701
119. Rowley, D. A., Fitch, F. W., Stuart, E. P. *et al.* (1973). Specific suppression of immune responses. *Science*, **181**, 1133
120. Waller, M. (1973). Correlation between diagnosis and results of serologic tests for antiglobulin antibodies. *Am. J. Med.*, **54**, 731
121. Lewis, M. G., Hartman, D. and Jerry, L. M. (1976). Antibodies and anti-antibodies in human malignancy: an expression of deranged immune regulation. In: *International Conference on Immunobiology of Cancer*, **276**, 316 (New York Academy of Sciences)
122. Eilber, F. R. and Morton, D. L. (1970). Impaired immunologic reactivity and recurrence following cancer surgery. *Cancer*, **25**, 362
123. Pinsky, C. M., Oettgen, H. F., El Domeiri, A., Old, L. J., Beattie, E. J. and Burchenal, J. (1971). Delayed hypersensitivity reactions in patients with cancer. *Proc. Am. Assoc. Cancer Res.*, **12**, 100
124. Pinsky, C. M., El Domeiri, A., Caron, A. S., Knapper, W. H. and Oettgen, H. F. (1974). Delayed hypersensitivity reactions in patients with cancer. Recent results. *Cancer Res.*, **47**, 37
125. Hersh, E. M., Gutterman, J. U. and Mavligit, G. M. (1976). Immunodeficiency in cancer and the importance of immune evaluation of the cancer patient. *Med. Clin. N. Am.*, **60**, 623
126. Hersh, E. M. and Friereich, E. J. (1968). Host defense mechanisms and their modification by cancer chemotherapy. In: *Methods in Cancer Research*, **IV**, 355 (New York: Academic Press)
127. Hersh, E. M., Gutterman, J. U., Mavligit, G. M., McCredie, K. B., Bodey, G. P. Sr, Freireich, E. J., Rossen, R. D. and Butler, W. T. (1973). Host defense, chemical immunosuppression and the transplant recipient, relative effects of intermittent versus continuous immunosuppression therapy with reference to the objectives of treatment. *Transplant. Proc.*, **5**, 1191
128. Sen, L. and Borella, L. (1973). Expression of cell surface markers and T- and B-lymphocytes after long-term chemotherapy of acute leukemia. *Cell. Immunol.*, **9**, 84

129. Heppner, G. H., Griswold, D. E., Lorenzo, J. D., Poplin, E. A. and Calabresi, P. Selective immunosuppression by drugs in balanced immune responses. *Fed. Proc.*, **33**, 1882
130. Old, L. J., Benacerraf, B., Clarke, D. A. and Goldsmith, M. (1960). The reticuloendothelial system and the neoplastic process. *Am. N.Y. Acad. Sci.*, **88**, 264
131. Dent, P. B. (1972). Immunodepression by ocogenic viruses. *Prog. Med. Virol.*, **14**, 1
132. Dent, P. B. (1975). Immunodepression by oncogenic viruses. In: *The Immune System and Infectious Diseases*, p. 95 (Basel: Karger)
133. Ceglowski, W. S. and Friedman, H. (1967). Suppression of primary antibody plague responses of mice following infection with Friend disease virus. *Proc. Soc. Exp. Biol. Med.*, **126**, 662
134. Ceglowski, W. S. and Friedman, H. (1968). Immunosuppression by leukemia viruses. I. Effect of Friend disease virus on cellular and humoral hemolysis responses of mice to a primary immunization with sheep erythrocytes. *J. Immunol.*, **101**, 594
135. Ceglowski, W. S. and Friedman, H. (1969). Immunosuppression by leukemia viruses. II. Cytokinetics of appearance of hemolysin forming cells in infected mice during arnanestic response to sheep erythrocytes. *J. Immunol.*, **102**, 338
136. Bennett, M. and Steeves, R. A. (1970). Immunocompetent cell functions in mice infected with Friend leukemia virus. *J. Natl. Cancer Inst.*, **44**, 1107
137. Borella, L. (1971). The immunosuppression effects of Rauscher leukemia virus upon spleen cells cultured in cell impermeable diffusion chambers. *J. Immunol.*, **107**, 464
138. Hayry, P., Rago, D. and Defendi, V. (1970). Inhibition of phytohemagglutinen and alloantigen-induced lymphocyte stimulation by Rauscher leukemia virus. *J. Natl. Cancer Inst.*, **44**, 1311
139. Strauss, R. R., Jacobs, A. A., Paul, B. B. and Sbarra, A. J. (1972). The role of the phagocyte in host-parasite interactions. XXXIV. The effect of phagocytizable particles and phyto-hemmagglutinin-P on DNA synthesis by spleen cells from leukemic and non-leukemic ADR mice. *J. Reticuloendoth. Soc.*, **11**, 277
140. Kamo, I., Kateley, J. and Friedman, H. (1975). Mastocytoma induced suppression of *in vivo* antibody formation. *Proc. Soc. Exp. Biol. Med.*, **148**, 833
141. Kamo, I., Patel, C., Kateley, J. and Friedman, H. (1975). Immunosuppression induced *in vitro* by mastocytoma tumor cells and cell-free extracts. *J. Immunol.*, **114**, 1749
142. Bendinelli, M. and Toniolo, A. (1976). Reversal of immunosuppression induced by Murine leukemia virus. In: *International Conference on Immunobiology of Cancer*, **276**, 431 (New York Academy of Sciences)
143. Siegel, B. V., Weaver, W. L. and Koler, R. D. (1964). Mouse erythroleukemia of viral etiology. *Nature (Lond.)*, **201**, 1042
144. Plescia, O. J., Smith, A. H. and Grinwich, K. (1975). Subversion of immune system by tumor cells and role of prostaglandins. *Proc. Natl. Acad. Sci. USA*, **72**, 1848
145. Strausser, H. and Humes, J. (1975). Prostaglandin synthesis inhibition: effect on bone changes and sarcoma tumor induction in balb/c mice. *Int. J. Cancer*, **15**, 724
146. Landsteiner, K. and Chase, M. W. (1942). Experiments on transfer of cutaneous sensitivity to simple chemicals. *Proc. Soc. Exp. Biol. Med.*, **49**, 688
147. Lawrence, H. S. (1949). The cellular transfer of cutaneous hypersensitivity to tuberculin in man. *Proc. Soc. Exp. Biol. Med.*, **71**, 716
148. Yonemoto, R. H. and Terasaki, P. I. (1972). Cancer immunotherapy with HLA compatible thoracic duct lymphocyte transplantation. *Cancer*, **30**, 1438
149. Yonemoto, R. H. (1976). Adoptive immunotherapy utilizing thoracic duct lymphocytes. In: *International Conference on Immunotherapy of Cancer*, **277**, 7 (New York Academy of Sciences)
150. Pisano, J. C. and Di Luzio, N. R. (1970). Purification of an opsonic protein fraction from rat serum. *J. Reticuloendoth. Soc.*, **7**, 386

151. Di Luzio, N. R. and Lindsey, E. S. (1973). Surgery-induced alterations in plasma recognition factor activity in normal renal donors and renal recipients. *Proc. Soc. Exp. Biol. Med.*, **142**, 715
152. Scovill, W. A. and Saba, T. M. (1973). Humoral recognition deficiency in the etiology of reticuloendothelial depression induced by surgery. *Ann. Surg.*, **178**, 59
153. Di Luzio, N. R., McNamee, R., Olcay, I., Kitahama, A. and Miller, R. H. (1974). Inhibition of tumor growth by recognition factors. *Proc. Soc. Exp. Biol. Med.*, **145**, 311
154. Mansell, P. W. A., Inchinose, H., Reed, R. J., Krementz, E. T., McNamee, R. and Di Luzio, N. R. (1975). Macrophage-mediated destruction of human malignant cells *in vivo*. *J. Natl. Cancer Inst.*, **54**, 571
155. Mansell, P. W. A., Krementz, E. T. and Di Luzio, N. R. (1975). *Beringwerk. Mitt.*, **56**, 256
156. Mansell, P. W. A. and Di Luzio, N. R. (1976). The *in vivo* destruction of human tumor by glucan activated macrophages. In: *Proc. N.C.I. Workshop Role of Macrophages in Neoplasia* (In press)
157. Di Luzio, N. R. and Riggi, S. J. (1970). The effects of laminarin, sulfated glucan and oligosaccharides of glucan on reticuloendothelial activity. *J. Reticuloendoth. Soc.*, **8**, 465
158. Masek, M. A., Rhoades, D. J. and Frenster, J. H. (1973). *In vivo* macrophage interaction with lymphocytes in Hodgkin's disease. *Proc. Am. Assoc. Cancer Res.*, **14**, 8
159. Kirchner, H., Glaser, M. and Herberman, R. B. (1975). Suppression of cell-mediated tumor immunity by Corynebacterium parvum. *Nature (Lond.)*, **257**, 396
160. Frenster, J. H. and Rogoway, W. M. (1970). Immunotherapy of human neoplasms with autologous lymphocytes activated *in vitro*. In: *Proceedings of the Fifth Leukocyte Culture Conference* (J. E. Harris, ed.), p. 359 (New York: Academic Press, Inc.)
161. Vetto, R. M., Burger, D. R., Nolte, J. E., Vandenbark, A. A. and Baker, H. W. (1976). Transfer factor therapy in patients with cancer. *Cancer*, **37**, 90
162. Eilber, F. R., Morton, D. L., Homes, E. C., Sparks, F. C. and Ramming, K. P. (1976). Immunotherapy with BCG for lymph node metastases from malignant melanoma. *N. Engl. J. Med.*, **294**, 237
163. Gutterman, J. U., Mavligit, G. M., Burgess, M. A., Cardenas, J. O., Blumenschein, G. R., Gottlieb, J. A., McBride, C. M., McCredie, K. B., Bodey, G. P., Rodriguez, V., Freireich, E. J. and Hersh, E. M. (1976). Immunotherapy of breast cancer, malignant melanoma and acute leukemia with BCG prolongation. *Cancer Immunol. Immunother.*, **1**, 99
164. Study Group for Bronchogenic Carcinoma (1975). Immunopotentiation with levamisole in resectable bronchogenic carcinoma: a double blind controlled trial. *Br. Med. J.*, **3**, 461
165. Bast, R. C. Jr., Bast, B. S. and Rapp, H. J. (1976). Critical review of previously reported animal studies of tumor immunotherapy with non-specific immunostimulants. In: *International Conference on Immunotherapy of Cancer*, **277**, 60 (New York Academy of Sciences)
166. Zbar, B., Bernstein, I. D., Bartlett, G. L., Hanna, M. G. Jr. and Rapp, H. J. (1972). Immunotherapy of cancer regression of intradermal tumors and prevention of growth of lymph node metastases after intralesional injection of living Mycobacterium bovis. *J. Natl. Cancer Inst.*, **49**, 119
167. Parr, I. (1972). Response of syngeneic Murine lymphomata to immunotherapy in reaction to the antigenicity of the tumor. *Br. J. Cancer*, **26**, 174
168. Mathé, G., Pouillart, P. and Lapeyraque, F. (1969). Active immunotherapy of L1210 leukemia applied after the graft of tumor cells. *Br. J. Cancer*, **23**, 814
169. Bansal, S. C. and Sjogren, H. O. (1973). Effects of BCG on virus facets of immune response against polyoma tumors in rats. *Int. J. Cancer*, **11**, 162

170. Fisher, B., Wolmark, N., Saffer, E. and Fisher, E. R. (1975). Inhibitory effect of prolonged Corynebacterium parvum and cyclophosphamide administration on the growth of established tumors. *Cancer*, **35**, 134
171. Hanna, M. G. Jr., Zbar, B. and Rapp, H. J. (1972). Histopathology of tumor regression after intralesional injection of Mycobacterium bovis. II. Comparative effects of Vaccinia virus, oxazolone, and turpentine. *J. Natl. Cancer Inst.*, **48**, 1697
172. Gutterman, J. U., Mavligit, G. M., Blumenshein, G., Burgess, M. A., McBride, C. M. and Hersh, E. M. (1976). Immunotherapy of human solid tumors with BCG: prolongation of disease-free interval and survival in malignant melanoma, breast and colorectal cancer. In: *International Conference on Immunotherapy of Cancer*, **27**, 9135 (New York Academy of Sciences)
173. Morton, D. L., Eilber, F. R., Holmes, E. C., Hunt, J. S., Ketcham, A. S., Silverstein, M. J. and Sparks, F. C. (1974). BCG immunotherapy of malignant melanoma: a seven-year experience. *Ann. Surg.*, **180**, 635
174. Mastrangelo, M. A., Berd, D. and Bellet, R. E. (1976). Critical review of previously reported clinical trials of cancer immunotherapy with non-specific immunostimulant. In: *International Conference on Immunotherapy of Cancer*, **277**, 94 (New York Academy of Sciences)
175. Zbar, B., Ribi, E. and Rapp, H. J. (1973). An experimental model for immunotherapy of cancer. *Natl. Cancer Inst. Monogr.*, **39**, 3
176. Yamamura, Y., Azuma, S., Taniyama, T., Sugimura, K., Hirao, F., Tokuzen, R., Okabe, M., Nakahara, W., Yasumoto, K. and Ohta, M. (1976). Immunotherapy of cancer with cell wall skeleton of Mycobacterium bovis-BCG: experimental and clinical results. In: *International Conference on Immunotherapy of Cancer*, **277**, 209 (New York Academy of Sciences)
177. Azuma, I., Ribi, E. E., Meyer, T. J. and Zbar, B. (1974). Biologically active components from mycobacterial cell walls. I. Isolation and composition of cell wall skeleton and component P3. *J. Natl. Cancer Inst.*, **52**, 95
178. Israel, L. (1974). Clinical results with Corynebacterium parvum. In: *Investigations and Stimulation of Immunity in Cancer Patients* (G. Mathé, ed.), **1**, 486 (New York: Springer Verlag)
179. Renoux, G. and Renoux, M. (1971). Effet immunostimulant d'un imidothiazole dans l'immunisation. Des souris contre l'infection par Brucella abortus. *Compt. Rend.*, **272**, 349
180. Symoens, J. and Brugmans, J. (1975). The effects of Levamisol on host defense mechanisms: a review. *Fogarty International Center Proceedings No. 28.* (Washington, D.C., U.S. Government Printing Office) (In press)
181. Editorial (1975). Immunological control of cancer. *Lancet*, **i**, 502
182. Spreafico, F. and Garattini, S. (1974). Selective anti-metastatic treatment: current status and future prospects. *Cancer Treat. Rev.*, **1**, 239
183. Sadowski, J. M. and Rapp, F. (1975). Inhibition by levamisole of metastases by cells transformed by herpes simplex virus type 1 (38776). *Proc. Soc. Exp. Biol. Med.*, **149**, 219
184. Amery, W. (1975). Double blind study with levamisole in resectable lung cancer. *London 9th International Congress of Chemotherapy*
185. Hirshant, Y., Pinsky, C. M. Wanebo, H. J. and Oettgen, H. F. (1976). Design of phase-I trials of immunopotentiators for cancer therapy: levamisole and Corynebacterium parvum. In: *International Conference on Immunotherapy of Cancer*, **277**, 252 (New York Academy of Sciences)
186. Bekesi, J. G., St-Arneault, G., Walter, L. and Holland, J. F. (1972). Immunogenicity of leukemia L1210 cells after neurominidase treatment. *J. Natl. Cancer Inst.*, **49**, 107

187. Sanford, B. H. and Codington, J. F. (1971). Further studies on the effect of neurominidase on the tumor cell transplantability. *Tissue Antigens*, **1**, 153
188. Simmons, R. L., Rios, A., Lundgren, G., Ray, P., McKhann, C. and Haywood, G. (1971). Immunospecific repression of methylcholanthrene fibrosarcoma with the use of neurominidase. *Surgery*, **70**, 38
189. Cunningham, T. J., Olson, K. B., Laffin, R., Horton, J. and Sullivan, J. (1969). Treatment of advanced cancer with active immunization. *Cancer*, **24**, 932
190. Simmons, R. L. and Rios, A. (1971). Immunotherapy of cancer: immunospecific rejection of tumors. *Science*, **174**, 591
191. Takita, H., Han, T. and Marabella, P. (1974). Immunotherapy in bronchogenic carcinoma: effects on cellular immunity. *Surg. Forum*, **25**, 235
192. Shibata, H. R., Jerry, L. M., Lewis, M. G., Wilkinson, R., Capek, A., Marquis, G. and Hartmann, D. (1976). Tumor immunotherapy with autologous irradiated tumor cells and oral BCG. *Cancer* (In press)
193. Takita, H., Minowada, J., Han, T., Takada, M. and Lane, W. W. (1976). Adjuvant immunotherapy in bronchogenic carcinoma. In: *International Conference on Immunobiology of Cancer*, **276**, 345 (New York Academy of Sciences)
194. Stewart, T. H. M., Hollingshead, A. C., Harris, J. E., Belanger, R., Crepran, A., Hooper, G. D., Sachs, H. J., Klaasen, D. J., Hirte, W., Rapp, E., Crook, A. F., Orizaga, M., Sengar, D. P. S. and Raman, S. Immunochemotherapy of lung cancer. In: *International Conference on Immunotherapy of Cancer*, **277**, 436 (New York Academy of Sciences)
195. Burton, R., Thompson, J. and Warner, N. L. (1975). *In vitro* induction of tumour-specific immunity. I. Development of optimal conditions for induction and assay of cytotoxic lymphocytes. *J. Immunol. Methods*, **8**, 133
196. Kall, M. A. and Hellstrom, I. (1975). Specific stimulatory and cytotoxic effects of lymphocytes sensitized *in vitro* to either alloantigens or tumor antigens. *J. Immunol.*, **114**, 1083
197. Rollinghoff, M. (1974). Secondary cytotoxic tumor immune response induced *in vitro*. *J. Immunol.*, **112**, 1718
198. Cerottini, J., Engers, H. D., MacDonald, H. R. and Brunner, K. T. (1974). Generation of cytotoxic T lymphocytes *in vitro*. I. Response of normal and immune mouse spleen cells in mixed leukocyte cultures. *J. Exp. Med.*, **140**, 703
199. Vandenbark, A. A., Burger, D. R. and Vetto, R. M. (1976). Human transfer factor: trials with an assay in guinea-pigs. In: *Transfer Factor: Basic Properties and Clinical Applications* (M. S. Ascher, A. A. Gottlieb and C. H. Kirkpatrick, eds.), p. 425 (New York: Academic Press)
200. Vandenbark, A. A., Burger, D. R. and Vetto, R. M. (1977). Human transfer factor activity in the guinea-pig. Absence of antigen specificity. *Clin. Immunol. Immunopathol.*, **8**, 7
201. Humphrey, L. J., Lincoln, P. M. and Griffin, W. O. Jr. (1968). Immunologic response in patients with disseminated cancer. *Ann. Surg.*, **168**, 374
202. Humphrey, L. J., Boehm, B., Jewell, W. R. and Boehm, O. R. (1972). Immunologic response of cancer patients modified by immunization with tumor vaccine. *Ann. Surg.*, **176**, 554
203. Seigler, H. F., Shingleton, W. W., Metzgar, R. S., Buckley, C. E. and Bergoc, P. M. (1973). Immunotherapy in patients with melanoma. *Ann. Surg.*, **178**, 352
204. Burger, D. R., Vetto, R. M. and Vandenbark, A. A. (1974). Preparation of human transfer factor: a time-saving modification for preparing dialyzable transfer factor. *Cell. Immunol.*, **14**, 332
205. Lawrence, H. S. (1974). Transfer factor in cellular immunity. In: *The Harvey Lectures Series 68*, p. 239 (New York: Academic Press)
206. Jeter, W. S., Tremaine, M. M. and Seebohm, T. M. (1954). Passive transfer of delayed

hypersensitivity to 2,4-dinitrochlorobenzene in guinea-pigs with leucocytic extracts. *Proc. Soc. Exp. Biol. Med.*, **86**, 251

207. Kirkpatrick, C. H. and Gallin, J. J. (1975). Suppression of cellular immune responses following transfer factor: report of a case. *Cell. Immunol.*, **15**, 470
208. Spitler, L. E., Wybran, J., Fudenberg, H. H. and Levin, A. S. (1973). Transfer factor therapy of malignant melanoma. *Clin. Res.*, **21**, 221
209. Lo Buglio, A. F. and Neidhart, J. A. (1974). A review of transfer factor immunotherapy in cancer. *Cancer*, **34**, 1563
210. Ascher, M. S. and Andron, L. A. (1976). *In vitro* properties of leukocyte dialysates containing transfer factor: micro method and recent findings. In: *Transfer Factor: Basic Properties and Clinical Applications* (M. S. Ascher, C. H. Kirkpatrick and A. A. Gottlieb, eds.), p. 3 (New York: Academic Press)
211. Burger, D. R., Wilson, B. J., Malley, A. and Vetto, R. M. (1974). The effect of anti-lymphocyte antibody on lymphocyte transformation: selective suppression of mitogen, MLC, and antigen stimulation of human lymphocytes. *Transplantation*, **17**, 541
212. Burger, D. R. (1973). Animal models for transfer factor. In: *Workshop on Basic Properties and Clinical Applications of Transfer Factor* (C. H. Kirkpatrick and D. Rifkind, eds.) (Washington: H.E.W.)
213. Kleisius, P., Burger, D. R., Malley, A. and Kramer, T. (1975). The passive transfer of coccidian and diptheria toxoid hypersensitivity across species barriers. *Transplant. Proc.*, **8**, 449
214. Vandenbark, A. A., Burger, D. R., Dryer, D. L., Daves, G. D. and Vetto, R. M. (1977). Human transfer factor: fractionation by electrofocusing and high pressure, reverse phase chromatography. *J. Immunol.*, **118**, 636
215. Burger, D. R., Vandenbark, A. A., Daves, R., Anderson, W. A. Jr., Vetto, R. M. and Finke, P. (1976). Human transfer factor: fractionation and biological activity. *J. Immunol.*, **117**, 789
216. Burger, D. R., Vandenbark, A. A., Daves, D., Anderson, W. A. Jr., Vetto, R. M. and Finke, P. (1976). Human transfer factor: identification of a suppressive component. *J. Immunol.*, **117**, 797
217. Burger, D. R., Vandenbark, A. A. and Vetto, R. M. Immunotherapy for cancer. In: *Proc. 3rd Internatl. Cong. Immunol., Sydney*. (In press)
218. *Transfer Factor: Basic Properties and Clinical Applications* (M. S. Ascher, A. A. Gottlieb and C. H. Kirkpatrick, eds.) (New York: Academic Press)
219. Byers, V. S., Levin, A. S., Le Cam, L., Johnston, J. O. and Hackett, A. J. (1976). Tumor specific transfer factor therapy in osteogenic sarcoma: a two-year study. In: *International Conference on Immunotherapy of Cancer*, **277**, 621 (New York Academy of Sciences)
220. Halliday, W. J. and Miller, S. (1972). Leukocyte adherence inhibition: a simple test for cell-mediated tumour immunity and serum blocking factors. *J. Cancer*, **9**, 477
221. Vetto, R. M., Burger, D. R., Vandenbark, A. A. and Finke, P. Changes in tumor immunity during therapy determined by leukocyte adherence inhibition and dermal testing. *Cancer* (In press)
222. Burger, D. R., Vandenbark, A. A., Finke, P., Malley, A., Frikke, M., Black, J., Acott, K., Begley, D. and Vetto, R. M. Assessment of reactivity to tumor extracts by leukocyte adherence inhibition and dermal testing. *J. Natl. Cancer Inst.* (In press)
223. Mannick, J. A. and Egdahl, R. H. (1962). Transformation of non-immune lymph node cells to state of transplantation immunity by RNA. *Ann. Surg.*, **156**, 356
224. Mannick, J. A. and Egdahl, R. H. (1964). Transfer of heightened immunity to skin homografts by lymphoid RNA. *J. Clin. Invest.*, **43**, 2166
225. Wilson, D. B. and Wecker, E. E. (1966). Quantitative studies on the behaviour of sensitized lymphoid cells *in vitro*. III. Conversion of 'normal' lymphoid cells to an immunologically

active status with RNA derived from isologous lymphoid tissues of specifically immunized rats. *J. Immunol.*, **97**, 512

226. Bondevik, H. and Mannick, J. A. (1968). RNA mediated transfer of lymphocytes v.s. target cell activity. *Proc. Soc. Exp. Biol. Med.*, **129**, 264
227. Klein, G. (1966). Tumor antigens. *Annu. Rev. Microbiol.*, **20**, 223
228. Alexander, P., Delorme, E. J. and Hall, J. G. (1966). The effect of lymphoid cells from the lymph of specifically immunized sheep on the growth of primary sarcomata in rats. *Lancet*, **i**, 1186
229. Ramming, K. P. and Pilch, Y. H. (1970). Mediation of immunity to tumor isografts in mice by heterologous ribonucleic acid. *Science*, **168**, 492
230. Ramming, K. P. and Pilch, Y. H. (1971). Transfer of tumor specific immunity with RNA: inhibition of growth of Murine tumor isografts. *J. Natl. Cancer Inst.*, **46**, 735
231. Deckers, P. J. and Pilch, Y. H. (1972). Mediation of immunity to tumor specific transplantation antigens by RNA: inhibition of isograft growth in rats. *Cancer Res.*, **32**, 839
232. Deckers, P. J. and Pilch, Y. H. (1971). Transfer of immunity to tumor isografts by the systemic administration of xenogeneic 'immune' RNA. *Nature New Biology*, **231**, 181
233. Pilch, Y. H., Ramming, K. P. and Deckers, P. J. (1971). Transfer of tumor immunity with RNA. *Isr. J. Med. Sci.*, **7**, 246
234. Pilch, Y. H., Fritze, D., de Kernion, J. B., Ramming, K. P. and Kern, D. H. (1976). Immunotherapy of cancer with immune RNA in animal models and cancer patients. In: *International Conference on Immunotherapy of Cancer*, **277**, 592 (New York Academy of Sciences)
235. Hellström, I., Hellström, K. E., Evans, C. A., Heppner, G. H., Pierce, G. E. and Yang, J. P. S. (1969). Serum-mediated protection of neoplastic cells from inhibition by lymphocytes immune to their tumor-specific antigens. *Proc. Natl. Acad. Sci. USA*, **62**, 362
236. Baldwin, R. W., Price, M. R. and Robins, R. A. (1972). Blocking of lymphocyte-mediated cytotoxicity for rat hepatoma cells by tumour-specific antigen-antibody complexes. *Nature New Biology*, **239**, 185
237. Law, L. W., Ting, R. and Stanton, M. (1968). Some biologic, immunogenic, and morphologic effects in mice after infection with a murine sarcoma virus. I. Biologic and immunogenic studies. *J. Natl. Cancer Inst.*, **40**, 1101
238. Pearson, G. R., Redman, L. W. and Bass, L. R. (1973). Protective effect of immune sera against transplantable Moloney virus-induced sarcoma and lymphoma. *Cancer Res.*, **33**, 171
239. Fefer, A. (1969). Immunotherapy and chemotherapy of Moloney sarcoma virus-induced tumors in mice. *Cancer Res.*, **29**, 2177
240. Hu, C. and Linna, T. J. (1976). Serotherapy of avian reticuloendothelosis virus-induced tumors. In: *International Conference on Immunotherapy of Cancer*, **277**, 634 (New York Academy of Sciences)
241. Pressman, D. (1958). In: *Second United Nations Geneva Conference*, p. 138 (London: Pergamon Press)
242. Davies, D. A. L. and O'Neill, G. J. (1973). *In vivo* and *in vitro* effects of tumour-specific antibodies with chlorambucil. *Br. J. Cancer*, **28 (Suppl. 1)**, 285
243. Vetto, R. M., Burger, D. R., Wilson, B. J. and Malley, A. (1973). Specific antilymphocyte antibody for use in transplantation. *Am. Surg.*, **39**, 429
244. Ghose, T., Norvell, S. T., Buclu, A., Cameron, D., Bodurtha, A. and MacDonald, A. S. (1972). Immunochemotherapy of cancer with chlorambucil-carrying antibody. *Br. Med. J.*, **3**, 495
245. Ghose, T., Tai, J., Guclu, A., Norvell, S. T., Bodurtha, A., Aquino, J. and MacDonald, A. S. (1976). Antibodies as carriers of radionuclides and cytotoxic drugs in the treatment and diagnosis of cancer. In: *International Conference on Immunotherapy of Cancer*, **277**, 671 (New York Academy of Sciences)

246. Mathé, G and TranBaLoc, B. J. (1958). Effect on mouse leukemia 1210 of a combination by diazo-reaction of amethopterin and gamma-globulins from hamsters inoculated with such leukemia by heterografts. *Acad. Sci. Paris*, **246**, 1626
247. Ghose, T., Cerini, M., Carter, M. and Nairn, R. (1967). Immunoradioactive agent against cancer. *Br. Med. J.*, **1**, 90
248. Hawthorne, M., Wiersma, R. and Takasugi, M. (1972). Preparation of tumor-specific boron compounds. I. *In vitro* studies using boron labelled antibodies and elemental boron as neutron targets. *J. Med. Chem.*, **15**, 449
249. Philpott, G., Bower, R. J. and Parker, C. W. (1973). Selective iodination and cytotoxicity of tumor cells with an antibody-enzyme conjugate. *Surgery*, **74**, 51

6
Bone Marrow Transplantation

D. W. van BEKKUM*, B. LÖWENBERG†
and H. M. VRIESENDORP*
*Radiobiological Institute TNO
†Erasmus University, Rotterdam

APPLICABILITY AND LIMITATIONS OF BONE MARROW TRANSPLANTATION

Among 200 bone marrow grafts performed before 1964 in patients with aplastic anaemia no survivors were obtained[1]. Currently, bone marrow transplantation has been established as a life-saving procedure in a number of clinical conditions. This is the outcome of the clinical application of laboratory research on various basic problems during the last 30 years. An increasing understanding of the pathophysiological aspects of graft-versus-host disease (GVHD) and of the mechanism of graft rejection, and advancing knowledge of the kinetics of proliferation and differentiation of haemopoietic stem cells (HSC) have contributed to this development. Especially by improved donor selection, significant progress has been made in the prevention and mitigation of GVHD. The exploration of the major histocompatibility complex (MHC) has led to the characterization of distinct loci (in man designated by HLA-A, HLA-B, HLA-C and HLA-D*) and has permitted the selection of donors who are identical to the recipient for these MHC determinants. At the same time preparative treatment schedules have been designed which suppress the anti-graft forces of the host and condition the recipient for accepting the allogeneic graft. Due to the primary disease, the preparation for engraftment or the presence of GVHD, nearly all

---

* HLA-A, HLA-B and HLA-C are defined by serological methods (SD antigens); HLA-D is usually defined in mixed lymphocyte culture (lymphocyte defined or LD antigens). The MHC of the mouse is designated H_2. The MHC of the dog and the rhesus monkey are in analogy to HLA identified with the letters DLA and RhLA, respectively.

recipients experience periods of greatly increased risk of infection and haemmorrhage, which require specific supportive care. Progress in granulocyte and thrombocyte transfusion methodology and in bacteriological decontamination with isolation in laminar air-flow systems seems to have resulted in better survival, although controlled studies are still lacking. Presently, bone marrow transplants are employed in patients with severe combined immunodeficiency (SCID), severe bone marrow aplasia and leukaemia (Table 6.1). The collected results indicate that the treatment of SCID—an otherwise fatal disease—by MHC identical bone marrow transplantation results in approximately 50% cures[2]. Bone marrow aplasia, if not improving spontaneously or following therapy with androgens and/or corticosteroids during the initial 3-month period, usually takes a fatal course[3–5] which can be prevented in approximately 50% of cases by treatment with an MHC identical bone marrow transplant[6–9]. The objective of bone marrow grafts in acute leukaemia patients is to obtain haemopoietic regeneration following a very aggressive course of anti-leukaemia therapy aimed at total eradication of the leukaemic cell population. The latter, inevitably, eliminates the normal haemopoietic cells. In acute leukaemia, refractory to chemotherapy, therapeutic regimens involving bone marrow transplantation have resulted in a 20% long-term survival rate[10,11]. In principle, bone marrow rescue would also apply to other tumours in which the disseminated malignant cells are to be wiped out by dosages of anticancer agents which in themselves may produce a lethal bone marrow aplasia. Bone marrow transplantation may thus enable the employment of more effective treatment modalities in primary bad risk patients with malignancies or in patients refractory to chemotherapy. This set of results roughly represents the clinical gain of transplanting haemopoietic cells derived from a healthy donor.

Table 6.1 Current applications of bone marrow transplantation

Condition	*Objective*	*Rate of survival*	*Present status*
Aplastic anaemia (including radiation accidents)	Haemopoietic regeneration	50–60%	First choice therapy
SCID	Immunological reconstitution	50%	First choice therapy
Leukaemia	Haemopoietic regeneration after intensive anticancer treatment	18% 50%*	Explorative
Dysfunctioning cell series, (e.g. granulocytic, erythrocytic)	Correction of abnormality	?	Preliminary
Disseminated malignancies	Haemopoietic regeneration after intensive anticancer treatment	?	Phase 1

* Monozygotic twin donor recipient pairs

Because of these advances, the restrictions interfering with bone marrow transplantation are of increasing concern (Table 6.2). As many as 30% of the grafts in patients with aplastic anaemia do not take[6,8,9] and thus fail to correct the disease. Despite sophisticated donor selection, GVHD still occurs in approximately half of the patients and has a fatal outcome in about 25%[6–8]. Failing engraftment or graft rejection, and GVHD taken together account for an approximately 50% failure rate in adult patients with aplastic anaemia.

Table 6.2 Major problems of clinical MHC identical bone marrow transplantation

Causative factors	*Incidence (%) in*		
	SCID	*Aplasia*	*Leukaemia*
Graft failure			
Insufficient cell numbers grafted Incomplete abrogation of host-versus-graft resistance (conditioning) Previous antidonor sensitization of host	0%	30%	5%
GVHD			
Inadequate donor selection Ineffective treatment	40%	50%	75%
Infections			
Underlying disease immunodeficiency in SCID patients granulocytopenia Application of immunosuppression in recipient (for conditioning; for GVHD prophylaxis or treatment) Secondary to GVHD	near 100%		

The following sections successively deal with an identification of the present problems in clinical bone marrow transplantation (in aplasia, SCID and leukaemia), and a discussion of the present status and perspectives of experimental research on marrow graft take and GVHD.

A PROBLEM ORIENTATION IN CLINICAL BONE MARROW TRANSPLANTATION

In aplastic anaemia and SCID the aim of the transplant manoeuvre is the repair of the underlying insufficiency of marrow function. In aplastic anaemia an analysis can be made of the recovery of thrombocytopoiesis, erythropoiesis and myelopoiesis from allografts in recipients who originally maintain normal immunological capacities. Allotransplantation in aplasia, therefore, lends itself conveniently to the study of the mechanism of allograft take and the effect of means to manipulate it. SCID on the other hand, represents a unique combination of B and T immunological incompetence.

In these patients, the occurrence of GVHD and lymphocytic regeneration can be adequately studied without the interfering factors associated with iatrogenic immunosuppression. In leukaemia the aim is to eradicate the malignant cells and substitute them by normal cells. The immunobiological aspects of bone marrow transplantation occurring in leukaemic patients are in essence the same as the ones in aplastic and SCID patients.

Aplastic anaemia

Almost half of the patients with aplastic anaemia subjected to MHC compatible marrow transplantation acquire and maintain good marrow function, resume normal life without the requirement of medication[12]. In young adults and particularly in infants the cure rate of bone marrow transplantation exceeds 70%[13]. A recently conducted prospective controlled trial has demonstrated that marrow transplantation is presently the therapy of choice in aplastic anaemia. Patients undergoing a marrow transplantation have a significantly superior survival rate as compared to those on transfusion and androgens/corticosteroids only[14]. This is the favourable side of the picture. The other side shows the approximately 50% of all recipients who do not benefit from the procedure.

Take failures in aplastic anaemia

In the compiled Seattle and Transplant Registry series, failing engraftment was experienced in 29 (28%) of a total of 103 evaluable patients[6–8]. Various factors have been analysed for prognostic significance of graft rejection, such as sex match or mismatch, donor age, donor recipient ABO groups, the extent of random donor transfusions and preceding prednisone or androgen treatment, none of which showed valid correlations with marrow graft failure. The administration of blood products of family members before transplantation appears to be correlated with a higher transplant failure rate than when unrelated donors are used for transfusion purposes[7]. Two parameters were found to be significantly associated with graft failure: (a) an increase in mixed lymphocyte culture (MLC) reactivity of the recipient against the donor; and (b) a transplant size below 3×10^8 cells per kg recipient body weight[15]. When both parameters were present, graft rejection occurred in eight out of 10 patients. If they were not involved, persistent takes were scored in all 16 patients. The slight increase in MLC response has been suggested to reflect a sensitization phenomenon of recipient against donor antigens by previous transfusions. This is indeed the most plausible explanation, although, failing a correlation between the elevated MLC reactivity and the number of previous transfusions, other possibilities are still open. It is conceivable, for example, that disease related factors (autoimmune features of the disease) determine the augmented MLC values in a proportion of the patients.

The association of take with the cell number grafted is not surprising, in view of the large body of experimental data in rodents, canines, and subhuman primates demonstrating this relationship[16–20]. Under the standard circumstances of recipient conditioning, most of the transplant failures have to be attributed to the inoculation of insufficient numbers of haemopoietic cells. One may predict that in man, as in animals, more specific conditioning regimens directed at the abrogation of allogeneic resistance[20] will be useful to promote a take. The development of effective means in overriding host-antigraft resistance is particularly important because the problems of engraftment are likely to be intensified when marrow transplantation will be advanced beyond MHC identity.

GVHD in aplastic anaemia

The improvement of transplantation results is equally dependent on avoidance of GVHD. Even when donor and recipient are matched for the MHC locus, GVHD evolves in approximately 50% of the cases and accounts for mortality in 25% of recipients[6–8]. In infants, the occurrence of GVHD is of the same order of magnitude (50%), but only 14% of them die[13]. This is not due to a different grading of the severity of GVH reactions in young recipients. It is most likely that infants tolerate the pathophysiological events associated with GVH reactions better. A sex mismatch between donor and host has been suggested to be predictive for post-graft GVHD[7,8]. An enumeration of those patients from the Seattle series who survived beyond at least 18 days post-transplantation and did have persisting grafts shows that 68% (of 25 patients) grafted with marrow from a sex mismatched donor, developed GVHD, whereas the occurrence of GVHD was 41% (of 22 patients) in sex identical donor–recipient pairs. From the considerable frequency of GVHD in spite of MHC and sex matching, it is apparent that other unknown variables between donor and recipient are involved. The immunogenetic details of the sex and MHC control of GVH are discussed below. Presently, these two parameters seem to provide the best available selection criteria for sibling donor–recipient pairs.

Early transplantation in aplastic anaemia

It may be expected that the results of bone marrow transplantation may further improve if those patients who have an unfavourable prognosis on conservative treatment are transplanted earlier. This may reduce the considerable pre-transplant mortality and also avoid interfering effects on the outcome of the transplantation (e.g. sensitization by transfusions). It has been computed that if account is taken of both the survival rate without transplantation (spontaneous recovery or recovery after drug and transfusion therapy) and that following marrow transplantation, an early transplantation protocol (at 3 weeks after presentation of the patient) may ensure a net gain of survival of almost 20% over transplantation at 4 months[3]. The same tendency was evident from a comparison of the survival rate after bone marrow transplantation undertaken at 3 months (55%) and at 9 months after diagnosis (only 13%)[6]. Attempts to delineate a bad risk group among patients with aplastic anaemia are desirable. Some recent studies indicate that patients with reticulocyte counts below 10 000 per μl[4,5] and with a post-hepatitis aplastic anaemia[21] are candidates for early marrow transplantation. There is no doubt that the same applies for any patient who has the exceptional opportunity of an identical twin sibling as the source of syngeneic marrow.

SCID

SCID is the result of a congenital differentiation anomaly of the HSC which prevents them proceeding along the lymphatic pathway to mature into B and T lymphocytes. The transfer of sufficient numbers of HSC with normal differentiation capacities may lead to a lasting immunological reconstitution. Due to the primary immunodeficiency SCID patients are theoretically ideal recipients from the point of view of graft acceptance. At the same time, they represent a special hazard because they are extraordinarily susceptible for developing GVHD. This is borne out by the present experience in SCID.

Take of graft in SCID

All genotypically MHC identical marrow transplantations in patients who survived long enough to be evaluated demonstrated evidence of engraftment[2]. Of the 24 evaluable patients who received marrow from a related donor identical for some of the MHC loci or a phenotypically MHC identical donor 21 (88%) showed a take. Engraftment occurred irrespective of the cell number given (even with cell numbers as small as 10^6 cells per kg).

GVHD in SCID

The original observation that a single blood transfusion was able to induce lethal GVH reactions in immunodeficient SCID patients[22–25] has caused great caution. It has generally led investigators to transplant smaller numbers of cells than are usual in aplastic anaemia, for example, and this has probably beneficially influenced the frequency of GVHD.

In genotypically MHC identical donor–recipient pairs, GVHD was evident in five out of 14 evaluable individuals and was probably the cause of death in one recipient. Of the collected patients (evaluable for GVHD) receiving marrow with an incomplete genotypical MHC match a proportion of 86% (18/21) manifested GVHD and the overall results of immune reconstitution and survival were poor[2].

Several approaches have been practiced in avoiding or mitigating the effects of GVHD (Table 6.3). The successful reconstitution of one SCID infant with HLA-D identical but HLA-A and B incompatible bone marrow from family members[26] has been thought to represent a lead for expansion of the category of useful donors. So far, nine transplantations with HLA-D identical marrow have been reported in SCID. All but one developed symptoms of GVHD. Six patients died from infections associated with the GVH reactions. The remaining three patients are surviving with recovery of immunological function. It is evident from these data that a partial genotypical MHC match for the HLA-D locus may suffice to avoid lethal GVH reactions, even in SCID, and permit survival in a small minority of recipients. Not enough data are available to demonstrate a statistically significant difference between HLA-D matched or HLA-D mismatched family donors. Reliable recommendations for donor selection when an MHC identical sibling is not available, cannot yet be given. In view of the fact that even marrow grafts from full-house MHC identical siblings induce GVH reactions in a considerably frequency, partial MHC matching cannot be expected to fulfil the needs of a generally preventive method.

Table 6.3 Approaches for the control of GVHD in severe combined immunodeficiency

Available
Donor selection (MHC identity)
Limitation of transplant size
Elimination of T lymphocytes from graft
Immunosuppression post-transplantation
Institution of gnotobiotic state
In development
Fetal liver cell transplantation
Improvement of donor selection (typing for GVHD controlling loci within and outside MHC)

The data of the Transplant Registry suggest that the risks of GVHD are greater when very large transplants are given[2], which is in agreement with the abundant experimental evidence in animals of the positive correlation of graft size and incidence and severity of GVHD. The excellent takeability of allogeneic marrow in SCID is another strong reason to administer limited numbers of cells. This notion has been substantiated in the approach to employ very small numbers of cells to start with and, if no take is accomplished, to stepwise increase this number with any subsequent attempt (the so-called 'sneak-in' approach)[27].

Another line of action aimed at the avoidance of GVHD in SCID patients has involved the separation of lymphocytes from the graft prior to transplantation by discontinuous albumin gradient centrifugation[28–31] (see below). Application of stem cell fractions from MHC *in*compatible donors selectively depleted of T cells has fully prevented the early appearance of acute GVHD[32,33], which is the rule under these conditions[34]. The method was applied in patients who were not decontaminated and did not preclude the more protracted GVH syndrome. The patients died of bacterial infections associated with GVHD. It is necessary to pursue and evaluate the latter method in combination with complete bacterial decontamination and isolation.

Fetal liver grafts in SCID

Fetal liver cell transplants have gained increased interest as an alternative for bone marrow transplantation, since it was shown in animals that these grafts do not evoke acute GVHD, and secondly, lead to less severe delayed GVH reactions than allogeneic marrow cells[35–42]. The absence of acute GVHD is due to the very low numbers of immunocompetent cells in fetal liver tissue, whereas the nature of the observed mitigation of the delayed GVH reaction has been traced back to the distinct differentiation properties of fetal HSC[33,38]. Significant problems have been encountered in accomplishing engraftment, however. In the three largest series comprising 19 patients, no definite engraftment or immunological reconstitution ensued[43–45]. This is a major obstacle to a routine applicability of fetal liver cell transplantation at present. Results of animal studies suggest that the lower cell concentration of HSC in fetal liver than in marrow and the higher susceptibility to allogeneic suppression, may play a role in these failures[46,47]. Also the employment of the less efficient intraperitoneal route of transplantation and the frequent usage of frozen fetal liver cells (without monitoring stem cell viability) may have interfered with successful engraftment[47].

After the many negative clinical results with grafts of fetal liver cells, recently immunological reconstitution has been obtained in six infants. These represent the first successful transplantations in man using fully MHC incompatible haemopoietic cells. These fetal livers were obtained from embryos of less than 12 weeks' gestation. Although the clinical results available are rather fragmentary, they suggest that fetal livers of a maturation age of 8–12 weeks provide better chances of immune reconstitution. This maturation of human fetal liver is in accordance with that of mouse embryo liver if account is taken of the comparative stage of ontogenetic development of both species[48]. Although long-term results of immune reconstitution are still unknown, the remarkably minor degree of GVHD in spite of full MHC incompatibility warrants continuing investigations directed at elucidating the nature of the difficulties with older fetal liver cell transplants.

Other deficiencies of the haemopoietic system

Bone marrow transplantation in SCID is an outstanding example of the approach that the deficiency of one haemopoietic cell line of differentiation may be restored by the inoculation of normal HSC. This approach may be of a more general applicability. It may not only apply to the reconstitution of an absent cell line, but perhaps also to the replacement of aberrant or dysfunctioning blood cell lineages. So far, little experience has been obtained with the latter approach. In individual cases of patients with a congenital selective red cell aplasia[49], severe neutrophil dysfunction and intractable infections[50], chronic granulomatous disease[51] and paroxysmal nocturnal haemoglobinuria (PNH)[52] corrections of the basic haematological abnormality following marrow engraftment were obtained. These initial efforts support the validity of the notion that as marrow transplantation is gradually becoming a safer procedure in itself, it may attain a broader applicability, not only in acute fatal haemopoietic cell line disorders, but also in diseases with a considerable morbidity.

Leukaemia

Bone marrow transplantation in leukaemia comprises a combined effort to extinguish the malignant cell population and restore normal haemopoiesis. The success of this kind of treatment depends both on the quality of antileukaemic therapy preceding the marrow graft and on that of the transplantation procedure itself. The procedure of marrow transplantation is not basically different from that in aplastic anaemia.

A large series of patients with leukaemia have been subjected to transplantation with MHC identical marrow[11]. They were end-stage patients and had previously been treated with multiple drug, high dose chemotherapy schedules. Due to the intensive antileukaemic treatment (chemotherapy combined with total body irradiation (TBI)) take failures seldom occur (5%), even with cell numbers as low as 5×10^7 cells per kg.

Presumably for the same reason, the incidence of GVHD in leukaemic patients is impressive and outnumbers that in aplastic anaemia. Of those patients with sustained engraftment 80% developed GVHD[11,53].

Infectious complications after transplantation in leukaemia

Infectious complications are an especially critical problem in marrow transplantation in acute leukaemia. More than half of the patients who died did so from interstitial pneumonia or other infections[53]. In most instances, these complications coincided with the presence of GVHD. Both the GVHD, the severe immunosuppressive effects of the conditioning and the intensive chemotherapy to which the recipients have been exposed predispose to infection. The patterns of infection are typical of the ones of compromised patients in that they are Gram-negative bacterial, fungal and also viral infections. One-third of the patients who survive the immediate post-transplantation period with repopulation by donor marrow, develop a fatal bilateral interstitial pneumonia. In the majority of patients, the pneumonia is caused by viral agents (predominantly cytomegalovirus), or *Pneumocystis carinii* but in others no pathogens are found. The adverse influence of GVHD is apparent from the far higher frequency of lethal interstitial pneumonitis in the patients with moderate-severe GVHD (52% fatal pneumonitis) as compared with those without GVHD (11%).

Recurrent leukaemia after transplantation

Another source of failure is the relapse or persistence of leukaemia. This occurs in 31% of patients[11]. It has been calculated that the relapse rate would be as high as 65% if all problems concerned with bone marrow transplantation *per se* would be overcome[54]. Intensification of the antileukaemia pretreatment has been tested in a small trial and seems effective in further suppressing the recurrence rate[55]. The data suggest an inverse relationship between the severity of GVHD and the relapse incidence. Of 19 patients without GVHD 63% relapsed, whereas of 50 patients with moderate-severe GVHD only 12% had recurrent leukaemia. The question as to whether this is due to a graft-versus-leukaemia reaction as a component of GVHD[56,57] cannot be answered. The lower frequency of leukaemia relapse in association with GVHD was largely determined by the significantly shorter observation period (shorter survival) of patients with GVHD.

The fact that 13% of end-stage leukaemia patients acquired a continuing long-term remission and remain disease-free for 1–4 years without maintenance chemotherapy demonstrates the potential value of bone marrow transplantation. A prospective identification of leukaemia patients who will become resistant to chemotherapy, would allow for an earlier application of bone marrow transplantation and perhaps decrease the complication rate. The recurrence of leukaemia, the high percentage of GVHD and, last but not least, the numerous infectious complications are presently the major determinants of the prospects of allogeneic marrow transplantation in leukaemia.

Isogeneic and autologous transplants in leukaemia

The detrimental role of GVHD in the fate of the recipients with leukaemia is also suggested by the comparatively superior results in a series of 23 patients treated with identical twin marrow[10]. In only two of them did late infectious problems occur. The long-term survivors were not subject to frequent infections and showed adequate recovery of humoral and cellular immune responses[58]. In these patients the major cause of failure was an insufficient antileukaemic effect (40% failure of remission induction or relapse). The merit of the combined leukaemia eradication treatment and marrow transplantation is illustrated by the survival of ten of these patients. Eight of them are surviving between 12 and 36 months. It should be mentioned that immunotherapy during the first 3 weeks after transplantation may have had a role in these results, and that long-term responses were obtained in the absence of maintenance therapy[58]. These data in monozygotic twins indicate that when immunobiological graft–recipient interactions can be overcome promising possibilities exist for an incorporation of bone marrow transplantation in anticancer treatment.

Theoretically, the infusion of autologous marrow (or remission marrow in leukaemic patients) aspirated and preserved before the exposure to anticancer therapy or during remissions, offers an interesting possibility for marrow regeneration[59,60]. This approach has, so far, not had a systematic trial so that its usefulness remains to be determined.

EXPERIMENTAL STUDIES OF THE TAKE OF ALLOGENEIC HAEMOPOIETIC STEM CELLS

Generally the purpose of a treatment with allogeneic haemopoietic cells is to obtain a lasting establishment (= 'take') of a new and functionally active haemopoietic system in the recipient[17]. A crucial role in the realization of this objective is played by the pluripotent HSC. The maintained production of sufficient numbers of donor type erythrocytes, granulocytes, monocytes, thrombocytes and lymphocytes is absolutely dependent on the combined capacities of HSC for extensive self-replication and differentiation into end cells. Initially, the low and different concentrations of HSC in the various available sources of haemopoietic tissues (such as bone marrow, fetal liver, blood) has severely limited progress in the analysis of the take process[61]. Better possibilities for a detailed quantitative analysis became available with the advent of new assays. The number of HSC in a cell suspension can be determined in rodents, by counting the number of haemopoietic spleen colonies formed in isogeneic irradiated mice or rats after injection of graded numbers of cells[33,62]. In other species spleen colony assays cannot be performed. However, *in vitro* bone marrow colony formation has been described for many species including man[63]. The cells enumerated in such an assay are commonly thought of as committed granulocyte progenitor cells[61,64]. The close proximity of these cells to HSC in the haemopoietic differentiation pathway makes them a reasonable alternative for a quantitative estimate of the HSC content of a given cell suspension.

Table 6.4 Take of allogeneic haemopoietic cells

1. Analysis of take process	*2. Obstacles to take*	*3. Abrogation of obstacles to take*
(a) Space	(a) 'Innate' resistance of host	(a) Conditioning of host
(b) Homing	(b) Acquired resistance of host	(b) Origin of haemopoietic cells
(c) Self-replication		(c) 'Contaminating' cells
(d) Differentiation		(d) Host–donor relationship

Three major areas of interest have been identified in studies of take problems. They are listed with more detailed subdivisions in Table 6.4 and will be discussed in the following paragraphs.

Analysis of the take process

Space

It has been suggested that the haemopoietic areas need to be emptied to enable allogeneic HSC to grow in a new recipient. In mice, smaller numbers of parental lymphocytes are needed to kill an F_1 recipient by a GVH reaction if the recipient is preconditioned with TBI[27,65]. One possible explanation for this increased efficiency of lymphocytes after TBI is that they do not have to compete with host lymphocytes for space and nutrients. This space factor is, however, probably of only minor importance in transplants of haemopoiesis. Effective bone marrow transplants can be performed from normal co-isogeneic donors in W^v/W^v anaemic mice without any conditioning[66]. Also, allogeneic bone marrow grafts are successful without prior TBI or other space creating treatments in SCID patients who have normal erythro-, granulo- and thrombopoiesis[2]. Moreover, bone marrow space seems to be sufficiently available in patients[7] or animals[17,67,68] suffering from aplastic anaemia, yet drastic immunosuppression is needed to achieve a take of allogeneic bone marrow. These data indicate that host reactivity towards the donor is a more important factor in transplant failure than lack of space for donor HSC. Current methods in preparing (= 'conditioning') recipients usually create bone marrow space as well as decrease the host resistance against allogeneic cells. The more bizarre events in bone marrow transplantation, e.g. late reversals[17,69], split chimeras[17,69,70] or late graft failures[17,71] may all be explained by assuming that the applied conditioning protocol was ineffective in removing the host bone marrow cells and/or suppressing recipient antidonor reactivity.

Homing

Intravenously injected HSC will, after a short stay in lung capillaries, migrate to the appropriate extravascular areas in the bone marrow and spleen[72,73]. It can be calculated that from i.v. injected isogeneic HSC, approximately one out of four reaches the bone marrow cavity to initiate haemopoiesis*[33].

---

* The spleen colony assay has been used to quantify the number of HSC that can be recovered from the haemopoietic tissues early after injection. This has provided a direct measure of the 'homing' fraction. It has been found that 0.4% homes in one femur and 4.1% in the spleen[82,92]. The content of one femur shaft represents approximately 1/60 of the total marrow cellularity. Thus it can be computed that $(60 \times 0.4) + 4.1 = 28\%$ of all HSC grafted settle in the appropriate sites of haemopoiesis.

The reasons for the loss of the other three-quarters of HSC are obscure. The homing behaviour of HSC precludes the necessity of finding ways to deposit HSC directly in the bone marrow cavity. The intravenous route of administering HSC is preferred over other ways of administration, because it has a higher efficacy. Compared to the i.v. route, the i.p. route has a 33% efficacy in monkeys[74] and 2% efficacy in mice[75]. Injections of haemopoietic cells in brain or testicles[17] were not effective at all. These latter injection sites were investigated, because they were reported to be 'immunologically privileged sites', where less rejection of allogeneic tissues would occur. The lack of proliferation of HSC in these sites might be due to the presence of unexpected host resistance mechanisms or to the absence of the appropriate stimuli for HSC to initiate a haemopoiesis (lack of haemopoietic inductive microenvironment, see below).

Self-replication and differentiation of HSC

After homing, an HSC can rest, self-replicate or differentiate into one of the four possible lines (i.e. the erythrocytic, granulocytic, thrombocytic or lymphocytic pathway). The mechanisms which control these options are largely unknown[33,61,64]. One of the current hypotheses, known by the term HIM (haemopoietic inductive microenvironment) postulates an important role for bone marrow stroma in the induction of differentiation and possibly of homing of HSC[76]. Practical implications of this concept cannot be foreseen until more fundamental knowledge of HIM has been obtained. More details have become available regarding the identification of factors stimulating later cell stages in haemopoiesis (e.g. colony stimulating factor (CSF)[64], erythropoietin[77] and factors for lymphocytic differentiation[78]). Some of these factors appear to be elevated in serum after TBI or after tissue damage by other agents[79] and might promote haemopoietic recovery in an irradiated recipient.

Obstacles to a take

The obstacles to a HSC take, discussed above, are active resistance mechanisms mediated by the host. It is not known in detail where these resistance phenomena interfere with the take of donor HSC.

'Innate' or allogeneic resistance of the recipient

Early studies[16] have shown that protection of animals against radiation or chemically induced bone marrow aplasia requires lower numbers of autologous than of allogeneic bone marrow cells. Results from a recent analysis[20] in mice are given in Figure 6.1. About 30 times more F_1 bone marrow cells and about 60 times more allogeneic or xenogeneic rat cells than autologous cells are required to provide radioprotection in 50% of the animals. This shows that histoincompatible HSC can be inactivated in recipients after supralethal TBI, and that the proportion of inactivated HSC is dependent on histocompatibility differences between donor and recipient. The wider the difference, the larger the proportion of inactivated injected HSC. This is one of the major limitations to a more general application of allogeneic bone marrow transplantation in human patients. If the same ratios in cell requirements hold true for man, not enough HSC can be obtained from a single living donor to secure a lasting take. Assuming 2×10^7 cells per ml bone marrow and a total need of 10^9 bone marrow cells per kg body weight, approximately 3.5 litres of bone marrow would be required for a 70 kg MHC incompatible recipient. Innate, or as it is usually named allogeneic, resistance appears to differ from induced humoral or cellular immune reactions in at least two ways:

(1) Suspensions of allogeneic erythrocytes or thrombocytes have roughly the same survival times as autologous cells, in *un*immunized recipients. This is apparently not the case for allogeneic HSC in lethally irradiated recipients where functional survival is only seen for a few days at best (see Figure 6.2) following grafting of suboptimal numbers of cells. In such cases, an abortive rise in peripheral leukocyte, reticulocyte and thrombocyte counts is found around day 10 after TBI. This is probably not due to classical organ graft rejection since after transplants of insufficient numbers of autologous bone marrow cells the same phenomenon is observed. This suggests that a large proportion of allogeneic HSC are inactivated soon after injection, in contrast to the fate of allogeneic end cells.

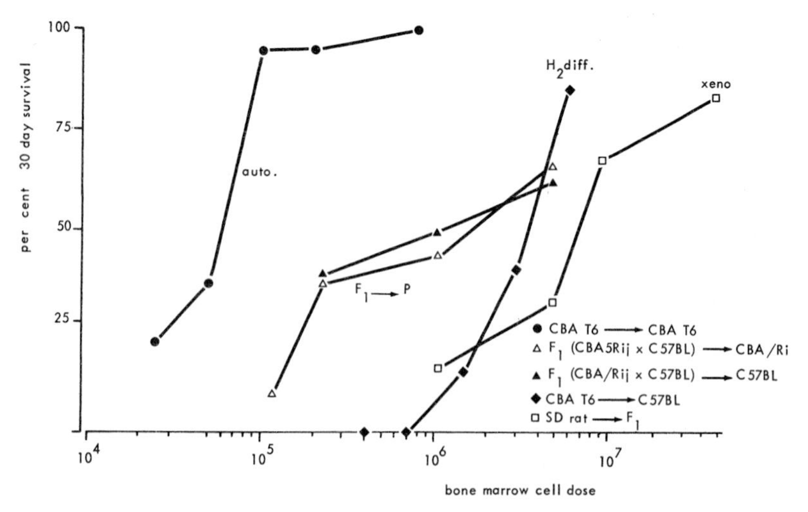

Figure 6.1 Thirty day survival of irradiated and bone marrow grafted mice. Fifteen to 20 mice per point

(2) It has been demonstrated that many immunological reactions such as skin graft rejection can be postponed by lethal TBI[80,81]. This is not the case for the resistance phenomenon. Other immunosuppressive agents have been found which do abolish induced or acquired immune reactivity against HSC but do not lower the *innate* resistance against HSC[82].

Allogeneic resistance to HSC may be effected by interference with homing, self-replication or differentiation of these cells. HSC from bone marrow show the same homing efficiency and self-renewal rate in allogeneic and isogeneic hosts, as measured by spleen colony assays. This suggests that inhibition of HSC differentiation is the most significant factor in allogeneic resistance against bone marrow HSC[33,47].

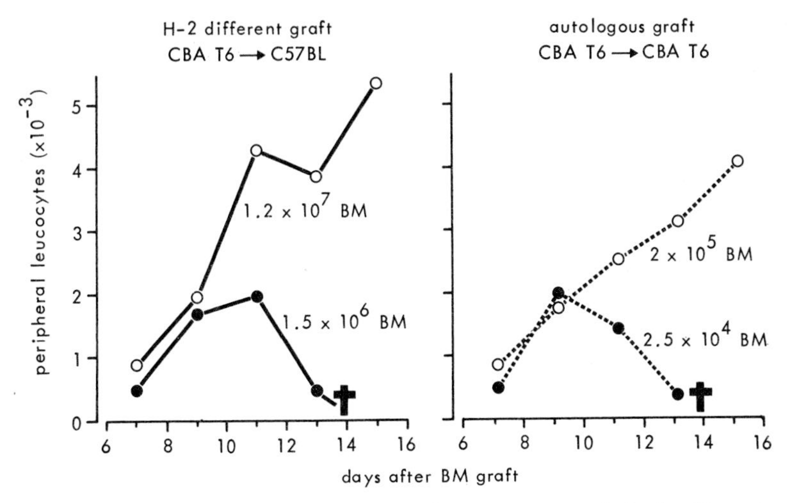

Figure 6.2 Peripheral leukocytes in irradiated and bone marrow grafted mice. Two mice per point

Combinations of silica particles and TBI[20] or of L-asparaginase and TBI as conditioning regimens[83,84] appear to lower the allogeneic resistance in dogs. Because silica particles are generally considered to inactivate macrophages and as L-asparaginase is known to suppress predominantly lymphocytes, these two cell populations are candidates for effector cells in allogeneic resistance. In this review survival after supralethal TBI and bone marrow transplantation has been taken as the assay for the presence or absence of resistance. In such investigations, the take of the injected cells can be established by immunogenetical, histological and haematological studies. Simplified procedures have been applied to the analysis of allogeneic resistance, such as spleen colony assays 10 days after TBI[62], or ^{125}IUDR uptake in the spleen 5 days after TBI[85]. The relevance of such models for survival of an individual animal after TBI and a bone marrow transplant is questionable in view of the poor correlation between these assays and survival[20] (van Bekkum, unpublished observations). A reliable *in vitro* assay for resistance is still lacking. It would facilitate further studies considerably, since it would allow for prospective genetic studies of this phenomenon in experimental animals, instead of the costly and cumbersome procedures of TBI and bone marrow transplantation in each individual animal. Moreover, it would enable a determination of the presence and strength of allogeneic resistance against human MHC mismatched haemopoietic cells.

Acquired resistance

Studies in monkeys[86], dogs[87,88] and man[7] have shown that the probability of a bone marrow graft take decreases when blood transfusions have been given to the recipient prior to grafting. Blood transfusions of the future bone marrow donor or his family induce a higher take failure rate than blood transfusions of third-party donors. Sensitization can also occur between host–donor pairs, which are identical for the MHC. In all probability the sensitized host will inactivate the HSC by its activated cellular and/or humoral immune mechanisms shortly after injection. This would be in contrast with the mode of action of innate resistance, which in all probability interferes with HSC in a later stage, i.e. with the differentiation of the HSC[33].

It has been difficult to demonstrate the presence of acquired host resistance (sensitization) prospectively *in vitro*. Recently, unilateral mixed lymphocyte cultures[15] and ^{51}Cr release assays[89] were reported to be of some, though not absolute, predictive value in this regard.

The acquired—extra—resistance to a bone marrow graft could be overcome in MHC mismatched dogs by the administration of procarbazine and antilymphocyte serum preceding the conditioning regimen of TBI[90].

Abrogation of obstacles preventing a take

Conditioning

Total body irradiation—TBI has been the oldest and most successful principle in conditioning recipients before the injection of HSC[17]. The highest tolerated dose of TBI is usually given to ensure a maximum suppression of antidonor reactivity. The upper limit to a TBI dose is set by gastrointestinal toxicity[17]. Total dose as well as dose rate influence the take of the graft[91–93]. The low dose rate irradiation (TBI of 1000 rad at 3.5 rad/min) originally introduced by the Seattle group has been adopted by several other clinics. In many radiological departments equipment is now available for delivering substantially higher dose rates, which permits shorter exposure times, to the convenience of the patients. However, if an equivalent TBI dose is to be given at a higher dose rate, a correction factor has to be applied. The value of the correction can be derived from the calculations of Liversage[94] and the extensive data available on the relation between LD 50/30d and dose rate from animal experimentation[95]. Employing this correction for the dose rate, the equivalent dose of 1000 rad at 3.5 rad/min can for instance be calculated to be 860 rad at 15 rad/min. Obviously, additional corrections for radiation quality and dose distribution need also to be applied when they differ significantly from the Seattle procedures. Lasting takes have been obtained using TBI for conditioning in donor–recipient pairs identical for the MHC in mice, dogs, and man[20,84,96], as specified in Table 6.5. In donor–recipient pairs, mismatched for MHC, higher numbers of HSC were required for takes in mice and dogs[17,19,20,97], but not in monkeys[18]. Therefore, TBI appears to be unable to suppress a major part of the host resistance against MHC *mismatched* HSC in some species of experimental animals. In man the use of MHC mismatched donors has not been systematically explored, due to the high risks of a rapidly fatal, acute GVH reaction[98].

Table 6.5 Relative bone marrow dose required for 50% survival rates after lethal total body irradiation*

Group	*Donor–recipient combination*	*Mice*[1]	*Dogs*[2]	*Monkeys*[3]	*Man*[4]
1	Autologous	$1(2\times10^6)$	$1(2.5\times10^7)$	$1(5\times10^7)$	$1(1\times10^8)$
2	$F_1\rightarrow$ parent	±30	—	—	—
3	MHC identical	3–4	3–4	?	3–4
4	MHC not identical	±60	±40	±4	?

* A comparable dose of approximately 800 rad X-ray was given
Dose rates differed per species
The absolute bone marrow dose per recipient kg body weight is given in brackets
[1] Reference 20
[2] References 84 and 97
[3] Reference 18
[4] Rough approximations from reference 96; evidently exact figures are lacking

Cyclophosphamide—Cyclophosphamide (Cy) conditioning was developed by Santos and co-workers[99]. It has been found to be less effective than TBI conditioning in terms of the number of HSC required for a take in MHC mismatched rodents[99], MHC matched dogs[69] and MHC mismatched monkeys[100,101]. The relative ineffectiveness in dogs of Cy conditioning can be explained by the low gastrointestinal tolerance for the drug in this species, which allows use of only a moderate Cy dose schedule. In humans, not sensitized to the allogeneic HSC donor a successful Cy conditioning regimen was found for MHC identical recipients[15]. In this species cardiotoxicity determines the maximum tolerated Cy dose[102].

Antilymphocyte serum—The use of antilymphocyte serum (ALS) as a conditioning agent was introduced by Seller and Polani[103] and by Mathé and co-workers[104,105]. Lasting *complete* takes have not been clearly demonstrated with the use of ALS alone in rodents or man[69,104–107]. The occurrence of split takes, sometimes of limited duration, was reported in both species: T lymphocytes were of recipient origin, while B lymphocytes and other blood elements were mainly of donor type. Further studies on the stability of this situation or its mechanism have not been reported. The minimal numbers of HSC required for a take after ALS conditioning have not been determined. The drawbacks of the use of ALS are the unpredictability of its potency, its thrombocytolytic activity and the possible contamination with anti-HSC antigen antibodies (see below). ALS has been used in combination with TBI or Cy as a conditioning regimen. An increased incidence of marrow takes from MHC mismatched donors was observed after ALS and TBI in some experiments with mice and dogs[108,109], but not in other dog studies[19,90]. The combination of ALS and Cy was about as effective as ALS alone in a small pilot study in human patients[105]. The conflicting data in the literature prohibit a conclusive statement on the usefulness of ALS as a conditioning agent in bone marrow transplantation.

Other chemotherapeutic agents—Chemotherapeutic agents which have been used for conditioning include thioguanine, nitrogen mustard, aminochloroambucil, busulphan, dimethylbusulphan and 6-mercaptopurine, and have been reviewed elsewhere[17,110]. With the exception of aminochloroambucil in rabbits[111], no successful suppression of host reactivity against donor bone marrow was reported. The possible combinations of TBI, Cy or ALS with other chemotherapeutic agents for conditioning purposes have received little attention, probably because of the severe toxicity problems expected in human patients. There is clearly a need for the development of a conditioning regimen of acceptable toxicity which will allow a realistic low number of MHC mismatched haemopoietic cells to take. Experiments in dogs have shown that TBI and i.v. injection of silica particles permit the take of low dose MHC mismatched bone marrow (4×10^8 cells/kg body weight)[19]. However, the applicability of this toxic conditioning method to humans is nil, due to the carcinogenic and fibrogenic properties of silica. The combination of TBI with L-asparaginase injections caused some improvement over TBI alone but a high percentage of graft failures is still observed[83,84]. Several conditioning regimens are known to be successful in breaking host resistance against HSC as measured in various modifications of the spleen colony assay[85,112]. Most of these regimens were ineffective, however, when survival was used as the end point in mice[20] and in dogs[19,82] (van Kessel and Vriesendorp, unpublished observations). Therefore, the relevance of the spleen colony assay to the study of allogeneic resistance is doubtful. In human leukaemic patients additional cytoreductive therapy has been introduced prior to the marrow transplantation with the purpose of eradicating a higher percentage of malignant cells. Three such regimens were clinically tested: (1) a combination of TBI + Cy[113], (2) a multidrug scheme abbreviated as BACT[2,114], and (3) a multidrug scheme + radiation therapy labelled SCARI[115]. Takes were observed in almost all of the patients. Therefore, the effect of such treatment schedules on the resistance to MHC *matched* transplants appears to be better than Cy conditioning alone where approximately a 30% take failure rate was observed[7,15]. Their effect on MHC mismatched grafts is unknown since they are currently hardly ever performed in man.

Source of the HSC

In mice, approximately twice as many HSC are required from fetal liver as from bone marrow to secure a take[33]. In contrast to HSC from bone marrow, the homing of HSC from fetal liver is depressed by a factor of two in allogeneic recipients[47]. This difference in homing between marrow and fetal liver might be caused by intrinsic differences between HSC from these two sources. One could speculate that distinct antigenic properties of embryonic HSC comparable to the carcinoembryonic antigen on digestive tract cells[116], evoke a stronger resistance. Another possible explanation for the difference in efficiency between HSC from bone marrow and fetal liver might be found in the presence of small numbers of immunocompetent cells in the bone marrow and their absence in fetal liver. The addition of large numbers of lymphocytes and leukocytes to bone marrow has been shown to decrease the number of HSC required for a take[117,118] (see also section below). It has not been determined whether small numbers of immunocompetent cells are capable of promoting a take.

The relative 'takeability' of HSC from the peripheral blood has not been determined in a strictly quantitative way. Studies in dogs have suggested that about 10^{10} nucleated cells from peripheral blood are needed per kg body weight to obtain a take in a MHC mismatched host[18]. This seems low in comparison to the number of similar bone marrow cells required for a take, i.e. 10^9 [119], when the concentration of HSC in the two sources is taken into account. In mice the proportion of HSC among nucleated cells from the peripheral blood is about 100 times lower than in bone marrow[61]. A similar difference was found in dogs when nucleated cells from blood and bone marrow were compared for their content of colony-forming cells *in vitro* (Vriesendorp, unpublished observations). If this 100 times lower concentration holds true for dog HSC in blood, 10 times less allogeneic HSC from blood would be required than from bone marrow to obtain a take in this species. Possible explanations for this difference are discussed in the next paragraph. It should be pointed out here, however, that this apparent increased 'takeability' of blood HSC is accompanied by an increased severity and incidence of acute GVH reactions due to the high number of immunocompetent cells in the blood.

Contaminating cells

In the previous paragraph the influence of cells other than HSC on the take of HSC has been introduced. Viable non-irradiated lymphocytes appear to be the most successful cells in suppressing the need for increasing numbers of HSC[82,117,118]. In principle, one of three mechanisms or a combination of them might explain this phenomenon. The most likely explanation is that an increased number of allogeneic lymphocytes in an AHC graft will induce a more severe GVH reaction and thereby, perhaps, decrease the innate allogeneic resistance of the host. Another possibility is that GVH reactions increase the efficiency of allogeneic HSC to repopulate a host by increasing the production of factors required for haemopoiesis. It is known for example that CSF can be found in the medium of mixed lymphocyte cultures[120] or in the serum of a bone marrow recipient during GVHD[121]. A third, more remote possibility is that larger numbers of immunocompetent cells in the graft offer the recipient better protection against opportunistic infections in the early post-conditioning period, thus prolonging the time available for the production of sufficient end cells by the allogeneic HSC. A further analysis of the role of donor lymphocytes in the take process might be worthwhile, since it could provide ways (a) to obtain a take of low (and clinically realistic) numbers of allogeneic HSC, and/or (b) to increase the rate of immunological reconstitution after conditioning in the host.

The host–donor relationship

TBI has been the most successful single agent method of conditioning so far (see above). When the maximum tolerable TBI is used, four different types of genetic relations between donor and recipient appear to have four different minimum requirements for bone marrow cells necessary to obtain a take. These genetic relations are (1) isogeneic or autologous, (2) F_1 hybrid into an inbred parent (only applicable in inbred strains of rodents), (3) allogeneic, matched for the MHC, and (4) allogeneic, mismatched for the MHC or xenogeneic. An estimate of the minimal number of bone marrow cells required for a take in a given donor–host relation is the one which will rescue 50% of the recipients, transplanted within 24 h of TBI, from death of the bone marrow syndrome. The importance of determining this minimum number of bone marrow cells is two-fold. Too low a number of bone marrow cells will lead to 'radiation-induced death of the recipient', too high a number will increase the risks of acute GVH reactions except in autologous and F_1 hybrid to parent transplants. Evidently these determinations can only be performed in experimental animals. A summary of the results obtained in mice, dogs and rhesus monkeys is given in Table 6.5. Mice and dogs appear to be similar in that in group 3 (MHC identical donors) about four times and in group 4 (MHC mismatched donors) about 50 times more bone marrow cells are required for a take, when compared to group 1 (autologous transplants). Whether the resistance against MHC identical and MHC mismatched bone marrow cells is determined by the same mechanism has so far not been investigated. Procedures allowing a decrease in the required number of MHC mismatched bone marrow cells have been described above. It is unknown whether these procedures will also decrease the numbers of MHC matched bone marrow cells required for take and, if so, whether these numbers are comparable to those required for an autologous graft. This would obviously facilitate the collection of sufficient numbers of allogeneic marrow cells for transplantation. Another advantage would be that it would decrease the number of lymphocytes transplanted with the HSC by a factor of four and thus lower the risk of acute GVH reactions. The data for man in Table 6.5 are incomplete. It remains to be seen whether man follows the mouse/dog pattern or the monkey pattern in the quantitative requirements for MHC mismatched bone marrow cells for takes. The reasons for a difference in effectivity of low numbers of MHC mismatched bone marrow cells between mice and dogs on the one hand and rhesus monkeys on the other hand are unknown. As a possible explanation it has been suggested that the higher number of immunocompetent cells in monkey bone marrow cell suspensions lower the amount of bone marrow cells required for a take (see above). An argument against this explanation is that only a minor increase in TBI dose is required for monkeys receiving lymphocyte-depleted allogeneic bone marrow cell suspensions to obtain takes (i.e. 50 rad)[119]. Other possible explanations include differences in radiosensitivity of the innate resistance between the different species or a low genetic polymorphism in rhesus monkeys for the factors controlling resistance. In the latter case all or most rhesus monkey host–donor pairs would be compatible for resistance factors. In dogs, immunogenetic studies have been performed to analyse the genetic control of innate resistance within the MHC[19,122]. Table 6.6 gives a summary of the results. The several subregions recognized in the canine MHC (DLA) are indicated here as LD or SD[123,124]. LD identity between a donor and a host is a negative unilateral MLC reaction, in which the host lymphocytes are not stimulated by the irradiated donor lymphocytes. SD identity indicates that a donor does *not* have antigens of the first, second or third SD series (officially called DLA-A, DLA-B, DLA-C) which are absent in the host. The first two lines in Table 6.6 indicate that low numbers of allogeneic bone marrow (4×10^8/kg body weight) usually take if they derive from a DLA identical sibling, while in DLA LD and SD different sibling pairs this does not occur. The single exception indicates that resistance is controlled by a locus or loci different from LD and SD. This is corroborated by the results obtained in non-related animals where identity for LD or SD alone appears to be insufficient for a take and where in two out of 25 unrelated, LD and SD different combinations a take was obtained. However, when both LD and SD were matched in unrelated animals lasting takes occurred, indicating that the genes controlling allogeneic resistance show a high degree of linkage disequilibrium with LD and SD genes. These data underline the present, unfavourable situation with regard to human MHC mismatched bone marrow grafts. The risk of take failure with ensuing mortality in such cases is so high that such a procedure is usually not undertaken. In a desperate situation, extrapolation from the dog data suggest that best chances exist with a conditioning regimen of TBI and the use of 4×10^8 bone marrow cells per kg body weight of an unrelated, LD and SD identical, donor. The low frequency of such donors in the random human population is an additional problem and will necessitate the use of large pools of tissue-typed donors with a computerized search for the most compatible donor. Evidently, more insights into the problems listed in Table 6.4 and discussed in the previous paragraphs are required to increase the applicability of MHC mismatched bone marrow transplants in man.

Table 6.6 Genetics of resistance against allogeneic dog bone marrow*

	DLA differences between donor and host		*Number of animals*	*Relation between donor and host*†	*Proportion of persisting take*
	LD	SD			
1	≠	≠	6	Sibs	0/6
2	=	=	40	Sibs	39/40
3	=	≠	6	Unrelated	0/6
4	≠	=	3	Unrelated	0/3
5	≠	≠	23	Unrelated	2/25
6	=	=	8	Unrelated	8/8

*Standard protocol 750–800 rad TBI followed 24 h later by 4×10^8 BM cells/kg body weight recipients. Group 6: the takes include animals which received BM after 72 or 120 h ($n = 6$) or which received split TBI
† Mainly beagles and a limited number of mongrel dogs of known pedigree were used

GRAFT-VERSUS-HOST DISEASE, THE MAIN COMPLICATION OF BONE MARROW GRAFTING

In those patients in whom a take of the bone marrow graft has been accomplished, GVHD is the most frequent and by far the most serious complication to occur. Even in patients treated with bone marrow from an HLA identical sibling donor, its morbidity and mortality is still considerable (see ref. 125). Apart from exhaustive descriptions of the symptomatology and the pathology of GVHD in humans[17,126–129] a wealth of information has been collected on GVHD in experimental animals, e.g. rodents[130,131] and monkeys[132,133]. Two main types of GVHD can be distinguished after transplantation of allogeneic haemopoietic cells (Figure 6.3). In both types immune competent T cells are the effective cells; in the acute form they are being grafted along with the bone marrow, whilst in the delayed form, the effective cells develop from primitive precursor cells under the influence of the thymus.

Delayed GVHD

In lethally irradiated mice a delayed form of GVHD occurs after grafting of allogeneic bone marrow cells. Its symptoms consist of diarrhoea with wasting, whilst in a proportion of the animals dermatitis begins to appear between 3 and 4 weeks after transplantation and may persist for as long as 2 months. The mortality varies according to the host–donor strain combination; in some it may be as high as 100%. A large proportion of the animals die with infections and septicaemia. As this type of GVHD starts well after the haemopoietic system has been repopulated, the term secondary disease has been widely used to distinguish it from the primary, radiation-induced, bone marrow aplasia.

Histological inspection of the tissues shows degenerated crypts and crypt abscesses scattered throughout the intestinal tract, as well as more extensive ulcerations especially in the colon, degeneration of hepatocytes and a quite characteristic dermatitis. The latter comprises hyperkeratosis, parakeratosis, dyskeratosis and basal cell degeneration which are reminiscent of those seen in lupus erythematosus. The affected tissues also show infiltration with lymphocytes. Another characteristic feature is the extreme atrophy of the lymphoid tissues[17,134] which is responsible for a protracted state of severe immune deficiency. The direct cause of death is septicaemia originating from the infectious processes in the gut, a point of view which is confirmed by the protective effect of treatment with antibiotics[135], and of so-called bacteriological decontamination[136,137].

Acute GVHD

The second form of GVHD in rodents is the acute type which develops after grafting of spleen cells or when lymph node cells are added to a marrow

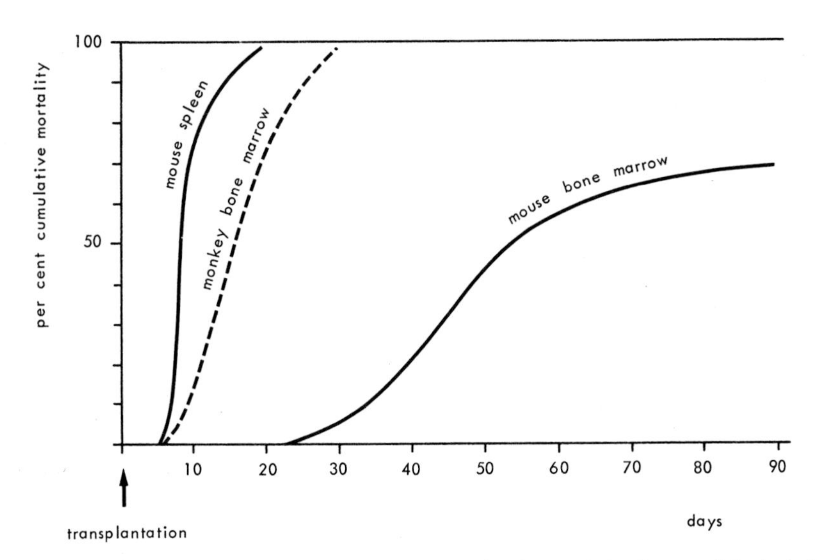

Figure 6.3 Acute and delayed GVHD in rodents and primates following conditioning with total body irradiation and grafting of haemopoietic cells

graft[96,138]. Under these conditions severe diarrhoea and rapid wasting begin at about 1 week after grafting. The lesions encountered in the gut are similar to but more severe than those of delayed type GVHD. A high incidence of mortality ensues between 10 and 20 days after grafting and is usually not associated with septicaemia. Surviving animals continue to suffer from delayed type GVHD and usually die later. Extensive crypt degeneration is also observed in germfree animals suffering from acute GVHD[139]. Mortality in germfree animals is somewhat delayed but not prevented, indicating that bacterial infection is not a decisive factor in acute GVHD mortality. Liver parenchyma cell necrosis and necrosis of the basal cell layer of the skin have also been observed in acute GVHD.

The difference in acute GVHD after allogeneic spleen cell transplantation as compared to delayed GVHD after allogeneic bone marrow grafting in rodents can be explained on the basis of the difference in the proportion of immune competent T cells in the two tissues. In rodents, the bone marrow contains few if any mature T cells; PHA response and GVH reactivity of bone marrow cells are low. In monkeys and man, bone marrow cells show a high mitogenic response to PHA. In the latter two species the GVHD which develops after grafting of incompatible bone marrow is essentially of the acute type. There is some preliminary evidence indicating that dog bone marrow occupies an intermediary position between that of rodents and primates.

The high PHA response of primate bone marrow cannot be ascribed to an admixture of peripheral blood because bone marrow pressed from the bones of exsanguinated monkeys induces a similarly severe acute GVHD as bone marrow obtained by puncture. Very small punctates of human bone marrow which presumably contain less peripheral blood, show the same response to PHA as large punctates[140]. In addition, it has been shown that transplantation of BSA density gradient fractions of monkey bone marrow, which are enriched in stem cells and depleted of T lymphocytes, no longer induce acute GVHD but instead the delayed type of the disease, similar to that observed in rodents after allogeneic bone marrow grafting[141].

Recovery from GVHD

While all available evidence points to pre-existing mature T cells of the graft being the direct inducers of acute GVHD, the delayed form is thought to be caused by T cells which have newly differentiated from the HSC during the first few weeks following transplantation. An essential requirement for such differentiation is the presence of a functional thymus[142]. It is postulated that during the process of maturation the T cells have an increased chance of becoming tolerant to the antigens of the host to which the developing T-cell population is exposed. When F_1 hybrid mice are irradiated and rescued with bone marrow from one of the parent strains, the delayed GVHD is generally not fatal and after recovery of the immune system of the chimera, its lymphocytes have been shown to be *specifically tolerant* towards the tissue antigens of the other parent strain[143,144]. On the other hand, parental *spleen* cells if grafted in sufficient numbers into lethally irradiated F_1 hybrid mice may produce violent and rapidly fatal acute GVHD.

Fetal liver cells induce less severe delayed GVHD than bone marrow cells, even when equal numbers of HSC—as measured with the spleen colony assay—are grafted[38]. This difference between HSC derived from fetal liver and those from adult bone marrow seems to be compatible with the higher susceptibility of newborn animals compared with adults regarding the induction of tolerance to a variety of antigens. The nature of the tolerance of the donor lymphocytes versus host tissue antigens observed in clinically normal long-term radiation chimeras is not precisely known. Hellström[145,146] has ascribed the absence of or recovery from GVHD to the presence of blocking factors in the serum of radiation chimeras, but his findings were not confirmed by others[147–149]. It remains intriguing that stable radiation chimeras seem to exert a certain resistance to reinduction of GVHD by injection of fresh donor type cells[150,151]. This resistance can be transferred to normal animals by parabiosis or cross-circulation[152]. The serum of 'tolerant' radiation chimeras when incubated with donor type spleen cells reduces their ability to mount a local GVH reaction[153]. Whether so-called suppressor T cells are also of importance has not adequately been investigated, but recent observations on rats made independently by Santos and by ourselves[54] seem to support this possibility.

Immunogenetic factors determining GVHD

After the first observations by Mathé[98] that severe acute GVHD is consequent upon a take of allogeneic non-matched bone marrow in man, a number of attempts were made to decrease the risk of inducing that complication by donor selection. Eventually, after HLA matching was introduced, it turned out that the results are far better when the donor is an MHC identical sibling of the recipient. As was mentioned before, in those optimally matched situations GVHD still occurs in a substantial proportion of patients. Although the disease is reminiscent of delayed type GVHD in the majority of the patients, a substantial number has been described in whom the early onset and extreme severity of GVHD are indistinguishable from those of the acute type seen after transplantation of HLA incompatible marrow.

Factors within MHC

The important role of the MHC in the control of GVHD has been confirmed in experimental animals as well as in man. In view of the many different polymorphic loci within the MHC it is of great practical importance to identify those loci, which are involved in the genetic control of GVH reactions. The smaller the number of loci involved and the lower the polymorphism per locus, the easier it will be to select a 'GVH compatible' donor from a pool of unrelated individuals. Studies in mice have shown that GVH control within the MHC is in all probability polygenic[140]. The notion that the degree of reactivity or absence of reactivity in mixed lymphocyte cultures might predict the severity of GVH reactions was proven to be incorrect in dog studies[130–132]. The observation that transplantation of bone marrow from HLA-D matched unrelated donors in SCID patients results in a high percentage of GVHD[133], is in accordance with the above findings. A prognostic test for GVHD which will identify unrelated donors with similarly favourable properties as MHC identical sibs, is therefore not yet available. It is possible that further insight into presently undefined areas of the MHC might provide such a test. Alternatively, the control of GVHD in man may be under such a complex multilocus control within the MHC that the selection of an unrelated, well-matched donor will prove to be impractical.

Factors outside MHC

The occurrence of GVHD in human host–donor combinations genotypically identical for the MHC is in accordance with the findings of Cantrell and Hildeman[154] who induced a GVH reaction of varying strength in newborn mice with spleen cells from donors differing only at non-H-2 loci from the recipients. It should be noted that this particular GVH reaction is not identical with acute GVHD developing in radiation chimeras, but that both are induced by immune-competent T cells present in the graft. So far, minor histocompatibility loci specifically involved in inducing GVHD in man have not been identified[155], although suggestive leads have been obtained[156]. Of the many factors that were retrospectively analysed in a series of grafted patients by Storb *et al.*[157,158], sex mismatch between recipient and donor was strongly correlated with the occurrence of GVHD. In a series of transplanted aplastic patients, the incidence of GVHD was 64% when recipient and donor were of different sex, and only 10% when sex was matched. The correlation was present for a sex mismatch, in either of the two directions, which implies that if these correlations are based on immunogenetic factors, histocompatibility loci have to be present on the Y as well as on the X chromosomes. Such a model could also explain the exceptions to the rule of a correlation between GVHD and sex mismatch. In mice, an influence of Y-linked histocompatibility on the development of GVHD has been reported by Lengerova and Chutna[159]. GVHD could be induced in irradiated C57BL male mice when bone marrow from females of the same inbred strain was grafted, but not in the reverse combination.

These results have been extended by Uphoff[160], who studied a number of different strains and found the Y effect on GVHD to be dependent on their

MHC genotype. Other investigators failed to observe GVHD in female-to-male mouse bone marrow grafting[161]. X chromosome-associated histo-incompatibility has been reported in mice using skin grafts[162], but its effect on GVHD induction has not been described so far. These sex chromosome histoincompatibilities in mice generally result in weak rejection reactions and it is therefore surprising that they appear to play a significant role in the development of GVHD in humans.

In outbred species, the only experimental animal in which data on the transplantation of clinically realistic numbers of bone marrow cells between MHC identical siblings are available, is the dog[84]. The incidence of GVHD in such dogs was about 50%, but its severity was less than seen in human patients and mortality seldom occurred. A search for parameters which may predict GVHD following transplantation of MHC identical marrow between dog littermates revealed the following: the third-party disparity ratio in MLC, as was originally recommended for this purpose by Park and Good *et al.*[163], did not correlate with GVHD[164]. Several red cell antigens and white blood cell enzymes were not associated with GVHD. A positive correlation was found between GVHD and phosphoglucomutase (PGM2) incompatibility (not absolute) and a negative correlation appeared between GVHD and incompatibility for the canine secretory alloantigen system (CSA) as defined by Zweibaum and co-workers[165].

In an immunogenetic approach to the prevention of GVHD in MHC identical sibs, it would be of relevance to identify the number of loci involved in the control of this phenomenon. It was noted earlier that when many polymorphic loci are involved, donor selection cannot be the solution for this problem. Such an analysis should be undertaken under conditions similar to those of clinical transplantation, because other factors, for example preimmunization of the donor, or unrealistically high cell doses, may exaggerate the influence of specific immunogenetic differences between donor and recipient[154]. In this respect it is of interest that weekly transfusions of irradiated blood from unrelated donors during the first month after grafting of compatible sibling bone marrow did not affect the *incidence* but increased the severity of GVHD in dogs[84]. The finding that the bone marrow from a single MHC matched donor produced GVHD in one sibling recipient and not in the other on several occasions, argues against a donor-specific determinant of GVHD (such as degree of lymphocyte contamination of the bone marrow).

Thus, it seems that genetic factors outside the MLC locus determine whether GVHD will occur and that the severity of this complication may be influenced by factors not directly associated with the immunogenetic difference between recipient and donor. The latter notion is supported by observations in mice, which suggest that the crypt lesions associated with acute GVHD in germ-free fetal gut implants are aggravated by the presence of enterobacteria in the intestinal tract of the chimeric animal carrying the implant. In fact, indirect evidence has been obtained for the presence of cross-reacting antigens which enforce GVHD on enterobacteria species and on the epithelial cells of the gut in mice[166].

Immune responses after bone marrow transplantation

The rate of recovery of many immune functions has been recorded in radiation chimeras. No attempt will be made to review this large body of data here, instead only the main trends will be described (see refs. 17, 167, 168). In general, it seems that the larger the degree of histoincompatibility between recipient and donor, the longer it takes for full immunological reconstitution (IR) to be attained. In particular the delayed type GVHD is characterized by severe atrophy of the lymphatic tissues and by pronounced immune deficiency. Accordingly, the occurrence of GVHD, even if of minor clinical importance, greatly delays IR in transplanted individuals. The time needed for IR to begin and the completeness of the recovery closely parallel the repopulation of the lymphatic system. In isologous chimeras histological recovery of the lymphatic tissues is usually completed after 12 months, and by that time substantial immune responses, both humoral and cellular, have been recorded[169,170].

In the allogeneic situation in mice *with* GVHD, the survivors begin to show a rise from their low levels of immunological functions after day 90, concomitant with the disappearance of GVHD symptoms, but subnormal responses may persist for a year and longer. T-cell deficiency in the spleens of allogeneic mouse chimeras was demonstrated 4–8 months after bone marrow transplantation[171], although high numbers of θ positive cells have been found in the spleen as early as 2–3 weeks after grafting[172]. For the allogeneic combinations without GVHD, that is F_1 hybrid marrow transplanted to one of the parent strains, no relevant information is available.

In non-inbred laboratory animals the most extensive data are available for dogs[168] and relate to allogeneic DLA compatible as well as to incompatible transplants following conditioning with TBI. Lymphocyte counts and lymph node histology took 100–200 days to normalize. All cellular immune functions except the tuberculin reaction were subnormal before day 200 and so was antibody formation against a variety of antigens. Strangely enough, no difference was noted between this group of 48 animals and five dogs grafted with autologous marrow.

The pattern of recovery of immunoglobulin formation was studied in rhesus monkeys grafted with autologous[173] or with allogeneic bone marrow[174]. In the autologous situation, the specific antibody production at 30 and 60 days after transplantation was slightly delayed as compared with normal monkeys. In the allogeneic chimeras only scattered data are available due to poor survival.

A limited number of leukaemic and aplastic patients have been investigated in a systematic way for IR following bone marrow grafting with syngeneic or allogeneic matched sibling marrow[175]. Immunoglobulin levels normalized between 100 and 150 days in most cases. Antibody formation against phage QX 174 remained absent or low for as long as 2 years in the allogeneic human chimeras. In most allogeneic cases skin tests with antigens and DNCB remained negative, although their lymphocytes responded to PHA and in MLC. These findings in general correlate with the clinical experience that syngeneic transplant patients develop significantly fewer infectious complications than allogeneic transplant recipients[176,177].

One of the most distressing complications after successful allogeneic bone marrow transplantation in leukaemic and aplastic patients is the occurrence of interstitial pneumonia 1 or 2 months after grafting (see above). A thorough analysis of this syndrome has been made by Neiman *et al.*[175]. Its occurrence is associated with poor condition of the patients before and after transplantation and patients with symptoms of GVHD are a particularly bad risk. Some transplant teams tend to attribute the pneumonia to a late effect of radiation on the lungs, but this interpretation is contradicted by the fact that it has not been observed following transplantation of isogeneic bone marrow from identical twin donors, who received the same conditioning regimen as the group treated with allogeneic bone marrow[176].

As the prolonged state of immune deficiency and its complications in bone marrow transplant patients may well be the most important problem of clinical bone marrow grafting in the future, more detailed experimental investigations of the factors which determine and those which may influence the recovery of the immune functions, are clearly needed. The presently available data do not permit a systematic comparison of the rate of IR as related to presence or absence of GVHD, nor to separate the effects of the allogeneic situation *per se* from the effects secondary to GVHD.

Prevention and treatment of GVHD

Since the discovery that GVHD is caused by immune competent cells of the donor marrow reacting against certain tissue components of the recipient, many attempts have been made to interfere with that reaction. Numerous ingenious methods have been devised for that purpose and a considerable number has been found to exert some beneficial effect in the most commonly employed experimental model, the mouse radiation chimera. At present it can safely be stated that the problem of how to prevent GVHD in the mouse and produce stable H-2 different radiation chimeras, has been solved, even when the most aggressive source of haemopoietic cells—the spleen—is employed for grafting. The situation is far less satisfactory in outbred animal species, the monkey and the dog, and in man. In these, GVHD is still a major and often fatal complication, even with presently available GVHD reductive measures. This suggests that the mouse is much more prone to develop 'tolerance' of donor cells towards the recipient than the other species. Although the acute GVHD induced in lethally irradiated mice by grafting of allogeneic spleen cells or a mixture of bone marrow and lymph node cells is an excellent model for screening, it serves only to select measures or agents which *may* have some value in the human. In general, the methods having relatively low protective action in the mouse model were found to be devoid of protection in monkeys and dogs. On the other hand, most agents which had a significant protective or curative action in monkeys (and dogs) have been found to be of value in clinical GVHD. Experimental GVHD reductive methods have been directed at the donor, at the recipient prior to transplantation, at the haemopoietic cell graft itself before it is injected into the recipient, and at the recipient after transplantation.

Donor treatment

Manipulation of the donor remains of theoretical interest only, since current clinical practice will generally not permit this type of interference. Passive immunization of donor mice against recipient antigens has reduced the ability of the donor spleen cells to produce splenomegaly in newborn recipients[178]. Active immunization of the donor with soluble MHC antigens of the recipient moderately reduced acute GVHD[179] as did immunization of the donor with bacterial polysaccharide[180]. A limited number of daily injections of high dose ALS completely prevented acute GVHD following the transplantation of spleen cells from these mice into lethally irradiated allogeneic recipients[181], but a similar treatment of monkey donors had no effect on acute GVHD in allogeneic recipients[182]. This discrepancy is possibly not due to a species difference but to differences in penetration of ALS into various tissues following systematic administration of ALS, as was demonstrated in the mouse by Tridente *et al.*[183]. Interference with the recipient or with the haemopoietic cell graft *in vitro* being more realistic, details of the various methods reported are presented in Table 6.7.

Treatment of recipient

Treatment of the recipient prior to grafting with a short course of high dose ALS or antilymphocyte globulin (ALG) has been found to be quite effective in the prevention of acute GVHD both in the mouse and in the monkey. For two reasons this treatment has not been advanced clinically: firstly, some ALG preparations contain antistem-cell activity so that their administration may compromise the take of the graft[184–186]. Secondly, a course of high dose ALG carries the risk of inducing fatal haemorrhages in thrombopenic patients. Nonetheless, pregrafting treatment with ALG—under protection of thrombocyte transfusions—is currently being employed as part of the conditioning regimen in combination with cyclophosphamide and procarbazide or with whole body irradiation, to promote the take of the graft in sensitized recipients[187]. It has not yet been established whether this application of ALS also reduces the incidence of GVHD.

In vitro *treatment of graft*

The experimental modification of the haemopoietic cell graft *in vitro* comprises a large variety of methods aimed at selective elimination or inactivation of the immune competent T cells, with concomitant sparing of the HSC. All manipulations are only partially specific, and, ideally, the specificity index, i.e. the relative reduction of T cells as compared to HSC, should be determined before conclusions regarding the practical value of the method are drawn[138]. In the majority of the investigations listed this has not been done. In all instances the optimal conditions of *in vitro* treatment of the graft are critical. In the mouse models these can be quite satisfactorily determined experimentally by the quantitative enumeration of T cells and of HSC. For human bone marrow, however, an assay for functional pluripotential stem cells does not exist. For certain *in vitro* manipulations such as the physical separation of T lymphocytes and HSC by density gradient fractionation, the measurement of colonies in soft agar (CFUc) provides a realistic indication for HSC, but this is not the case for exposures to antibodies directed against lymphoid cells. HSC and CFUc have been found in the mouse to possess different surface antigens[188] so that the absence of cytotoxicity of an antiserum for CFUc does not guarantee that it will leave HSC undamaged. In fact, many antisera which were active in suppressing GVHD by *in vitro* incubation with the cells to be grafted, were also found to inactivate HSC[184,185,189]. In some instances the toxicity for HSC could be removed by exhaustive absorptions with liver, spleen, plasmacytoma cells, etc.[190,191], but the final specificity of these preparations can only be estimated accurately in animal systems thus far. An additional complication is that CFUc are in cycle and HSC are mostly in G_0—at least in mouse bone marrow—so that these two cell types may be expected to show different sensitivity to incubation parameters. This makes it extremely difficult to extrapolate complicated treatments, e.g. the absorption of reactive donor lymphocytes on monolayers of host type cells, to the practical clinical situation, with some degree of reliability.

It can be seen in Table 6.7 that the *in vitro* exposure to antisera directed to lymphoid cells or their products has been extremely popular. Positive results have been reported with antilymph node or antithymus type antibodies, as well as antitheta serum, antimouse brain serum, antimouse Ig serum, and antimouse whole serum. These results are not always reproducible, which may depend on variations in the quality of the antisera. In many instances the selectivity of these antibodies for GVH-inducing cells has not been adequately demonstrated. The group of Thierfelder has systematically advanced the *in vitro* application of ALS and has prepared purified antibodies which seem to cause selective inactivation of lymphoid cells in human bone

Table 6.7 Experimental and clinical mitigation of GVHD

1. Treatment of recipient prior to grafting

Agent	*Animal system*	*Efficacy*	*Clinical data*
High dose ALG 4–48 h before grafting	mouse: acute GVHD	high[208,209]	Not attempted in combination with effective conditioning permitting take
	monkey: acute GVHD	high[198,210]	
	dog: acute GVHD	low[199]	

2. Manipulation of haemopoietic cells *in vitro*

Incubation treatment	*Animal system*	*Efficacy*	*Clinical data*
ALS, ATS, ALG, ATG	mouse: acute GVHD	high[211]	One case—no take[219]
		moderate[182,191]	
		none[212]	
	rat: GVHD	high[213]	
	monkey: acute GVHD	variable[182]	
A-θ serum, A-serum serum	mouse: acute GVHD	high[214]	
A-mouse brain globulin (AMBG)	mouse: acute GVHD	high[190]	
A-Ig serum	mouse: acute GVHD	high[189]	
	mouse: delayed GVHD	moderate[215]	
A-light chain serum	splenomegaly in newborn mice	high[193]	
A-recognition serum	splenomegaly in newborn mice	moderate[216]	
Fab (from ALG)	mouse: acute GVHD	high[192,197,217]	
(from ATG, AMBG, A-Ig)	mouse: acute GVHD	none[212]	
$F(ab')_2$ (from ALS, AMBG, A-Ig)	mouse: acute GVHD	none[218]	
37 °C—2 h	mouse: acute GVHD	moderate[207,220]	No systematic investigations
40 °C—1 to 3 days	mouse: acute GVHD	moderate[72]	
Thymic chalone	mouse: acute GVHD	slight[212]	
Concanavalin A	mouse: acute GVHD	high[177]	
H2 antigens of host	mouse: acute GVHD	moderate[221,222]	
Absorption of donor cells on host cell monolayers	splenomegaly in newborn mice	partial[223], none or adverse[196]	
	splenomegaly in irradiated mice	only effective with sensitized lymphocytes[194]	
		high[195]	
Culture with host cells and [^{3}H]thymidine suicide	mouse: acute GVHD	moderate[224]	
Culture with host cells and BUDR-light suicide	local GVH response	moderate[225]	No effect[227,228], 2 cases
Separation of immune competent cells by density gradient centrifugation	mouse: acute GVHD	high[28]	Encouraging results in treatment of SCID[32]
	monkey: acute GVHD	high[32]	
Velocity gradient separation	mouse: acute GVHD	postulated[226]	Few attempts, negative[125]

Table 6.7—*continued*

3. Treatment of recipient after transplantation

Treatment	*Animal model*	*Efficacy*	*Clinical data*
Active enhancement	GVH reaction in non-irradiated F_1 mice	moderate[229]	
Passive enhancement (antihost serum)	GVH reaction in non-irradiated F_1 mice	moderate or adverse[229,230]	No obvious effect (see ref. 231)
	GVH reaction in sublethally irradiated F_1 rats	none or adverse[231]	
ALS	mouse: acute GVHD	moderate[181,232]	Effective in treatment of established GVHD[15,113]
	dog: acute GVHD	low[199,212]	
	monkey: GVHD	high[233]	
Methotrexate	mouse: acute GVHD	high[201,234]	Routinely administered post-grafting; but efficacy in preventing GVHD not proven
	dog: GVHD prolonged treatment	high[235–237]	
high dose	monkey: acute GVHD	high[201]	
Cyclophosphamide	mouse: acute GVHD	high[201,200,238]	Not investigated
high dose	dog: GVHD	none[237]	
	monkey: acute GVHD	high[201]	
Hydroxyurea	mouse: acute GVHD	moderate[200]	
Procarbazine (natulan)	mouse: acute GVHD	moderate[200,238]	
Cytosine arabinoside	mouse: acute GVHD	moderate/high[239,240]	
Corticosteroids	mouse: delayed GVHD	adverse[238,240]	Occasionally used[9], no evaluation
	mouse: acute GVHD	none	
	mouse: GVH reaction in unirradiated hybrids	none, adverse[241]	
Thymic chalone	mouse: acute GVHD	moderate[212]	
Soluble host H2 antigens	mouse: acute GVHD	slight[221]	
Donor lymph node or spleen cells	mouse: delayed type GVHD	low/moderate[151]	

A- = anti

marrow. The value of this technique in clinical use still has to be established. The results with $F(ab')_2$ and Fab fragments have been controversial, in that Fab fragments of ALG were reported to be effective *in vitro* only by the groups of Trentin and Rietmüller[191,192]. Others have not observed any activity of either Fab or $F(ab')_2$ fragments from ALG and other antibodies. Of particular interest are the findings of Mason and Warner[193] that pre-incubation with antisera directed against the heavy chains of IgM, IgA and IgG did not reduce the ability of mouse spleen cells to induce a GVH reaction (splenomegaly in newborn mice), while such abolition could consistently be produced by incubation of the cells with antiserum directed against light chains. Several authors have explored the possibility of pre-absorption of the GVH reactive lymphocytes on cells genotypically identical with the future recipient. So far, encouraging experimental results have been obtained but it seems that absorption of non-sensitized lymphocytes is non-specific. Sensitization can take place to a certain degree *in vitro* which may explain the fact that Clark and Kimura[194] did not observe specificity with an absorption of 3 h while Lonai *et al.*[195] using an 18 h absorption period, scored positive effects, and also why short periods of contact may even lead to an enhancement of GVH reactivity[196]. Apart from the logistic problems associated with this technique, the uncertainties concerning specificity and the questionable survival of HSC during relatively long culture periods, have precluded its clinical application so far.

Density gradient separation has been successfully carried out through all stages of preclinical testing and was used for human bone marrow on several occasions in the treatment of SCID patients, where the amount of donor marrow available is usually not limiting. Purified stem cells from HLA identical sibling donors were capable of reconstituting SCID patients just as well as whole bone marrow. In a series of similar grafts of purified stem cells from incompatible donors, three patients could be fully evaluated. None of these developed acute GVHD as is the rule following grafting of unmodified bone marrow. The patients died with severe infections of the intestinal tract, suggesting that further attempts along these lines have to include bacteriological decontamination, since this prevents mortality from delayed-type GVHD in rodents[197] and, to some extent, in monkeys[190]. In the treatment of aplastic anaemia, purified stem cells have been employed only occasionally, so that an evaluation cannot yet be made. In view of the requirement for larger amounts of donor marrow and the uncertainties concerning the takeability of purified stem cells in man, a systematic clinical investigation will be justified only when recipients with a high risk of developing GVHD can be identified.

Treatment of recipient after grafting

As regards the treatment of the recipient during the period after transplantation, some measures which proved to be very effective in laboratory experiments and have become established in the clinical GVHD. Post-transplantation treatment with moderate doses of methotrexate (MTX) has become standard practice, after it was shown to be effective in mitigating GVHD in dogs. It should be noted that a control series of patients not receiving MTX is not available and that it is by no means excluded that this treatment may adversely influence take of the graft, or delay recovery of the immune responsiveness in patients. After treatment with high doses of ALG was shown to be an effective means of treating overt GVHD in monkeys[182,198] and in dogs[199], it was also introduced clinically with encouraging results. ALG is now an accepted part of the therapeutic arsenal available in bone marrow transplant centres.

Many other chemotherapeutic agents have been screened in the Radiobiological Institute for their efficacy in preventing the occurrence of acute GVHD. The screening method[200,201] has consisted of their administration during one or more days before grafting and/or during one or more days (up to five) after grafting. The only very effective components found thus far are methotrexate and cyclophosphamide, which have to be given in high doses. Both were equally active in the monkey when administered during the first few days after bone marrow transplantation. When given later, GVHD is effectively suppressed, but so is haemopoietic activity, so that the end result is failure of the graft. Although there is no convincing evidence that corticosteroids suppress GVHD of the type which occurs in haemopoietic chimeras, there are recurring reports of their application in clinical GVHD[9]. Corticosteroids are anti-inflammatory agents and this may explain some of their effects seen in the treatment of patients suffering from GVHD, especially with regard to the skin lesions. On the other hand, these drugs are also known to be immunosuppressive and to increase the risk of infection. Furthermore, they have an adverse influence on the mortality of mouse radiation chimeras suffering from acute GVHD (van Bekkum, unpublished observations). Therefore, this treatment cannot be considered as sound and rational and should be discouraged until solid experimental support is provided.

An interesting observation has been made by Thompson *et al.*[151] which has never been further analysed. They could diminish the delayed mortality of radiation chimeras by the administration of large numbers of donor type lymph node or spleen cells on day 21 after the bone marrow transplant. Although the protection was moderate, it is most surprising that the donor lymphoid cells did not aggravate the GVHD. The latter did occur when the donor mice had been preimmunized with recipient tissue. Similar observations were recently reported by Storb *et al.*[202] in dog radiation chimeras, which were given 5×10^8 lymphocytes per kg body weight at 200–1400 days after bone marrow transplantation. In view of the serious problems associated with prolonged immune deficiency in many human transplant patients, a more thorough investigation along these lines has to be recommended.

Gnotobiotic conditions are of major importance in the control of delayed GVHD mortality. No beneficial effect has been documented in the treatment of acute GVHD. However, enterobacteria-free mice and germ-free mice show very little or no mortality at all under conditions of allogeneic bone marrow transplantation which usually results in a high percentage of delayed death. It is of practical interest that the reintroduction of a conventional gut microflora as early as 4 weeks after grafting, does not reinduce the diarrhoea and the concomitant wasting[136]. This observation suggests that crypt lesions associated with delayed GVHD are induced soon after transplantation, and that they may heal rapidly and permanently, if infection with enterobacteria is prevented. Bacteriological decontamination has also been shown to prolong the survival of monkeys suffering from the delayed type of GVHD, following the transplantation of lymphocyte depleted stem cell concentrates from random non-matched donors[203].

Total bacteriological decontamination, which can only be achieved under nursing conditions of reverse isolation, is presently being practised at a few clinical transplant centres[204–206]. The experience so far seems to be encouraging, but the number of evaluable patients is insufficient to permit valid comparisons with conventional patients.

Prevention of GVHD after transplantation of marrow from non-genotypically HLA identical donors

When the most effective technique for the prevention of GVHD, namely, purification of stem cells combined with bacteriological decontamination of the recipients, was applied to the most demanding model, i.e. the irradiated rhesus monkey grafted with random mismatched marrow, the survival time was increased from an average of 13 days for the conventional monkeys receiving unmodified marrow to over 60 days[190]. The eventual mortality in the latter group was not due to overt GVHD but was associated with generalized virus infections[207]. These viruses were endogenous and their secondary invasiveness is attributed to the extreme immune depression which is prevalent in these allogeneic monkey chimeras. A similar approach for the clinical mitigation of GVHD has not been made thus far, and for good reasons. The experiments with monkeys described above suggest the existence of important differences between rodents and primates in the rate of recovery of immune competence of allogeneic bone marrow chimeras. Humans are more likely to conform to the patterns found in monkeys than those seen in mice. Therefore, another mitigating factor has to be added before a serious attempt at the use of non-sibling donors for bone marrow transplantation in human patients is justified. At present the most profitable approach seems to be the selection of HLA-A, -B, -C and if possible HLA-D compatible donors from other relatives or unrelated individuals and to combine this selection with stem cell separation and bacteriological decontamination.

CONCLUSIONS

When one overlooks the clinical achievements with bone marrow transplantation over the past 10 years, the most striking feature is the relative negligence on the part of clinicians to take into account the wealth of useful information emerging from the research with experimental animal models. If the guidelines which have emerged from the latter results had been more carefully adopted, the outcome of clinical transplants could have reached higher levels much sooner.

Foremost examples are the convincing evidence that a minimal cell number is required to achieve a take of the bone marrow graft, that sensitization of the recipient counteracts graft take, that small marrow cell numbers are preferred in SCID if GVHD is to be avoided and that treatment with ALG is effective in suppressing GVHD. For many years it has been known that cyclophosphamide is not a very effective conditioning agent, yet large series of patients had to be conditioned that way before other conditioning regimens developed.

In addition, TBI is employed to condition patients for bone marrow grafting in a very inconvenient regimen of low dose irradiation, and sometimes partial body irradiation is used. These procedures have no scientific rationale and ignore the existence of exhaustive experience with the production of animal radiation chimeras and with radiation biology as a whole.

A sound understanding of the processes occurring in lethally irradiated mice following a bone marrow graft will warrant a high-level scientific approach to the problems of clinical bone marrow transplantation. As a rule, significant modifications of the clinical transplantation regimen should be adopted only after their value has been thoroughly demonstrated in other outbred species, e.g. the monkey or the dog.

The argument that one is dealing with treatment of otherwise fatal disease cannot be accepted to justify unnecessary experimentation with human patients, since perfectly adequate preclinical models are available to unravel the majority, if not all of the problems at hand. There can be no doubt that the most pressing questions of the present, namely the abrogation of allogeneic resistance, the improvement of donor selection and the enhancement of immunological recovery after a take has been established, can all be satisfactorily investigated in appropriate animal models and eventually solved, if the laws of biology will permit a solution.

References

1. Bortin, M. M. (1970). A compendium of reported bone marrow transplants. *Transplantation*, **9**, 571

2. Bortin, M. M. and Rimm, A. A. (1977). Severe combined immunodeficiency disease. Characterization of the disease and results of transplantation. *Transplant. Proc.*, **9**, 169
3. Camitta, B. M., Rappaport, J. M., Parkman, R. *et al.* (1975). Selection of patients for bone marrow transplantation in severe aplastic anemia. *Blood*, **45**, 355
4. Hellriegel, K. P., Züger, M. and Gross, R. (1977). Prognosis in acquired aplastic anemia. An approach in the selection of patients for allogeneic bone marrow transplantation. *Blut*, **34**, 11
5. Lohrmann, H. P., Niethammer, D. and Kern, P. (1976). The identification of high-risk patients with aplastic anemia in selection for allogeneic bone marrow transplantation. *Lancet*, **ii**, 647
6. Advisory Committee of the Bone Marrow Transplant Registry (USA). (1976). Bone marrow transplantation from donors with aplastic anemia. *J. Am. Med. Assoc.*, **236**, 1113
7. Storb, R., Thomas, E. D., Buckner, C. D. *et al.* (1974). Allogeneic marrow grafting for treatment of aplastic anemia. *Blood*, **43**, 157
8. Storb, R., Thomas, E. D., Weiden, P. L. *et al.* (1976). Aplastic anemia treated by allogeneic bone marrow transplantation. A report on 49 new cases from Seattle. *Blood*, **48**, 817
9. UCLA Bone Marrow Transplant Team (1976). Bone marrow transplantation in severe aplastic anemia. *Lancet*, **ii**, 921
10. Thomas, E. D., Buckner, C. D., Cheever, M. A. *et al.* (1976). Marrow transplantation for leukemia and aplastic anemia. *Transplant. Proc.*, **7**, 603
11. Thomas, E. D., Buckner, C. D., Bonaji, M. *et al.* (1977). One hundred patients with acute leukemia treated by chemotherapy, total body irradiation, and allogeneic marrow transplantation. *Blood*, **49**, 511
12. Storb, R., Thomas, E. D., Buckner, C. D. *et al.* (1976). Allogeneic marrow grafting for treatment of aplastic anemia. A follow-up on long-term survivors. *Blood*, **48**, 485
13. Johnson, F. L., Hartmann, J. R., Thomas, E. D. *et al.* (1976). Marrow transplantation in treatment of children with aplastic anemia or acute leukaemia. *Arch. Dis. Child.*, **51**, 403
14. Camitta, B. M., Thomas, E. D., Nathan, D. G. *et al.* (1976). Severe aplastic anemia. A prospective study of the effect of early bone marrow transplantation on acute mortality. *Blood*, **48**, 63
15. Storb, R., Prentice, R. L. and Thomas, E. D. (1977). Marrow transplantation for treatment of aplastic anemia. *N. Engl. J. Med.*, **296**, 61
16. van Bekkum, D. W. and Vos, O. (1957). Immunological aspects of homo- and heterologous bone marrow transplantation in irradiated animals. *J. Cell. Comp. Physiol.*, **50**, 139
17. van Bekkum, D. W. and de Vries, M. J. (1967). *Radiation Chimaeras* (New York/London: Academic Press/Logos Press)
18. Crouch, B. G., van Putten, L. M., van Bekkum, D. W. *et al.* (1961). Treatment of total body X-irradiated monkeys with autologous and homologous bone marrow. *J. Nat. Cancer Inst.*, **27**, 53
19. Vriesendorp, H. M., Zurcher, C. and van Bekkum, D. W. (1975). Engraftment of allogeneic dog bone marrow. *Transplant. Proc.*, **7**, 465
20. Vriesendorp, H. M., Löwenberg, B., Visser, T. P. *et al.* (1976). Influence of genetic resistance and silica particles on survival after bone marrow transplantation. *Transplant. Proc.*, **8**, 483
21. Camitta, B. M., Nathan, D. G. *et al.* (1974). Postoperative severe aplastic anemia—an indication for early bone marrow transplantation. *Blood*, **43**, 473
22. Hathaway, W. E., Githens, J. H., Blackburn, W. R. *et al.* (1965). Aplastic anemia histocytosis and erythrodermia in immunologically deficient children. *N. Engl. J. Med.*, **273**, 953
23. Hathaway, W. E., Brangle, R. E., Nelson, Th. L. *et al.* (1966). Aplastic anemia and alymphocytosis in an infant with hypogammaglobulin anemia: Graft-versus-host reaction? *J. Pediatr.*, **68**, 713

24. Hathaway, W. E., Fulginiti, V. A., Pierce, C. W. *et al.* (1967). Graft-versus-host reaction following a single blood transfusion. *J. Am. Med. Assoc.*, **201**, 1015
25. Rosen, F. S., Gastoff, S. P., Craig, J. M. *et al.* (1966). Further observations on the Swiss type of agammaglobulinemia (alymphocytosis) the effect of syngeneic bone marrow cells. *N. Engl. J. Med.*, **274**, 18
26. Copenhagen Study Group of Immunodeficiencies. (1973). Bone marrow transplantation from an HLA nonidentical but mixed lymphocyte culture identical donor. *Lancet*, **i**, 1146
27. van Bekkum, D. W. (1972). Use and abuse of hemopoietic cell grafts in immune deficiency diseases. *Transplant. Rev.*, **9**, 3
28. Dicke, K. A., van Hooft, J. I. M. and van Bekkum, D. W. (1968). The selective elimination of immunocompetent cells from bone marrow and lymphatic cell mixtures. II. Mouse spleen cell fractionation on a discontinuous albumin gradient. *Transplantation*, **6**, 562
29. Dicke, K. A., Tridente, G. and van Bekkum, D. W. (1969). The selective elimination of immunocompetent cells from bone marrow and lymphatic cell mixtures. III. *In vitro* test for detection of immunocompetent cells in fractionated mouse spleen cell suspensions and primate bone marrow suspensions. *Transplantation*, **8**, 422
30. Dicke, K. A., Lina, P. H. C. and van Bekkum, D. W. (1970). Adaptation of albumin density gradient centrifugation to human bone marrow fractionation. *Rev. Eur. d'études Clin. Biol.*, **15**, 305
31. Dicke, K. A. and van Bekkum, D. W. (1972). Preparation and use of stem cell concentrates for restoration of immune deficiency diseases and bone marrow aplasia. *Rev. Eur. Études Clin. Biol.*, **17**, 645
32. van Bekkum, D. W. and Dicke, K. A. (1971). Treatment of immune deficiency disease with bone marrow stem cell concentrates. In: *Ontogeny of Acquired Immunity*. A Ciba Foundation Symposium, pp. 233–47 (Amsterdam: Elsevier/North-Holland)
33. Löwenberg, B. (1975). Fetal liver cell transplantation. (Thesis, Rotterdam University)
34. Buckley, R. H. (1971). Reconstitution: Grafting of bone marrow and thymus. In: *First Int. Congress of Immunology* (B. Amos, ed.), p. 1061 (New York/London: Academic Press)
35. Barnes, D. W. H., Loutit, J. F. and Micklem, H. S. (1961). 'Secondary disease' in lethally irradiated mice restored with syngeneic or allogeneic foetal liver cells. In: *Mechanisms of Immunology* (M. Hasek, A. Lengerova and M. Vojskova, eds.), pp. 371–7 (Prague: Czechoslovak Academy of Sciences)
36. Crouch, B. G. (1959). Transplantation of fetal hemopoietic tissues into irradiated mice and rats. In: *Proc. Seventh Congress of the Eur. Soc. for Haematology*, pp. 973–8, London
37. Lengerova, A. (1959). Comparison of the therapeutic efficiency of homologous and heterologous embryonic haematopoietic cells administered to lethally irradiated mice. *Folia Biol.*, **5**, 18
38. Löwenberg, B., de Zeeuw, H. M. C., Dicke, K. A. *et al.* (1977). Nature of the delayed graft-versus-host reactivity of fetal liver cell transplants. *J. Nat. Cancer Inst.*, **58**, 959
39. van Putten, L. M., van Bekkum, D. W. and de Vries, M. J. (1968). Transplantation of foetal haemopoietic cells in irradiated rhesus monkeys. In: *Radiation and the Control of the Immune Response*, pp. 41–9 (Vienna: IAEA)
40. Uphoff, D. E. (1958). Preclusion of secondary phase of irradiation syndrome by inoculation of fetal hematopoietic tissue following lethal total body X-irradiation. *J. Nat. Cancer Inst.*, **20**, 625
41. Uphoff, D. E. (1959). Alteration of survival pattern by homologous fetal haematopoietic tissue in lethally irradiated mice. *Radiat. Res.*, **11**, 474
42. Urso, I. S., Congdon, C. C. and Owen, R. D. (1959). Effect of foreign fetal and newborn blood-forming tissues on survival of lethally irradiated mice. *Proc. Soc. Exp. Biol. Med.*, **100**, 395
43. Githens, J. H., Fulginiti, V. A., Suvatte, V. *et al.* (1973). Grafting of fetal thymus and hematopoietic tissue in infants with immune deficiency syndromes. *Transplantation*, **15**, 427

44. Löwenberg, B., Vossen, J. M. J. J. and Dooren, L. J. (1977). Transplantation of fetal liver cells in the treatment of severe combined immunodeficiency disease. *Blut*, **34**, 181
45. Soothill, J. F., Kay, H. E. M. and Batchelor, J. R. (1971). Graft restoration of primary immunodeficiency. In: *Cell Interaction and Receptor Antibodies in Immune Responses* (O. Makelo, A. Cross and T. E. Kosmer, eds.), pp. 41–52 (New York: Academic Press)
46. Löwenberg, B., Dicke, K. A. and van Bekkum, D. W. (1975). Quantitative studies on the take of fetal liver haemopoietic transplants. *Transplant. Proc.*, **7**, 1965
47. Löwenberg, B., Dicke, K. A., van Bekkum, D. W. *et al.* (1976). Quantitative aspects of fetal liver cell transplantation in animals and man. *Transplant. Proc.*, **8**, 527
48. Rugh, R. (1958). X-irradiation effects of the human fetus. *J. Pediatr.*, **52**, 531
49. August, C. S., King, E., Githens, J. H. *et al.* (1976). Establishment of erythropoiesis following bone marrow transplantation in a patient with congenital hypoplastic anemia (Diamond–Blackfan Syndrome). *Blood*, **48**, 491
50. Camitta, B. M., Quesenberry, P. J., Parkman, R. *et al.* (1977). Bone marrow transplantation for an infant with neutrophil dysfunction. *Exp. Hematol.*, **5**, 109
51. The Westminster Hospitals Bone-Marrow Transplant Team (1977). Bone marrow transplant from an unrelated donor for chronic granulomatous disease. *Lancet*, **i**, 210
52. Storb, R., Evans, R. S., Thomas, E. D. *et al.* (1973). Paroxysmal nocturnal haemoglobinuria and refractory marrow failure treated by marrow transplantation. *Br. J. Haematol.*, **24**, 743
53. Johnson, F. L., Thomas, E. D., Buckner, C. D. *et al.* (1974). The current status of bone marrow transplantation in cancer treatment. *Cancer Treatm. Rev.*, **1**, 81
54. Second International Symposium on the Immunobiology of Bone Marrow Transplantation, Los Angeles, 27–29th June, 1977. *Transplant. Proc.* (In press)
55. UCLA Bone Marrow Transplant Team (1977). Bone marrow transplantation with intensive combination chemotherapy/radiation therapy (SCARI) in acute leukemia. *Ann. Intern. Med.*, **86**, 155
56. Boranic, M. (1968). Transient graft-versus-host reaction in the treatment of leukemia in mice. *J. Nat. Cancer Inst.*, **41**, 421
57. Bortin, M. M., Rimm, A. A., Saltzstein, E. C. *et al.* (1973). Graft versus leukemia. III. Apparent independent antihost and antileukemic activity of transplanted immunocompetent cells. *Transplantation*, **16**, 182
58. Fefer, A., Thomas, E. D., Buckner, C. D. *et al.* (1974). Marrow transplants in aplastic anemia and leukemia. *Sem. Hematol.*, **11**, 353
59. Buckner, C. D., Clift, R. A., Fefer, A. *et al.* (1974). Treatment of blastic transformation of chronic granulocytic leukemia by high dose cyclophosphamide, total body irradiation and infusion of cryopreserved autologous marrow. *Exp. Hematol.*, **2**, 138
60. Dicke, K. A., McCredie, K. B., Stevens, E. E. *et al.* (1977). Autologous bone marrow transplantation in a case of acute adult leukemia. *Transplant. Proc.*, **9**, 193
61. Metcalf, D. and Moore, M. A. S. (1971). Haemopoietic cells, their origin, migration and differentiation. In: *Frontiers of Biology*, Vol. 24 (Amsterdam: North-Holland Publ. Co.)
62. McCulloch, E. A. and Till, J. E. (1963). Repression of colony-forming ability of C57BL hematopoietic cells transplanted into non-isologous hosts. *J. Cell. Comp. Physiol.*, **61**, 301
63. Pike, B. L. and Robinson, W. A. (1970). Human bone marrow colony growth in agar-gel. *J. Cell. Physiol.*, **76**, 77
64. van den Engh, G. J. (1976). Early events in haemopoietic cell differentiation. (Thesis, Leiden University)
65. Vos, O., de Vries, M. J., Collenteur, J. C. *et al.* (1959). Transplantation of homologous and heterologous lymphoid cells in X-irradiated and non-irradiated mice. *J. Nat. Cancer Inst.*, **23**, 53
66. Bernstein, S. E. and Russell, E. S. (1959). Implantation of normal blood-forming tissue in

genetically anemic mice, without X-irradiation of host. *Proc. Nat. Acad. Soc. Exp. Biol.*, **101**, 769
67. Kolb, H. J., Storb, R., Weiden, P. L. *et al.* (1974). Immunologic, toxicologic and marrow transplantation studies in dogs given dimethyl myleran. *Biomedicine*, **20**, 342
68. Santos, G. W. and Tutschka, P. J. (1974). Marrow transplantation in the busulfan treated rat: Preclinical model of aplastic anemia. *J. Nat. Cancer Inst.*, **53**, 178
69. Storb, R., Epstein, R. B., Rudolph, R. H. *et al.* (1969). Allogeneic canine bone marrow transplantation following cyclophosphamide. *Transplantation*, **7**, 378
70. Mathé, G., Schwarzenberg, L., Amiel, J. L. *et al.* (1972). Bone marrow transplantation after antilymphocyte globulin conditioning split lymphocyte chimerism. *Transplant. Proc.*, **4**, 551
71. Storb, R. and Thomas, E. D. (1972). Bone marrow transplantation in randomly bred animal species and in man. In: *Proc. 6th Leukocyte Culture Conference*, p. 805 (New York: Academic Press)
72. Balner, H., Simmel, E. B. and Clarke, D. A. (1962). Proliferation and rejection of transplanted tritium labelled bone marrow cells in mice. *Transplant. Bull.*, **29**, 427
73. Nowell, P. C., Cole, L. J., Roan, P. L. *et al.* (1956). The distribution and *in situ* growth pattern of rat marrow cells in X-radiated mice. *Cancer Res.*, **16**, 258
74. Schaefer, U. W., Snel, D. P. B. M. and Boorman, G. A. (1972). Intraperitoneal administration of allogeneic bone marrow cells in lethally irradiated rhesus monkeys. *Exp. Hematol.*, **22**, 98
75. van Bekkum, D. W., Vos, O. and Weijzen, W. W. H. (1956). Homo- et hétérogreffe de tissus hématopoietiques chez la souris. *Rev. Hématol.*, **11**, 477
76. Trentin, J. J. (1971). Determinations of bone marrow stem cell differentiation by normal hemopoietic inductive microenvironments (HIM). *Am. J. Pathol.*, **65**, 621
77. Wagemaker, G. (1976). Erythropoietine, enkele aspecten van de humorale regulatie van de erythropoiese. (Thesis, Erasmus University, Rotterdam)
78. van Bekkum, D. W. (ed.) (1975). *The Biological Activity of Thymic Hormones* (Rotterdam: Kooyker Scientific Publications/New York: Wiley)
79. Robinson, W., Bradley, T. R. and Metcalf, D. (1967). Effect of whole body irradiation on colony production of bone marrow cells *in vitro*. *Proc. Soc. Exp. Biol. Med.*, **125**, 388
80. van Bekkum, D. W. (1974). Use of ionizing radiation in transplantation. *Transplant. Proc.*, **6**, 59
81. Makinodan, T. and Price, G. B. (1972). In: *Transplantation* (J. S. Najarian and R. L. Simmonds, eds.), p. 251 (Philadelphia: Lea and Febiger)
82. Weiden, P. L., Storb, R., Graham, T. C. *et al.* (1977). Resistance to DLA-nonidentical marrow grafts in lethally irradiated dogs. *Transplant. Proc.*, **9**, 285
83. Herzig, G., Carolla, R., Alvegard, T. *et al.* (1972). Allogeneic bone marrow transplantation (BMTX) following total body irradiation (TBI) and L-asparaginase (L-asp). *Clin. Res.*, **20**, 490
84. Vriesendorp, H. M., Zurcher, C., Bull, R. W. *et al.* (1975). Take and graft-versus-host reactions of allogeneic bone marrow in tissue-typed dogs. *Transplant. Proc.*, **7**, Suppl. 1, 849
85. Cudkowicz, G. and Bennett, M. (1971). Peculiar immunobiology of bone marrow allografts. I. Graft rejection by irradiated responder mice. *J. Exp. Med.*, **134**, 83
86. van Putten, L. M., van Bekkum, D. W., de Vries, M. J. *et al.* (1967). The effect of preceding blood transfusions on the fate of homologous bone marrow grafts in lethally irradiated monkeys. *Blood*, **30**, 749
87. Storb, R., Epstein, R. B., Rudolph, R. H. *et al.* (1970). The effect of prior transfusion on marrow grafts between histocompatible canine siblings. *J. Immunol.*, **105**, 627
88. Storb, R., Rudolph, R. H., Graham, T. C. *et al.* (1971). The influence of transfusions from unrelated donors upon marrow grafts between histocompatible canine siblings. *J. Immunol.*, **107**, 409

89. Warren, R. P., Storb, R., Weiden, P. L. *et al.* (1977). Direct and antibody dependent cell-mediated cytotoxicity against HLA-identical sibling lymphocytes. Correlation with marrow graft rejection. *Transplantation* (In press)
90. Storb, R., Floersheim, G. L., Weiden, P. L. *et al.* (1974). Effect of prior blood transfusions on marrow grafts: abrogation of sensitization by procarbazine and antithymocyte serum. *J. Immunol.*, **112**, 1508
91. Bull, M. I., Herzig, G. P. and Graw, R. G. (1976). Canine allogeneic bone marrow transplantation. Technique and variables influencing engraftment. *Transplantation*, **22**, 150
92. Courtenay, U. D. (1963). Studies on the protective effect of allogeneic marrow grafts in the rat following whole body irradiation at different dose rates. *Br. J. Radiol.*, **36**, 440
93. Gengozian, N., Carlson, D. E. and Allen, E. M. (1969). Transplantation of allogeneic and xenogeneic (rat) marrow in irradiated mice as effected by radiation exposure rates. *Transplantation*, **7**, 259
94. Liversage, W. E. (1969). A general formula for equating protracted and acute regimens of radiation. *Br. J. Radiol.*, **42**, 432
95. UN Report of the United Nations Scientific Committee on the Effects of Atomic Radiation, New York (1962). Official records of the General Assembly, Seventeenth Session, Supplement No. 16 (A/5216)
96. van Bekkum, D. W. (1968). Hostile grafts. In: *Advance in Transplantation* (J. Dausset, J. Hamburger and G. Mathé, eds.), pp. 565–72 (Copenhagen: Munksgaard)
97. Thomas, E. D., Ashley, C. A., Lochte, H. L. *et al.* (1959). Homografts of bone marrow in dogs after lethal body irradiation. *Blood*, **14**, 720
98. Mathé, G., Bernard, J., de Vries, M. J. *et al.* (1960). Nouveaux essais de greffe de moelle osseuse homologue après irradiation totale chez des enfants atteints de leucémie aiguë en rémission. *Rev. Hématol.*, **15**, 115
99. Santos, G. W. and Owens, A. H. Jr. (1968). Syngeneic and allogeneic marrow transplants in the cyclophosphamide pretreated rat. *Adv. Transplant.*, **28**, 431
100. van Bekkum, D. W., Dicke, K. A., Balner, H. *et al.* (1970). Failure to obtain take of allogeneic bone marrow grafts in monkeys following pretreatment with cyclophosphamide. *Exp. Hematol.*, **20**, 27
101. Storb, R., Buckner, C. D., Dillingham, L. A. *et al.* (1970). Cyclophosphamide regimens in rhesus monkeys with and without marrow infusion. *Cancer Res.*, **30**, 2195
102. Appelbaum, F. R., Strauden, J. A., Graw, R. G. Jr. *et al.* (1976). Acute lethal carditis caused by high-dose combination chemotherapy. A unique clinical pathological entity. *Lancet*, **i**, 58
103. Seller, M. J. and Polani, P. E. (1969). Transplantation of allogeneic haemopoietic tissue in adult anaemic mice of the W series using antilymphocytic serum. *Lancet*, **i**, 18
104. Mathé, G., Amiel, J. L., Schwarzenberg, L. *et al.* (1968). Greffe de moelle osseuse allogénique chez l'homme prouvée par six marqeurs antigéniques après conditionnement du receveux et du donneur par le serum antilymphocytaire. *Rev. Eur. Études Clin. Biol.*, **13**, 1025
105. Mathé, G. and Schwarzenberg, L. (1974). Bone marrow transplantation in France 1958–1973. *Transplant. Proc.*, **4**, 335
106. Mathé, G., Amiel, J. L., Schwarzenberg, L. *et al.* (1971). Bone marrow graft in man after conditioning by antilymphocytic serum. *Transplant Proc.*, **3**, 325
107. Speck, B. and Kissling, M. (1971). Successful bone marrow grafts in experimental aplastic anemia using antilymphocyte serum for conditioning. *Rev. Eur. Études Clin. Biol.*, **16**, 1047
108. Bau, J. and Thierfelder, S. (1973). Antilymphocytic antibodies and marrow transplantation. I. The effect of antilymphocytic serum on xenogeneic engraftment. *Transplantation*, **15**, 564
109. Corneci, I., Adrian, T., Costachel, O. *et al.* (1971). Antilymphoid globulin in the therapy of secondary disease. *Transplant. Proc.*, **3**, 422

110. van Bekkum, D. W. (1974). The double barrier in bone marrow transplantation. *Sem. Hematol.*, **11**, 325
111. Cree, I. C. (1962). Homografting of haemopoietic tissue after cytotoxic drugs. *Lancet*, **i**, 1104
112. Rauchweyer, J. M., Gallagher, M. T., Monié, H. J. *et al.* (1976). 'Xenogeneic resistance' in rat bone marrow transplantation. III. Maturation and abrogation with cyclophosphamide, *Corynebacterium parvum* and fractionated irradiation. *Biomedicine*, **24**, 20
113. Storb, R., Thomas, E. D., Buckner, C. D. *et al.* (1974). Transplantation of bone marrow in refractory marrow failure and neoplastic diseases. *Am. J. Clin. Pathol.*, **62**, 212
114. Graw, R. G. Jr., Lohrmann, H. P., Bull, M. I. *et al.* (1974). Bone marrow transplantation following combination chemotherapy immunosuppression (BACT) in patients with acute leukemia. *Transplant. Proc.*, **6**, 349
115. Gale, R. P., Fey, S. A. and Varna, G. (1977). A cytoreductive conditioning program for bone marrow transplantation in resistant leukemia (SCARI). *Transplant. Proc.*, **9**, 177
116. Gold, P. and Freeman, S. O. (1965). Demonstration of tumour-specific antigens in human colonic carcinomata by immunological tolerance and absorption techniques. *J. Exp. Med.*, **121**, 439
117. Goodman, J. W. and Shrinpock, S. G. (1972). Further studies on the relationship of the thymus to hemopoiesis. *Transplantation*, **13**, 203
118. Storb, R., Epstein, R. B., Bryant, J. *et al.* (1968). Marrow grafts by combined marrow and leukocyte infusions in unrelated dogs selected by histocompatibility typing. *Transplantation*, **6**, 587
119. Dicke, K. A. (1970). Bone marrow transplantation after separation by discontinuous albumin density gradient centrifugation. (Thesis, Leiden University)
120. Parker, J. W. and Metcalf, D. (1974). Production of colony stimulating factor (CSF) in mixed leukocyte cultures. In: *Lymphocyte Recognition and Effector Mechanisms* (K. Lindahl-Kiessling and D. Osoba, eds.), pp. 445–550 (New York/London: Academic Press)
121. Singer, J. W. and Thomas, E. D. (1976). Colony stimulating factor as a marker for graft-versus-host disease in man. *Exp. Hematol.*, **4**, Suppl. 1976, p. 197
122. Vriesendorp, H. M., Bijnen, A. B., Westbroek, D. L. *et al.* (1977). Genetics and transplantation immunology of the DLA complex. *Transplant. Proc.*, **9**, 293
123. Vriesendorp, H. M. (1973). The major histocompatibility complex of the dog. (Thesis, Erasmus University, Rotterdam)
124. Vriesendorp, H. M., Grosse Wilde, H. and Dorf, M. E. (1978). The major histocompatibility system of the dog. In: *Organization of the Histocompatibility System* (D. Götze and J. Klein, eds.) (Heidelberg: Springer Verlag) (In press)
125. Amato, D., Bergsagel, D. E., Clarysse, A. M. *et al.* (1971). Review of bone marrow transplants at the Ontario Cancer Institute. *Transplant. Proc.*, **3**, 397
126. Glucksberg, H., Storb, R., Fefer, A., Buckner, C. D. *et al.* (1974). Clinical manifestations of graft-versus-host disease in human recipients of marrow from HL-A matched sibling donors. *Transplantation*, **18**, 295
127. Krüger, G. R. F., Berad, C. W., DeLellis, R. A. *et al.* (1971). Graft-versus-host disease. *Am. J. Pathol.*, **63**, 179
128. Mathé, G., Schwarzenberg, L., de Vries, M. J. *et al.* (1965). Les divers aspects du syndrome secondaire compliquant les transfusions allogéniques de moelle osseuse ou de leucocytes chez des sujets atteints d'hémopathies malignes. *Eur. J. Cancer*, **1**, 75
129. Slavin, R. E. and Santos, G. W. (1973). The graft-versus-host reaction in man after bone marrow transplantation: Pathology, pathogenesis, clinical features, and implication. *Clin. Immunol. Immunopathol.*, **1**, 472
130. Balner, H. (1964). Secondary disease in rat radiation chimeras. *J. Nat. Cancer Inst.*, **32**, 419
131. de Vries, M. J. and Vos. O. (1959). Delayed mortality of radiation chimeras. A pathological and hematological study. *J. Nat. Cancer Inst.*, **23**, 1403

132. de Vries, M. J., Crouch, B. G., van Putten, L. M. *et al.* (1961). Pathologic changes in irradiated monkeys treated with bone marrow. *J. Nat. Cancer Inst.*, **27**, 67
133. Woodruff, J. M., Eltringham, J. R. and Casey, H. W. (1969). Early secondary disease in the rhesus monkey. I. A comparative histopathologic study. *Lab. Invest.*, **20**, 499
134. Mathé, G. and Amiel, J. L. (1961). Études sur le tissu lymphoid des radio-chimères hématologiques. *Pathol.-Biol.*, **9**, 894
135. van Bekkum, D. W. and Vos, O. (1961). Treatment of secondary disease in radiation chimeras. *Int. J. Radiat. Biol.*, **3**, 173
136. van Bekkum, D. W., Roodenburg, J., Heidt, P. J. *et al.* (1974). Mitigation of secondary disease of allogeneic mouse radiation chimeras by modification of the intestinal microflora. *J. Nat. Cancer Inst.*, **52**, 401
137. Heit, H., Wilson, R., Fliedner, T. M. *et al.* (1972). Mortality of secondary disease in antibiotic-treated mouse radiation chimeras. In: *Germfree Research, Biological Effect of Gnotobiotic Environments* (J. B. Heneghan, ed.), pp. 477–83 (New York/London: Academic Press)
138. van Bekkum, D. W. (1964). The selective elimination of immunologically competent cells from bone marrow and lymphatic cell mixtures. I. Effect of storage at 4 °C. *Transplantation*, **2**, 393
139. van Bekkum, D. W., de Vries, M. J. and van der Waaij, D. (1967). Lesions characteristic of secondary disease in germfree heterologous radiation chimeras. *J. Nat. Cancer Inst.*, **38**, 223
140. Dicke, K. A., Löwenberg, B. and Nieuwerkerk, H. T. M. (1975). Elimination of lymphocytes from human marrow suspensions: Gradient versus small marrow aspirates. *Transplant. Proc.*, **7**, Suppl. 1, 863
141. Dicke, K. A. and van Bekkum, D. W. (1971). Allogeneic bone marrow transplantation after elimination of immunocompetent cells by means of density gradient centrifugation. *Transplant. Proc.*, **3**, 666
142. van Putten, L. M. (1964). Thymectomy: Effect on secondary disease in radiation chimeras. *Science*, **145**, 935
143. van Bekkum, D. W. (1963). Determination of specific immunological tolerance in radiation chimeras. *Transplantation*, **1**, 39
144. Sprent, J., Boehmer, H. von and Nabholz, M. (1975). Association of immunity and tolerance to host H-2 determinants in irradiated F_1 hybrid mice reconstituted with bone marrow cells from one parental strain. *J. Exp. Med.*, **142**, 321
145. Hellström, I., Hellström, K. E., Storb, R. *et al.* (1970). Colony inhibition of fibroblasts from chimeric dogs mediated by the dogs' own lymphocytes and specifically abrogated by their serum. *Proc. Nat. Acad. Sci. USA*, **66**, 65
146. Hellström, I. and Hellström, K. E. (1973). Cellular immunity and blocking serum activity in chimeric mice. *Cell. Immunol.*, **7**, 73
147. Grant, C. K., Leuchars, E. and Alexander, P. (1972). Failure to detect cytotoxic lymphoid cells or humoral blocking factors in mouse radiation chimaeras. *Transplantation*, **14**, 722
148. Schroeder, M. L., Storb, R., Graham, T. C. *et al.* (1975). Canine radiation chimeras: an attempt to demonstrate serum blocking factors by an *in vivo* approach. *J. Immunol.*, **114**, 540
149. Tsoi, M. S., Storb, R. Weiden, P. L. *et al.* (1975). Canine marrow transplantation: are serum blocking factors necessary to maintain the stable chimeric state? *J. Immunol.*, **114**, 531
150. Field, E. O. and Gibbs, J. E. (1966). Reduced sensitivity of F_1 hybrid rats to re-challenge with parental strain spleen cells. *Clin. Exp. Immunol.*, **1**, 195
151. Thompson, J. S., Simmons, E. L., Moy, R. H. *et al.* (1967). Studies on immunologic unresponsiveness during secondary disease. II. The effect of added donor and host immunologically competent cells. *J. Immunol.*, **98**, 179

152. Field, E. O., Cauchi, M. N. and Gibbs, J. E. (1967). The transfer of refractoriness to G-V-H disease in F_1 hybrid rats. *Transplantation*, **5**, 241
153. Cauchi, M. N. and Dawson, K. B. (1975). Serum-mediated inhibition of graft-versus-host reaction. *J. Exp. Med.*, **142**, 248
154. Cantrell, J. L. and Hildemann, W. H. (1972). Characteristics of disparate histocompatibility barriers in congenic strains of mice. I. Graft-versus-host reactions. *Transplantation*, **14**, 761
155. van Rood, J. J. and van Leeuwen, A. (1976). Major and minor histocompatibility systems in man and their importance in bone marrow transplantation. *Transplant. Proc.*, **8**, 429
156. Parkman, R., Rosen, F. S., Rappaport, J. *et al.* (1976). Detection of genetically determined histocompatibility antigen differences between HL-A identical and MLC nonreactive siblings. *Transplantation*, **21**, 110
157. Storb, R., Weiden, P. L., Prentice, R. L. *et al.* (1977). Aplastic anemia (AA) treated by allogeneic marrow transplantation: the Seattle experience. *Transplant. Proc.*, **9**, 181
158. Storb, R., Prentice, R. L. and Thomas, E. D. (1977). *J. Clin. Invest.* (In press)
159. Lengerova, A. and Chutna, J. (1959). The therapeutic efficiency of isologous bone marrow cells in lethally irradiated mice C57BL in different donor-recipient sex combinations. *Folia Biol.*, **5**, 24
160. Uphoff, D. E. (1975). Comparative survival of lethally irradiated inbred male mice inoculated with marrow from virgin or multiparous female donors. *J. Nat. Cancer Inst.*, **54**, 1343
161. de Vries, M. J. and Vos, O. (1958). Treatment of mouse lymphosarcoma by total body X-irradiation and by injection of bone marrow and lymph node cells. *J. Nat. Cancer Inst.*, **21**, 1117
162. Bailey, D. W. (1963). Histoincompatibility associated with the X-chromosome in mice. *Transplantation*, **1**, 70
163. Park, B. H. and Good, R. A. (1972). Third party mixed leukocyte culture test. A potential new method of histocompatibility testing. *Proc. Nat. Acad. Sci. USA*, **69**, 1490
164. Vriesendorp, H. M., Bijnen, A. B., Zurcher, C. *et al.* (1975). Donor selection and bone marrow transplantation in dogs. In: *Histocompatibility Testing, 1975* (F. Kismeyer-Nielsen, ed.), pp. 963–71 (Copenhagen: Munksgaard)
165. Zweibaum, A., Oriol, R., Feingold, N. *et al.* (1974). Studies on canine secretory alloantigens. *Tissue Antigens*, **4**, 115
166. van Bekkum, D. W. and Knaan, S. (1977). Role of bacterial microflora in development of intestinal lesions from graft-versus-host reaction. *J. Nat. Cancer Inst.*, **58**, 787
167. van Bekkum, D. W. (1977). Perspectives of immunological reconstitution. In: *Proc. 9th Int. Congress of Allergology, 24–30 October, 1976, Buenos Aires* (Amsterdam: Exerpta Medica) (In press)
168. Ochs, H. D., Storb, R., Thomas, E. D. *et al.* (1974). Immunologic reactivity in canine marrow graft recipients. *J. Immunol.*, **113**, 1039
169. Gengozian, N., Makinodan, T., Congdon, C. C. *et al.* (1958). The immune status of long-term survivors of lethally X-irradiated mice protected with isologous, homologous, or heterologous bone marrow. *Proc. Nat. Acad. Sci. USA*, **44**, 560
170. Makinodan, T., Gengozian, N. and Congdon, C. C. (1965). Agglutinin production in normal, sublethally irradiated, and lethally irradiated mice treated with mouse bone marrow. *J. Immunol.*, **77**, 250
171. Urso, P. and Gengozian, N. (1973). T-cell deficiency in mouse allogeneic radiation chimeras. *J. Immunol.*, **111**, 712
172. Trier, L. and Rubin, B. (1974). Bone marrow transplantation in inbred strains of mice. I. The failure of development of normal T-cell function following allogeneic transplantation. *Acta Pathol. Microbiol. Scand., Sect. B*, **82**, 724

173. van der Berg, P., Rádl, J., Löwenberg, B. *et al.* (1976). Homogeneous antibodies in lethally irradiated and autologous bone marrow reconstituted Rhesus monkeys. *Clin. Exp. Immunol.*, **23**, 355
174. Rádl, J., van den Berg, P., Voormolen, M. *et al.* (1974). Homogeneous immunoglobulins in sera of rhesus monkeys after lethal irradiation and bone marrow transplantation. *Clin. Exp. Immunol.*, **16**, 259
175. Fass, L., Ochs, H. D., Thomas, E. D. *et al.* (1973). Studies of immunological reactivity following syngeneic or allogeneic marrow grafts in man. *Transplantation*, **16**, 630
176. Fefer, A., Einstein, A. B., Thomas, E. D. *et al.* (1974). Bone-marrow transplantation for hematologic neoplasia in 16 patients with identical twins. *N. Engl. J. Med.*, **290**, 1389
177. Tyan, M. L. (1975). Modification of graft-versus-host disease with Con A and pre-immunization (39093). *Proc. Soc. Exp. Biol. Med.*, **150**, 628
178. Safford, J. W. and Tokuda, S. (1970). Suppression of the graft-versus-host reaction by passive immunization of donor against recipient antigens (34537). *Proc. Soc. Exp. Biol. Med.*, **133**, 2
179. Halle-Pannenko, O., Martyre, M. C. and Mathé, G. (1971). Prevention of graft-versus-host reaction by donor pretreatment with soluble H-2 antigens. *Transplantation*, **11**, 414
180. Liacopoulos, P., Merchant, B. and Harell, B. E. (1967). Effect of donor immunization with somatic polysaccharides on the graft-versus-host reactivity of transferred donor splenocytes. *Proc. Soc. Exp. Biol. Med.*, **125**, 958
181. Ledney, G. D. and van Bekkum, D. W. (1968). Suppression of acute secondary disease in the mouse with antilymphocyte serum. In: *Advance in Transplantation* (J. Dausset, J. Hamburger and G. Mathé, eds.), pp. 441–7 (Copenhagen: Munksgaard)
182. van Bekkum, D. W., Ledney, G. D., Balner, H. *et al.* (1967). Suppression of secondary disease following foreign bone marrow grafting with antilymphocyte serum. In: *Anti-lymphocytic serum*, CIBA Foundation Study Group no. 29, pp. 97–110 (London: Churchill)
183. Tridente, G. and van Bekkum, D. W. (1969). Effect of anti-lymphocyte serum on mouse lymphoid tissues *in vivo* and *in vitro*. In: *Lymphatic Tissue and Germinal Centers in Immune Response*, pp. 371–86 (New York: Plenum Press)
184. DeMeester, T. R., Anderson, N. D. and Shaffer, Ch. F. (1968). The effect of heterologous anti-lymphocyte serum on mouse hemopoietic stem cells. *J. Exp. Med.*, **127**, 731
185. Field, E. O. and Gibbs, J. E. (1968). Cross-reaction of anti-lymphocyte serum with haemopoietic stem cells. *Nature (Lond.)*, **217**, 561
186. Mookerjee, B. K., Azzolina, L. and Poultar, L. (1974). Interaction of anti-lymphocyte serum with hematopoietic stem cells. I. Effects *in vitro* and *in vivo*. *J. Immunol.*, **112**, 822
187. Storb, P., Gluckman, E., Thomas, E. D. *et al.* (1974). Treatment of established human graft-versus-host disease by antithymocyte globulin. *Blood*, **44**, 57
188. van den Engh, G. J. and Golub, E. S. (1974). Antigenic differences between hemopoietic stem cells and myeloid progenitors. *J. Exp. Med.*, **139**, 1621
189. Tyan, M. L. (1971). Modification of bone marrow induced GVH disease with heterologous antisera to gamma-globulin or whole serum. *J. Immunol.*, **106**, 586
190. Rodt, H., Thierfelder, S. and Eulitz, M. (1974). Anti-lymphocytic antibodies and marrow transplantation. III. Effect of heterologous anti-brain antibodies on acute secondary disease in mice. *Eur. J. Immunol.*, **4**, 25
191. Trentin, J. J. and Judd, K. P. (1973). Prevention of acute graft-versus-host (GVH) mortality with spleen-absorbed antithymocyte globulin (ATG). *Transplant. Proc.*, **5**, 865
192. Rietmüller, G., Rieber, E.-P. and Seeger, I. (1971). Suppression of graft-versus-host reaction by univalent anti-immunoglobulin antibody. *Nature New Biology*, **230**, 248
193. Mason, S. and Warner, N. L. (1970). The immunoglobulin nature of the antigen recognition site on cells mediating transplantation immunity and delayed hypersensitivity. *J. Immunol.*, **104**, 762

194. Clark, W. R. and Kimura, A. K. (1973). Effect of monolayer fractionation of lymphocytes on graft-versus-host reactivity. *Transplantation*, **16**, 110
195. Lonai, P., Eliraz, A., Wekerle, H. *et al.* (1973). Depletion of specific graft-versus-host reactivity following adsorption of non-sensitized lymphocytes on allogeneic fibroblasts. *Transplantation*, **15**, 368
196. Rubin, B. (1975). Studies on the adsorbability of graft-versus-host reactive lymphocytes. *Clin. Exp. Immunol.*, **20**, 513
197. Richie, E. R., Gallagher, M. T. and Trentin, J. J. (1973). Inhibition of the graft-versus-host reaction. II. Prevention of acute graft-versus-host mortality by Fab fragments of antilymphocyte globulin. *Transplantation*, **15**, 486
198. van Bekkum, D. W., Balner, H., Dicke, K. A. *et al.* (1972). The effect of pretreatment of allogeneic bone marrow graft recipients with antilymphocytic serum on the acute graft-versus-host reaction in monkeys. *Transplantation*, **13**, 400
199. Kolb, H. J., Storb, R., Graham, T. C. *et al.* (1973). Antithymocyte serum and methotrexate for control of graft-versus-host disease in dogs. *Transplantation*, **16**, 17
200. van Bekkum, D. W. (1969). The prevention and control of secondary disease following allogeneic bone marrow transplantation. In: *Bone-Marrow Conservation, Culture and Transplantation*, pp. 35–45 (Vienna: IAEA)
201. Muller-Bérat, C. N., van Putten, L. M. and van Bekkum, D. W. (1966). Cytostatic drugs in the treatment of secondary disease following homologous bone marrow transplantation: extrapolation from the mouse to the primate. *Ann. N.Y. Acad. Sci.*, **129**, 340
202. Storb, R., Tsoi, M. S. and Thomas, E. D. (1976). Studies on the mechanism of stable graft host tolerance in canine and human radiation chimeras. *Transplant. Proc.*, **8**, 561
203. van Bekkum, D. W. (1975). Current developments in bone marrow transplantation. *Transplant. Proc.*, **7**, Suppl. 1, 805
204. Vossen, J. M. and van der Waay, D. (1972). Reverse isolation in bone marrow transplantation: ultra-clean room compared with laminar flow technique. II. Microbiological and clinical results. *Rev. Eur. Études Clin. Biol.*, **16**, 564
205. Vossen, J. M. and van der Waay, D. (1972). Reverse isolation in bone marrow transplantation: ultra-clean room compared with laminar flow technique. I. Isolation systems. *Rev. Eur. Études Clin. Biol.*, **17**, 457
206. Vossen, J. M., Dooren, L. J. and van der Waay, D. (1972). Clinical experience with the control of the microflora. In: *Germfree Research, Biological Effect of Gnotobiotic Environments* (J. B. Heneghan, ed.), pp. 97–105 (New York/London: Academic Press)
207. Mathé, G., Amiel, J. L., Schwarzenberg, L. *et al.* (1963). A method of reducing the incidence of the secondary syndrome in allogeneic marrow transplantation. *Blood*, **22**, 44
208. van Bekkum, D. W. (1970). Mitigation of acute secondary disease by treatment of the recipient with antilymphocytic serum before grafting of allogeneic hemopoietic cells. *Exp. Hematol.*, **20**, 3
209. van Bekkum, D. W., Balner, H., van Putten, L. M. *et al.* (1970). Suppression of immune competent cell reactivity by antilymphocyte serum. In: Proceedings of the White Cell Transfusion Congress, June 1969, Paris, p. 153 (Paris: CNRS)
210. Merritt, C. B., Darrow, C. C., II, Vaal, L. *et al.* (1972). Bone marrow transplantation in rhesus monkeys following irradiation. Modification of acute graft-versus-host disease with antilymphocyte serum. *Transplantation*, **14**, 9
211. Gallagher, M. T., Harrod, F., Kulkarni, S. S. *et al.* (1977). Effect on GVH disease of *in vitro* donor cell pretreatment with rabbit antisera against various mouse lymphoid tissues. *Transplant. Proc.*, **9**, 1045
212. Mathé, G., Halle-Pannenko, O., Kiger, N. *et al.* (1976). Prevention and treatment of secondary disease. I. Effects of three non-specific agents: anti-thymocyte serum, antigen binding fragment extracted from anti-thymocyte serum and thymic chalone. *Int. J. Radiat. Oncol. Biol. Phys.*, **1**, 447

213. Müller-Ruchholtz, W., Wottge, H. U. and Müller-Hermelink, H. K. (1976). Bone marrow transplantation in rats across strong histocompatibility barriers by selective elimination of lymphoid cells in donor marrow. *Transplant. Proc.*, **8**, 537
214. Tyan, M. L. (1973). Modification of severe graft-versus-host disease with antisera to the θ antigen or to whole serum. *Transplantation*, **15**, 601
215. Cole, L. J. and Maki, S. E. (1971). Differential inactivation of lymphocytes and bone marrow stem cells by heterologous anti-mouse gamma-globulin serum. *Nature New Biology*, **230**, 244
216. Joller, P. W. (1972). Graft-versus-host reactivity of lymphoid cells inhibited by anti-recognition structure serum. *Nature New Biology*, **240**, 214
217. Gallagher, M. T., Richie, E. R., Heim, L. R. *et al.* (1972). Inhibition of the graft-versus-host reaction. I. Reduction of the graft-versus-host potential of mouse spleen cells (with a sparing of stem cells) by treatment with antilymphocyte globulin-derived Fab fragments. *Transplantation*, **14**, 597
218. Rodt, H., Thierfelder, S. and Eulitz, M. (1974). Antilymphocytic antibodies and marrow transplantation. IV. Comparison of the effects of antibody fragments directed against immunoglobulin or lymphocyte antigens on acute secondary disease. *Exp. Hematol.*, **2**, 195
219. Rodt, H., Netzel, B., Niethammer, D. *et al.* (1977). Specific absorbed antithymocyte globulin for incubation treatment in human marrow transplantation. *Transplant. Proc.*, **9**, 187
220. Bortin, M. M., Rimm, A. A. and Saltzstein, E. C. (1971). Graft-versus-host inhibition. IV. Production of allogeneic radiation chimeras using incubated spleen and liver cell mixtures. *J. Immunol.*, **107**, 1063
221. Halle-Pannenko, O., Zalc-Gouget, C., Kuroiwa, A. *et al.* (1976). Prevention and treatment of secondary disease. II. Effects of four specific agents: Anti-recognition-structure serum, host and donor-directed sera and host soluble H-2 antigens. *Int. J. Radiat. Oncol. Biol. Phys.*, **1**, 927
222. Bonavida, B. and Kedar, E. (1974). Transplantation of allogeneic lymphoid cells specifically depleted of graft-versus-host reactive cells. *Nature (Lond.)*, **249**, 658
223. Mage, M. G. and McHugh, L. L. (1975). Specific partial depletion of graft-versus-host activity by incubation and centrifugation of mouse spleen cells on allogeneic spleen cell monolayers. *J. Immunol.*, **115**, 911
224. Cheever, M. A., Einstein, A. B. Jr., Kempf, R. A. *et al.* (1977). Reduction of fatal graft-versus-host disease by [^{3}H]thymidine suicide of donor cells cultured with host cells. *Transplantation*, **23**, 299
225. Rich, R. R., Kirkpatrick, C. H. and Smith, T. K. (1972). Simultaneous suppression of responses to allogeneic tissue *in vitro* and *in vivo*. *Cell. Immunol.*, **5**, 190
226. Phillips, R. A. and Miller, R. G. (1970). Physical separation of hemopoietic stem cells from cells causing graft-versus-host disease. I. Sedimentation properties of cells causing graft-versus-host disease. *J. Immunol.*, **105**, 1168
227. Salmon, S. E., Smith, B. A., Lehrer, R. I. *et al.* (1970). Modification of donor lymphocytes for transplantation in lymphopenic immunological deficiency. *Lancet*, **ii**, 149
228. Sandberg, J. S., Owens, A. H. Jr. and Santos, G. W. (1971). Clinical and pathologic characteristics of graft-versus-host disease produced in cyclophosphamide-treated adult mice. *J. Nat. Cancer Inst.*, **46**, 151
229. Voisin, G. A., Kinsky, R. and Maillard, J. (1968). Protection against homologous disease in hybrid mice by passive and active immunological enhancement–facilitation. *Transplantation*, **6**, 187
230. Batchelor, J. R. and Howard, J. G. (1965). Synergic and antagonistic effects of isoantibody upon graft-versus-host disease. *Transplantation*, **3**, 161
231. van Bekkum, D. W. (1977). Bone marrow transplantation. *Transplant. Proc.*, **9**, 147

232. Ledney, G. D. (1969). Antilymphocyte serum in the therapy and prevention of acute secondary disease in mice. *Transplantation*, **8**, 127
233. Balner, H., van Bekkum, D. W., de Vries, M. J. *et al.* (1967). Effect of anti-lymphocyte sera on homograft reactivity and G-v-H reactions in rhesus monkeys. *Adv. Transplant.*, **29**, 449
234. Uphoff, D. E. (1958). Alteration of homograft reaction by A-methopterin in lethally irradiated mice treated with homologous marrow (24450). *Proc. Soc. Exp. Biol. Med.*, **99**, 651
235. Thomas, E. D., Collins, J. A., Herman, E. C. *et al.* (1962). Marrow transplants in lethally irradiated dogs given methotrexate. *Blood*, **19**, 217
236. Storb, R., Epstein, R. B., Graham, T. C. *et al.* (1970). Methotrexate regimens for control of graft-versus-host disease in dogs with allogeneic marrow grafts. *Transplantation*, **9**, 240
237. Storb, R., Graham, T. C. and Thomas, E. D. (1974). Treatment of canine graft-versus-host disease with methotrexate and cyclophosphamide following bone marrow transplantation from histoincompatible donors. *Transplantation*, **10**, 165
238. Glucksberg, H. and Fefer, A. (1973). Combination chemotherapy for clinically established graft-versus-host disease in mice. *Cancer Res.*, **33**, 859
239. Floersheim, G. L. (1972). Treatment of hyperacute graft-versus-host disease in mice with cytosine arabinoside. *Transplantation*, **14**, 325
240. van Bekkum, D. W. (Unpublished observations)
241. Schwartz, R. S. and Beldotti, L. (1965). The treatment of chronic murine homologous disease: A comparative study of four 'immunosuppressive' agents. *Transplantation*, **3**, 79
242. Storb, R., Weiden, P. L. and Thomas, E. D. (1976). Use of antithymocyte serum in clinical and experimental marrow transplantation. *Postgrad. Med. J.*, **52**, Suppl. 5, 96

7
Histocompatibility in Clinical Renal Transplantation

GERHARD OPELZ

Department of Surgery, School of Medicine,
University of California at Los Angeles, Los Angeles, California 90024, USA

The last decade has witnessed the rapid development of a true area of biological engineering in clinical medicine: the replacement of malfunctioning kidneys in patients with end-stage renal disease by healthy organs from living or cadaveric donors. Since the pioneer days[1–3] some 30 000 human kidneys, most of them from cadaveric donors, have been transplanted worldwide and the growing number of patients with renal allografts is testimony that this treatment is now clinically accepted. With our current knowledge of the complexity of immunological mechanisms one cannot help but feel some degree of amazement over the relative success of renal transplantation which, in spite of vigorous immunological research, remains to a large extent unexplained. In view of the fact that even primitive organisms such as sea corals are able to mount an effective immune response against transplanted allogeneic tissue[4] the success rates obtained with the much more complex human kidneys are certainly remarkable. Studies on the genetics of transplantation antigens have served to explain the better survival of related donor grafts compared to cadaver donor grafts. The survival of approximately half of all tissue-incompatible cadaver transplants for at least a year is explained in part by the suppression of the recipient's immune system with drugs; however, that about half of the grafts fail within the first year illustrates the limitation of non-specific immunosuppression. Only recently has attention been focused on factors such as the strength of a recipient's immunological responsiveness and effects of antigenic pretreatment of the host. Although many questions remain to be answered, it appears now that four, at times seemingly competing, areas of transplantation research, namely histocompatibility matching, immunoresponsiveness, immunosuppression and immunological manipulation of the recipient by means of pretreatment with alloantigen, are all relevant to the final outcome of renal transplantation.

GENETICS OF TRANSPLANT HISTOCOMPATIBILITY

The early clinical studies[1–3] established the fact that human kidney grafts from donors who were blood relatives of the recipients were more successful than when the donors were unrelated. Subsequently, it was discovered that compatibility for ABO blood group antigens prolonged skin graft survival[5] and matching for ABO was generally adopted in clinical renal transplantation. (It should be noted though that some of the few transplants have been done against an ABO barrier have functioned for several years, indicating that the strength of ABO antigens in renal transplantation must be variable.) Evidence that human leukocyte-locus A (HLA) antigens are renal transplantation antigens was first produced by Singal *et al.*[6] and subsequently confirmed by numerous authors. A recent survey of North American transplants by the UCLA Transplant Registry confirmed the important influence of the HLA chromosome (haplotype) on transplant outcome (Table 7.1).

Table 7.1 Influence of matching for HLA haplotype on kidney graft survival

Recipient/donor HLA haplotype match	*Transplant category*	*No. patients studied*	*1-year graft survival rate* (% ± SE)
Both haplotypes matched	Identical twins	12	100
	HLA-identical siblings	765	85 ± 1
One haplotype matched, one haplotype mismatched	Siblings	562	70 ± 2
	Parent-to-child	1291	68 ± 1
Both haplotypes mismatched	Siblings	72	55 ± 6
	Cadaver	4851	46 ± 1

HLA antigens

Currently, four genetic loci within the HLA region (on chromosome 6) can be typed for: the A, B, C, and D loci. A series of allelic antigens are known to be controlled by each of these loci and the currently recognized specificities are summarized in Table 7.2. These antigens are expressed on the surface of most tissue cells; they are commonly typed for on lymphocytes. Antigens of the A, B, and C loci are typed for by serological methods[7,8], whereas antigens of the D locus are typed for in the mixed leukocyte culture (MLC) assay with the use of D-locus homozygous typing cells. For details and review see refs. 9–13.

Within a family, each child inherits one HLA chromosome (haplotype) from the mother and one from the father. Thus, only four different HLA types are possible among children (Figure 7.1). A simple calculation tells us that, by chance, 25% of all siblings will be HLA identical, 50% will have one haplotype in common and one different, and 25% will have no haplotype in common. Determination of HLA identity may be difficult when parents share

Table 7.2 Currently recognized HLA antigen specificities

Locus A	*Locus B*	*Locus C*	*Locus D*
HLA-A1	HLA-B5	HLA-CW1	HLA-DW1
HLA-A2	HLA-B7	HLA-CW2	HLA-DW2
HLA-A3	HLA-B8	HLA-CW3	HLA-DW3
HLA-A9	HLA-B12	HLA-CW4	HLA-DW4
HLA-A10	HLA-B13	HLA-CW5	HLA-DW5
HLA-A11	HLA-B14		HLA-DW6
HLA-A28	HLA-B18		
HLA-A29	HLA-B27		
HLA-AW19	HLA-BW15		
HLA-AW23	HLA-BW16		
HLA-AW24	HLA-BW17		
HLA-AW25	HLA-BW21		
HLA-AW26	HLA-BW22		
HLA-AW30	HLA-BW35		
HLA-AW31	HLA-BW37		
HLA-AW32	HLA-BW38		
HLA-AW33	HLA-BW39		
HLA-AW34	HLA-BW40		
HLA-AW36	HLA-BW41		
HLA-AW43	HLA-BW42		

Antigens with a prefix 'W' are provisional 'workshop' designations. The other specificities are officially recognized by the World Health Organization

antigens or when one or both parents are homozygous for one or more antigens (i.e. the same specificity is present in both chromosomes of an individual), or in cases of genetic crossovers within the HLA region, which are estimated to occur at a frequency of about 1%.

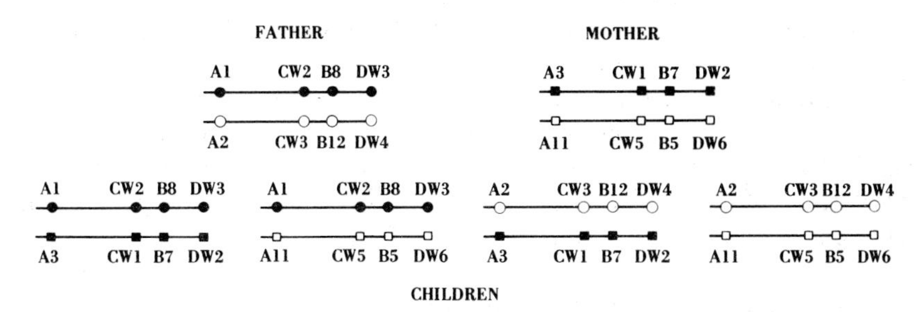

Figure 7.1 HLA chromosomes (haplotypes) in a family. Each child inherits one haplotype from the mother and one from the father. Only four different HLA types are possible among children. In a family with five children, at least two of them must be HLA identical

Recently, much attention has been focused on antigens that can be serologically detected on B (bone marrow-derived) lymphocytes but not on T (thymus-derived) lymphocytes[14–19]. These antigens appear to be controlled by (probably two) loci on the HLA chromosome. Preliminary data suggest that antigens of the D locus are closely linked to and may even be identical with these B cell-specific antigens[16]. This is further supported by findings that the stimulator cells in MLC are B cells[20–22].

The similarities of human B-cell specific antigens with murine immune response loci associated (Ia) antigens have led to speculation that these two antigen systems may be analogous. The importance of this for human genetic research is indicated by the recent discovery of a very close association of one of the B-cell specific antigens with multiple sclerosis[23–25]. The relevance in organ transplantation of B-cell antigens is still unknown.

HLA in renal transplantation

Table 7.1 illustrates the dominating role of the HLA chromosome in renal transplantation. There is a clear differentiation in graft survival rates depending on the number of HLA haplotypes shared between donor and recipient. That this relationship has held up over the years in spite of changes in transplantation techniques, the use of various treatment protocols, contribution of data by over 100 different transplant centres throughout North America, etc., is proof that the HLA chromosome *is the major histocompatibility chromosome* in renal transplantation.

From the difference in graft survival between identical twins and HLA-identical siblings (100% versus 85% at 1 year) we can deduct that non-HLA antigens contribute about 15% to the 1-year failure rate of kidney grafts. These antigens may be controlled by loci outside the HLA region but still on the same chromosome, distant enough from HLA to allow for frequent genetic crossovers, or they may be controlled by loci on other chromosomes.

Similarly, from the difference in graft survival rates between HLA two-haplotype different siblings (55% at 1 year) and cadaver donor transplants (46% at 1 year), we can deduct that about 9% of the cadaver transplant failures within the first year are caused by factors other than HLA, such as kidney preservation failures, etc.

The strength of one HLA haplotype is reflected in a difference in the 1-year graft survival rate of about 15%. This is shown best by the decline in survival rates from HLA-identical siblings (85% at 1 year) to parent-to-child grafts (68% at 1 year) and further to HLA two-haplotype different sibling transplants (55% at 1 year). (Table 7.1.)

HLA matching in cadaver donor transplants

This area has been controversial for several years. Matching for the HLA-A and B loci has resulted in a significant improvement of graft survival in

France and England[26], a moderate improvement in Scandinavia[27] and North America[28], improvement in presensitized recipients in the Eurotransplant data[29], but no improvement at all in a series of transplants reported from San Francisco[30]. Figure 7.2 shows an update of data collected by the UCLA Transplant Registry. The correlation of graft survival with the number of mismatched HLA antigens is statistically highly significant. However, the modest improvement of only 11% from the worst to the best matched category is clinically unsatisfactory. A cut-off whereby transplants with a given number of mismatches would be acceptable and those with more mismatches unacceptable is difficult to set.

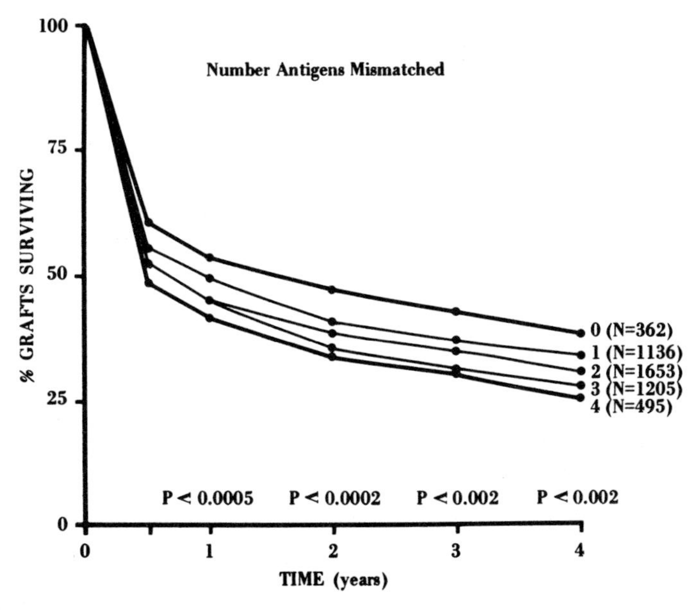

Figure 7.2 Correlation of HLA matching with cadaver transplant survival in North America. Numbers of HLA antigens that were mismatched (= present in the donor but absent in the recipient) and number of patients studied in each subset are indicated. Survival rates were calculated by actuarial methods. P values were estimated by regression analysis

Effect of ABO blood type and sex on HLA matching

Recently, two factors that strongly influence the effect of HLA matching in cadaver transplantation have been described: the recipient's ABO blood type[31] and the recipient's sex[32]. Figure 7.3 illustrates the difference between blood type O and non-O patients in a series of over 5700 cadaver transplants. Whereas HLA matching results in a striking correlation in non-O recipients, there is no significant effect in patients of blood type O. Because of the large number of patients that was studied it is highly unlikely that this dramatic difference is due to sampling error.

The influence of the recipient's sex is about as strong as that of ABO. Overall, male and female recipients have similar graft survival rates (Figure 7.4). When the effect of HLA matching is analysed in the four combinations of donor/recipient sex, a striking correlation is obtained in male-to-male and

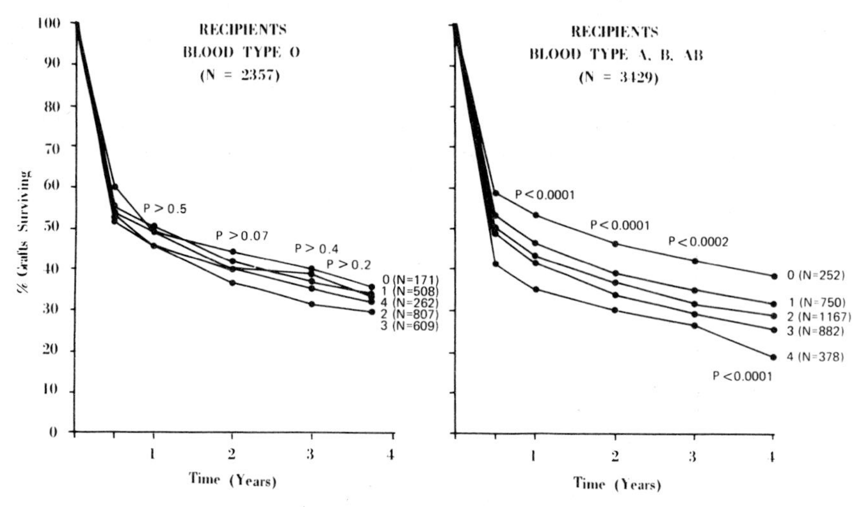

Figure 7.3 Comparison of HLA matching in blood-type O and non-type O recipients. Only in non-O patients was HLA of significant influence

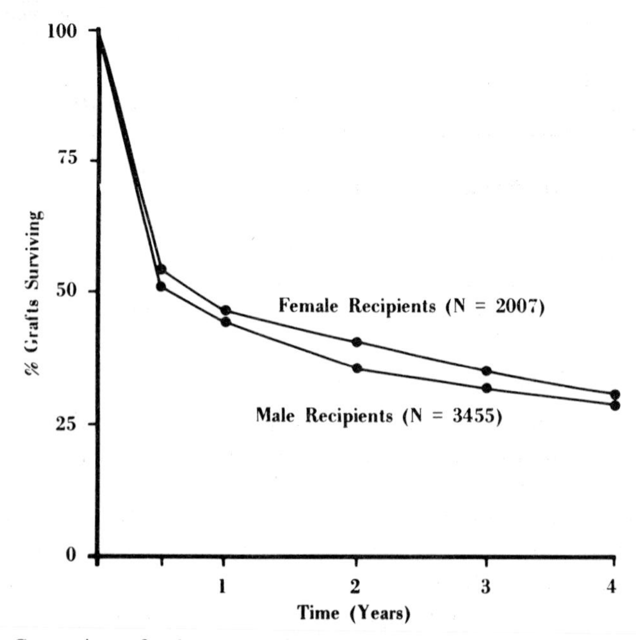

Figure 7.4 Comparison of cadaver transplant survival rates in female and male recipients

female-to-male grafts (Figure 7.5) whereas there is no correlation in female-to-female and male-to-female transplants (Figure 7.6). Thus, this effect is

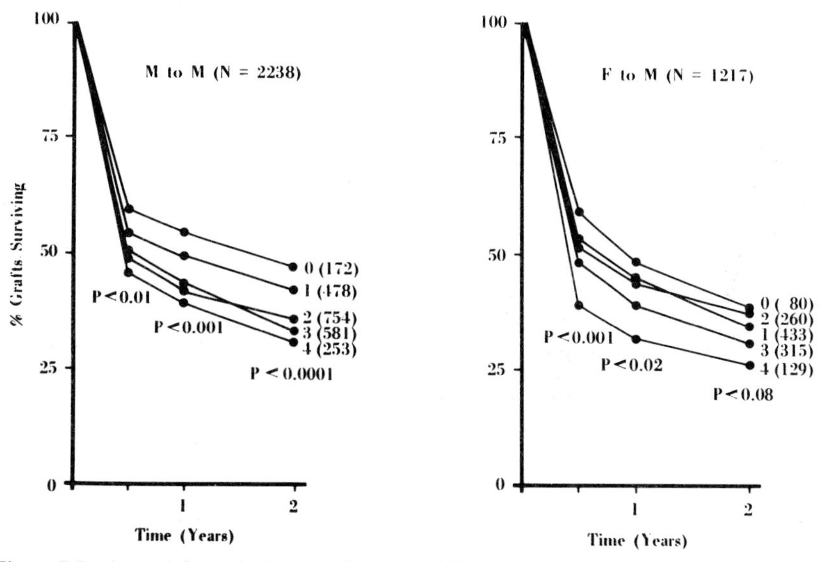

Figure 7.5 Actuarial survival rates of cadaver kidney grafts for different subsets of HLA matches in male recipients. There was a significant correlation with outcome regardless of the donor's sex (F = female, M = male)

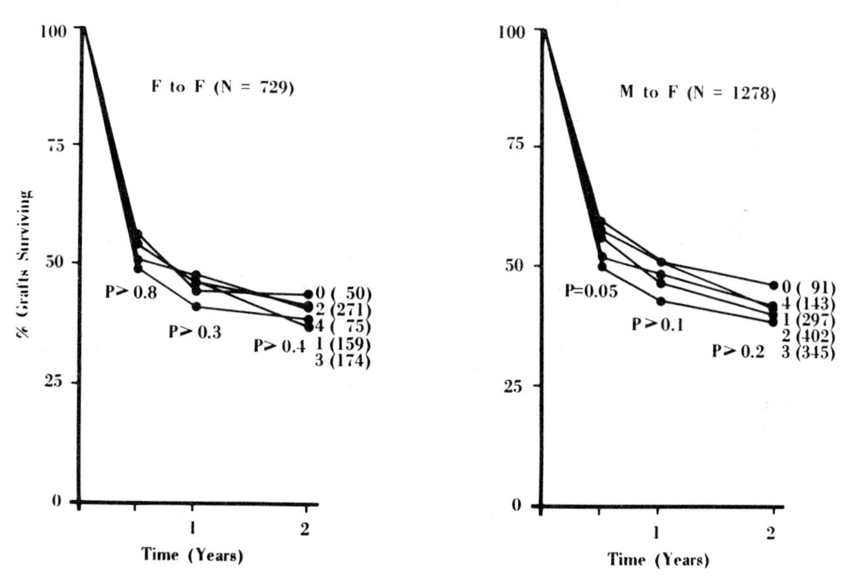

Figure 7.6 Actuarial survival rates of cadaver kidney grafts by HLA match in female recipients. There was no significant correlation of matching with graft outcome, whether the donors were female or male (F = female, M = male)

entirely dependent on the recipient's sex and not on that of the donor. The difference in HLA matching between female and male recipients is statistically highly significant as shown in Caucasian patients in Figure 7.7.

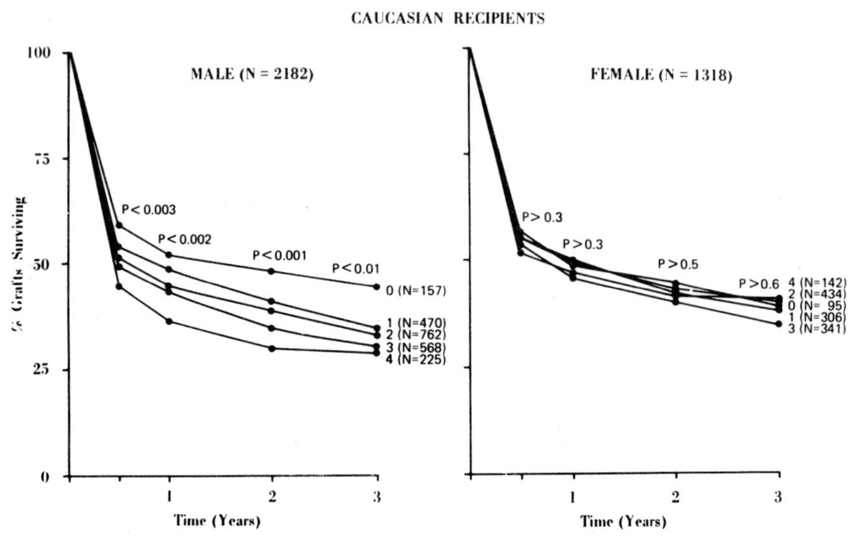

Figure 7.7 Correlation of HLA matching with cadaver graft survival in female and male Caucasian patients. The correlation in male recipients and the absence of correlation in females is striking. P values were calculated by regression analysis

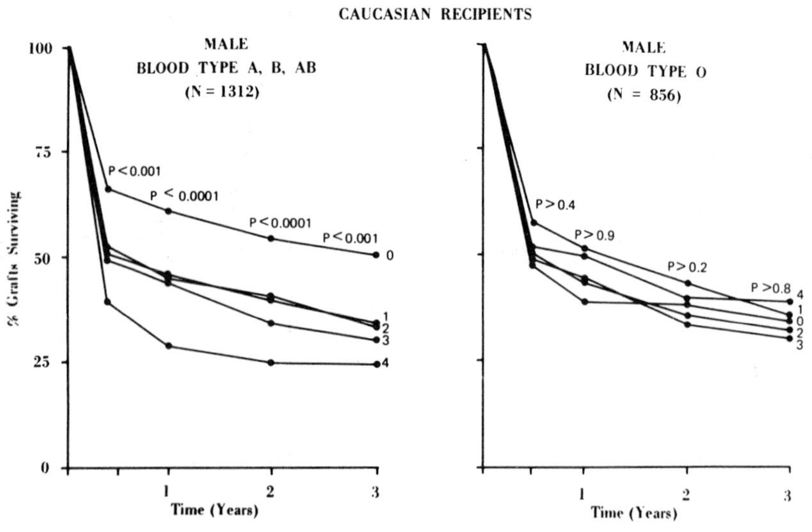

Figure 7.8 Combined effect of ABO blood type and sex on HLA matching in cadaver transplants. Male patients of non-blood-type O benefit greatly from HLA matching. Numbers of mismatched HLA antigens are indicated at the end of each curve

When combined, the effects of ABO blood type and sex appear to be additive, though overlapping to some extent. The difference in graft survival rates between transplants with the best versus the worst HLA match grades is an impressive 30% in male recipients of blood types A, B, or AB (Figure 7.8). Apparently it is this category of transplants that contributes the main share to the moderate overall correlation of matching with outcome shown in Figure 7.2. That the effects of ABO and sex are *independent* is further illustrated by the absence of a significant effect of HLA matching in females of non-O blood type (Figure 7.9).

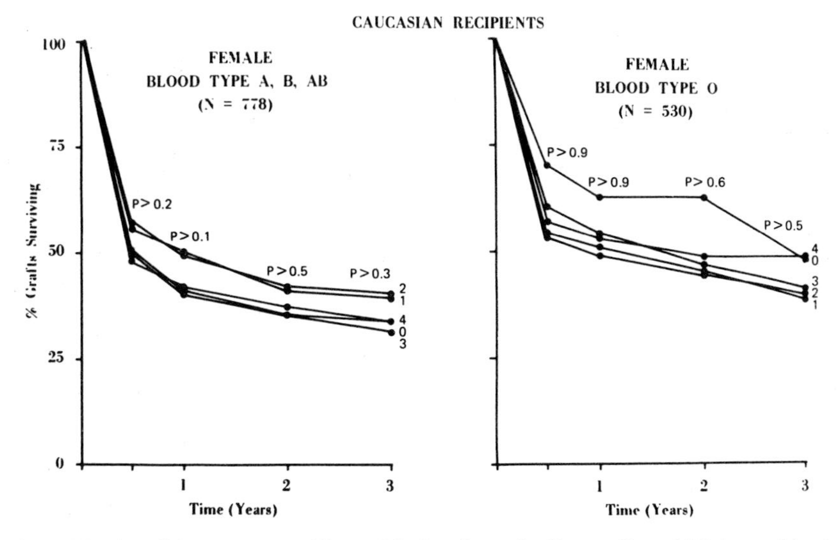

Figure 7.9 In striking contrast to Figure 7.8, there is no significant effect of HLA matching in females, regardless of the recipient's ABO blood type

With our limited understanding of histocompatibility in renal transplantation, this influence of blood type and sex on HLA matching is difficult to explain. A direct interrelation of ABO and HLA antigens, ABO or sex-linked regulator genes, an influence of sex hormones, differences in immunological responsiveness, all have to be considered. One hypothesis that would lend a common denominator to the influence of both ABO and sex is the possibility that prior exposure to allogeneic histocompatibility antigens may be the cause for the difference in results. Evidence that exposure to blood transfusions can prolong graft survival has been reported[33–38] and will be discussed later. It is known that blood type O patients have on an average much longer pretransplant waiting times on haemodialysis compared to patients of other blood types[39] and it is therefore likely that type O patients receive more blood transfusions before they are transplanted. The reduction of transfusion requirements by androgen treatment[40] often has unwanted side-effects in females and discontinuance of androgens often necessitates transfusions to stabilize the patient's haematocrit. In addition, exposure to fetal histocompatibility antigens in females who have undergone pregnancies may have altered their immune response toward allogeneic kidney grafts. Since poorly matched grafts would benefit the most from a decrease of immunological reactivity against incompatible transplants, the absence of a significant effect of HLA matching in patients with more frequent pretransplant alloantigen exposure could be plausibly explained.

Effect of preformed cytotoxic antibodies on HLA matching

It has been demonstrated that patients whose serum contains antibodies that kill lymphocytes of random donors prior to transplantation have a decreased chance of graft survival compared to patients who are not 'presensitized[34,41,42]. This is again confirmed for patients with broadly reacting antibodies in Table 7.3. Whereas Eurotransplant reported that the effect of HLA matching was particularly strong in presensitized patients[42], a recent analysis of North American data did not confirm this (Figure 7.10). There was a good correlation of matching with outcome in non-sensitized patients (< 5% reactivity against the random lymphocyte panel), a clear differentiation of O- and 1-mismatched grafts from the remaining transplants in moderately sensitized recipients (5–50% reactivity), but no correlation in recipients with broadly reactive antibodies (> 50% reactivity) (Figure 7.10).

Table 7.3 Influence of preformed lymphocytotoxic antibodies on cadaver transplant survival

Reactivity of recipient's serum against random panel	*No. patients studied*	*Graft survival rates* (% ± SE)	
		1 year	*2 years*
<5%	1620	50 ± 1	43 ± 1
5–50%	308	48 ± 3	40 ± 3
>50%	105	34 ± 5	29 ± 5

Strength of HLA-A locus versus HLA-B locus

Several European groups have reported that HLA-B locus antigens have a stronger effect on renal transplants than A-locus antigens[26,35]. In the North American data such an effect has not been demonstrable as summarized for related and cadaver donors in Table 7.4.

HLA-C and HLA-D locus antigens

Data on the relevance in clinical transplantation of these rather recently discovered loci is sparse. Antigens of the HLA-C locus have been found weakly immunogenic with respect to antibody production in immunized volunteers[43]. Preliminary data on the HLA-D locus suggest a significant role in cadaver transplantation. Cochrum *et al.*[44] reported an improved survival rate of cadaver grafts with weak MLC stimulation between recipient

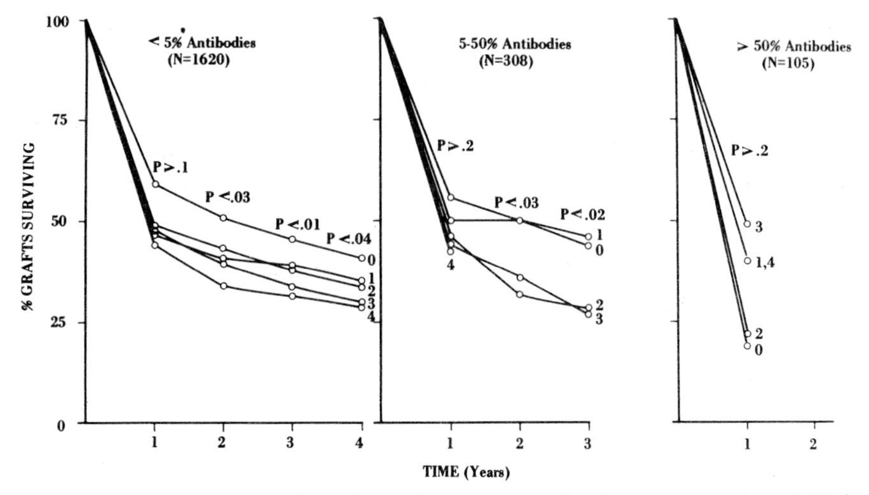

Figure 7.10 Influence of preformed lymphocytotoxic antibodies on correlation of HLA matching with cadaver transplant survival. Interestingly, there was no correlation in highly sensitized patients (>50% reactivity against the random panel); however, the number of patients studied was smallest in this subset

and donor, and presumably D-locus matched grafts did exceptionally well in a small series of grafts reported from London[35]. Among 131 cadaver donor transplants studied in Los Angeles the degree of MLC stimulation also correlated with transplant survival[45] (Figure 7.11). All these studies were

Table 7.4 Relative strength of HLA-A locus versus HLA-B locus

Transplant category	*Mismatch*	*No. patients studied*	*1-year graft survival rate (% ± SE)*
Sibling donors	0 on A-locus 1 on B-locus	253	74 ± 3
	0 on B-locus 1 on A-locus	192	72 ± 3
Parental donors	0 on A-locus 1 on B-locus	324	70 ± 3
	0 on B-locus 1 on A-locus	240	69 ± 3
Cadaveric donors	0 on A-locus 1 on B-locus	663	50 ± 2
	0 on B-locus 1 on A-locus	473	47 ± 2

done retrospectively, that is the MLC results were not utilized for the selection of donors. A major obstacle for the clinical application of these encouraging findings is that the MLC technique is time consuming; it takes approximately 5 days to perform D-locus typing or direct MLC tests between donors and recipients—longer than cadaver kidneys currently can be preserved. Modifications of the technique, such as the primed lymphocyte typing (PLT) technique, which utilizes *in vitro* sensitized lymphocytes to perform D-locus typing within 48 h[46], may prove to be more useful for clinical matching. Recent data, however, indicate that the PLT and MLC assays yield a disturbingly high fraction of discrepant results, thus suggesting that results obtained with these two techniques are probably not interchangeable[47].

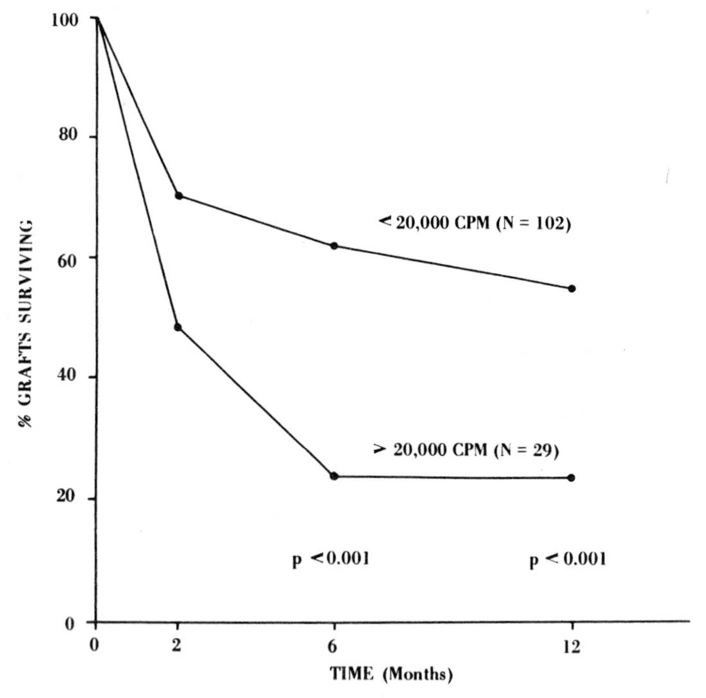

Figure 7.11 Actuarial graft survival rates for cadaver transplants with strong (>20 000 CPM) or weak (<20 000 CPM) stimulation between recipient and donor cells in MLC. The cultures were done in a bidirectional fashion with addition of the recipient's plasma. *P* values were estimated by Student's *t*-test

IMMUNORESPONSIVENESS AND RENAL TRANSPLANTATION

The immunological response status of the recipient appears to be an important factor in renal cadaver transplantation. Patients with preformed lymphocytotoxic antibodies have an increased risk of failure[34,41,42]. Of course, if these antibodies are directed against the actual kidney donor the result is frequently hyperacute rejection of the graft[48,49]. That rejection occurs more frequently in presensitized patients even if the antibodies are not directed against the donor's HLA antigens (i.e. the 'crossmatch' is negative) suggests that the antibodies are an indicator for the patient's general status of immunological reactivity. In the current North American data a decreased survival in presensitized patients is only demonstrable in recipients with broadly reactive antibodies (Table 7.3). Some centres have reported good results even in highly sensitized patients[50,51]; this may be related to treatment with anti-thymocyte immunoglobulin or other refined methods of immunosuppression. Recent data indicate that a recipient's status of cellular immunoresponsiveness as measured in *in vitro* lymphocyte proliferation assays also predicts graft outcome[51,52]. The absence of demonstrable lymphocytotoxic antibodies in spite of blood transfusions has been shown to correlate with very good graft survival[53], a further indication that the recipient's immune response status plays an important role in renal transplantation.

All these findings are of clinical significance because they indicate that a separation of poor and good transplant candidates should be possible prior to transplantation. Moreover, since we have reason to believe that a patient's status of responsiveness is alterable (see section on blood transfusions), *in vitro* and *in vivo* monitoring of a patient's immunological reactivity may provide means of selecting the 'right time' for grafting. Refinement of methods for *in vitro* monitoring and further clinical studies are therefore needed.

Retransplantation and immunoresponsiveness

Although it might be expected that a patient who has already rejected one kidney graft should be a poor-risk candidate for another transplant, second transplants were found to do almost as well as first grafts, and only third or fourth transplants had substantially decreased survival rates[54,55]. Lymphocytotoxic antibodies develop frequently following graft rejection[56,57] and their deleterious effect on graft survival is more pronounced in retransplants than in primary grafts[55].

The most important knowledge gained from the study of retransplants is the intriguing relationship between the duration of first grafts and the outcome of second grafts[54,55,58]. Patients whose first grafts had functioned for over a year were found to have second grafts that did extremely well; in fact their survival rate was better than the overall rate of first cadaver transplants (Figure 7.12). In contrast, patients who had rejected their first grafts between 1 and 3 months had a retransplant survival rate that was 30% lower at one year ($58 \pm 3\%$ versus $28 \pm 3\%$, $p < 0.0001$). Interestingly, patients whose first grafts had failed within the first months or between the third month and a year had a similar second graft outcome (Figure 7.12). The most plausible explanation for this unexpected survival rate in the < 1 month category is that early graft failures are often the result of preservation and other technical failures; the intermixture of non-immunological and acute immunological first graft failures results in the intermediate survival rate of second grafts shown in Figure 7.12.

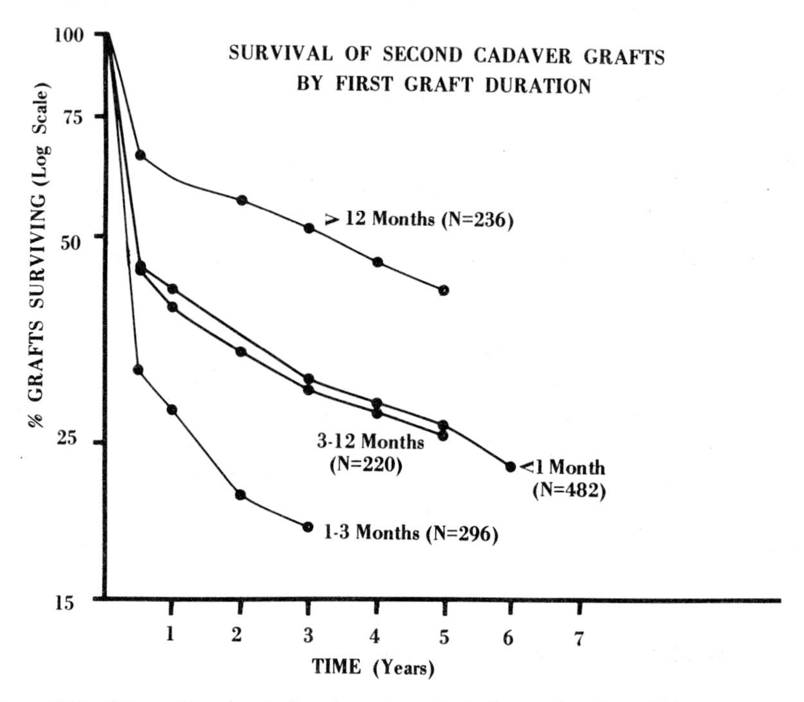

Figure 7.12 Effect of first graft duration on survival of second cadaver kidney transplants. There is a dramatic difference between the survival rates in patients whose first graft had lasted for more than a year compared to patients who had lost their first graft between the first and third month following transplantation ($P < 0.0001$)

The striking difference in second graft survival depending on first graft duration provides very valuable information with respect to studies on immunoresponsiveness. Since slow rejection of a primary graft is commonly followed by long duration of a second graft, these patients can be classified as genuine 'low responders'. Alternatively, a chronic rejection process may actively decrease the patient's ability to reject a second graft by inducing tolerance or enhancement. Acute immunological rejection of a first graft is commonly followed by acute rejection of a second graft. Accurate methods to determine whether the loss of a graft was immunological or not are needed to allow more accurate prediction of retransplant success chances. For the clinician these data are of obvious practical significance since they aid in his assessment whether a patient should be retransplanted or whether it might be advisable to maintain him on haemodialysis because of his poor risk for a second graft.

BLOOD TRANSFUSIONS AND KIDNEY GRAFTS

After some initial controversy, it seems now fairly well established that pretransplant blood transfusions have a prolonging influence on the survival of cadaver kidney grafts. The initial scepticism had been provoked by the theoretical danger of presensitization to histocompatibility antigens, particularly since preformed lymphocytotoxic antibodies are associated with an increase in failure rates (Table 7.3). However, the first report on the surprising finding that transplant patients who had never been transfused did very poorly[33] was confirmed in several independent retrospective[34–36,38] and prospective[55] studies. Overall, it appears that the beneficial effect of transfusions on graft survival outweighs the deleterious effect associated with antibody production[55] (Table 7.5).

Table 7.5 Effect of blood transfusions on cadaver transplant survival

No. pretransplant transfusions	*No. patients studied*	*1-year graft survival rate (% ± SE)*
0	143	31 ± 4
1–5	124	49 ± 5
>5	66	48 ± 6

Although an explanation for the graft prolongation following transfusions has yet to be found, it appears likely that exposure to transfused blood cells that carry allogeneic histocompatibility antigens alters the immune response of the host against a kidney graft. Induction of tolerance or enhancement have been suggested as possible mechanisms. The argument that the correlation of transfusions with prolonged graft survival may only be coincidental and reflect selection of patients with different types of diseases or pretransplant conditions is difficult to defend in light of experiments in dogs[59] and monkeys[60]. In these studies, outbred animals that were otherwise treated identically showed a strikingly better kidney graft outcome when pretreated with blood of the actual kidney donor. Whereas this form of pretreatment may seem risky in humans, success with donor cell pretreatment has been reported in at least one study[61]. Certainly, future studies in humans must be conducted with extreme caution.

Restriction of blood transfusions in potential renal transplant recipients does not seem indicated from an immunological standpoint. The greatest hazards associated with transfusions are hyperimmunization and hepatitis transmission. A patient who develops lymphocytotoxic antibodies against 95% or 99% of the random test panel will be extremely difficult to transplant since he will be crossmatch positive with most potential donors. From the available data it would seem that sensitization to this high degree should be rare with transfusions in the range of 10 units[57,62,63]. The use of blood from known hepatitis-free donors, possibly family members, would reduce the risk of hepatitis transmission. Eventually, pretreatment with purified antigenic products may eliminate the hepatitis hazard; however, since the exact mechanism whereby graft survival is prolonged is as yet unknown, this approach has to be viewed as a long-term goal.

From a clinical viewpoint it is now urgent to develop specific guidelines for the use of blood transfusions in potential transplant recipients. For example, it is unknown how many units of blood would give optimal results, whether whole blood, packed cells, or frozen blood should be given, at what intervals blood should be transfused, etc. In addition, it will be important to study whether this type of induction of unresponsiveness is under genetic control and whether the degree of HLA compatibility of transfused blood is of influence. Most importantly, methods have to be developed to measure changes in a patient's immunological status following transfusions; currently it is impossible to determine whether a patient has been 'sufficiently' pretreated or not.

Uncontrolled transfusions into patients waiting for transplants cannot be advocated. In order to explore the best possible methods of pretreatment, only careful follow-up in limited series of patients is acceptable. Testing of new transfusion protocols in large animals such as dogs and monkeys certainly has to be advocated to minimize the risk to patients in actual clinical studies.

PERSPECTIVES

Two main directions of histocompatibility research seem most promising at this time: the development of better methods to match donors and recipients, and the exploration of the nature of immunological responsiveness and of methods to alter responsiveness in a way favourable to the kidney graft.

With regard to histocompatibility matching, we can conclude that the HLA-A and -B antigens have a significant, although limited effect on cadaver graft survival (Figure 7.2). This effect appears to be strongest among male patients of blood types other than O (Figure 7.8). In this category of patients matching for the HLA-A and -B loci is of immediate clinical significance, with a possible improvement in survival rates of about 30%. The variable correlation of matching with graft outcome in other subsets of patients shows that the effect of the A and B loci is *relative*. For example, it was recently noted that matching had a stronger influence at transplant centres with poor overall results than at centres with good overall results[64] and that matching correlated with outcome in kidneys that had been preserved by simple cold storage but not in kidneys that had been preserved on pulsatile perfusion machines[65]. Obviously, many factors influence the effect of HLA matching on cadaver kidney graft survival. Furthermore, it is clear from the available data that poorly HLA-matched grafts can survive for prolonged periods under certain circumstances. If the gains that can be expected from HLA-A and -B matching are viewed realistically, HLA is a useful tool for the selection of donors in clinical renal transplantation.

In the near future we can expect answers as to the importance of other loci within the HLA region. There is plenty of room for improvement in the cadaver graft survival rates and it will be interesting to see if matching for the HLA-C and -D loci will provide a significant improvement. Furthermore, typing and matching for B-cell specific antigens should shortly become clinically evaluable. A key question with respect to these new loci is whether they will turn out to be stronger transplantation loci than the HLA-A and -B loci, or whether they will be of intermediate strength (like the HLA-A and -B loci) and only have an additive effect. Should the latter be the case, because of the great polymorphism at the various loci, it will be logistically very difficult to provide well-matched cadaver donors for a substantial fraction of all waiting recipients. Nationwide and international sharing of cadaver kidneys would have to be intensified.

In addition to testing these loci within the HLA region, research will have to focus on non-HLA antigens. Whereas these antigens were initially believed to be negligible in renal transplantation because of the 'nearly ideal' success rate of HLA-identical sibling grafts, it is now recognized that about 15% of all failures within the first year are attributable to antigens outside the HLA region[66]. Organ-specific antigens, such as antigens expressed on vascular endothelial cells[67] may be important in this context. Cellular techniques may be particularly suitable for research in this area of non-HLA transplantation antigens[68].

Perhaps the most promising area in transplantation research is that of induction of unresponsiveness. While significant prolongation of graft survival following pretreatment with alloantigen has been reported in numerous animal models, only the recent data on blood transfusions have shown that this approach is indeed feasible in humans without unacceptable risk to that patient. In fact, it can be deduced from the clinical results that the commonly quoted 50% graft survival rate at 1 year for cadaver kidney grafts is already a result of improvement by blood transfusions; patients without any transfusions were found to have graft survival rates of 30% or lower. In the coming years we can expect controlled clinical trials with planned transfusion protocols to improve cadaver transplant results. A crucial area that needs improvement is the measurement of a patient's immunological responsiveness status. While antibody levels and response to mitogens *in vitro* are a starting point, these measures have to be considered rather crude. Measurement of specific reactivity against histocompatibility antigens is needed, not only for assessment of the general responsiveness status of a patient, but more importantly for monitoring changes in reactivity following transfusions. Progress in this entire area of active induction of unresponsiveness will depend heavily on the development of suitable *in vitro* assays.

Pretreatment of transplant candidates with allogeneic histocompatibility antigens is not without risk to the patients and strict precautions have to be taken to protect the patient's interests. Hopefully, methods will be developed that will allow administration of alloantigens with full graft prolongation effect, but without the hazards of recipient hyperimmunization and hepatitis transmission.

Related donor transplantation has benefited substantially from histocompatibility matching. Limited tissue matching has already been of some benefit in cadaver donor transplants; extended matching including new histocompatibility loci will hopefully result in a further improvement of survival rates. The manipulation of the recipient's immune system by pretreatment with allogeneic histocompatibility antigens is a more hazardous, but potentially more powerful direct approach for immunological engineering. It can be anticipated that further developments in these two areas will greatly influence clinical renal transplantation.

References

1. Hamburger, J. J. *et al.* (1962). Renal homotransplantation in man after radiation of the recipient: Experience with six cases since 1959. *Am. J. Med.*, **32**, 854
2. Starzl, T. E. (1964). Experience in renal transplantation (W. B. Saunders Co.)
3. Hume, D. M., Lee, H. M., Williams, G. M., White, H. J. O., Ferre, H., Wolf, J. S., Prout, G. R. Jr., Slapak, M., O'Brien, J., Kilpatrick, S. J., Kauffman, H. M. Jr. and Cleveland, R. J. (1966). The comparative results of cadaver and related donor renal homografts in man, and the immunological implications of the outcome of second and paired transplants. *Ann. Surg.*, **164**, 352
4. Hildemann, W. H., Raison, R. L., Hull, C. G., Akaka, L. K., Okamoto, J. and Cheung, J. P. (1977). Tissue transplantation immunity in corals. In: *Proc. Third International Symposium on Coral Reefs.* (In press)
5. Ceppellini, R., Curtoni, E. S., Mattiuz, P. L., Leigheb, G., Visetti, M. and Colombani, A. (1966). Survival of test skin grafts in man: Effect of genetic relationship and of blood groups in compatibility. *Ann. N.Y. Acad. Sci.*, **129**, 421
6. Singal, D. P., Mickey, M. R. and Terasaki, P. I. (1969). Serotyping for homotransplantation. XXIII. Analysis of kidney transplants from parental versus sibling donors. *Transplantation*, **7**, 246
7. Terasaki, P. I. and McClelland, J. D. (1964). Microdroplet assay of human serum cytotoxins. *Nature (Lond.)*, **204**, 998
8. Mittal, K. K., Mickey, M. R., Singal, D. P. and Terasaki, P. I. (1968). Serotyping for homotransplantation. XVIII. Refinement of microdroplet lymphocyte cytotoxicity test. *Transplantation*, **6**, 913

9. H. Balner, F. J. Cleton and J. G. Ernisse, eds. (1965). *Histocompatibility Testing* (Copenhagen: Munksgaard)
10. E. S. Curtoni, P. L. Mattiuz and R. M. Tosi, eds. (1967). *Histocompatibility Testing* (Baltimore: Williams and Wilkins)
11. P. I. Terasaki, ed. (1970). *Histocompatibility Testing* (Copenhagen: Munksgaard)
12. J. Dausset and J. Colombani, eds. (1972). *Histocompatibility Testing* (Copenhagen: Munksgaard)
13. F. Kissmeyer-Nielsen, ed. (1975). *Histocompatibility Testing* (Copenhagen: Munksgaard)
14. Winchester, R. J., Fu, S. M., Wernet, P., Kunkel, H. G., Dupont, B. and Jersild, C. (1975). Recognition by pregnancy serums of non-HLA alloantigens selectively expressed on B lymphocytes. *J. Exp. Med.*, **141**, 924
15. Terasaki, P. I., Opelz, G., Park, M. S. and Mickey, M. R. (1975). Four new B lymphocyte specificities. In: *Histocompatibility Testing* (F. Kissmeyer-Nielsen, ed.) (Copenhagen: Munksgaard)
16. van Rood, J. J., van Leuwen, A., Keunig, J. J. and Blusse van Oud Alblas, A. (1975). The serological recognition of the human MLC determinants using a modified cytotoxicity technique. *Tissue Antigens*, **5**, 73
17. Arbeit, R. D., Sachs, D. H., Amos, D. B. and Dickler, H. B. (1975). Human lymphocyte alloantigen(s) similar to murine Ir-region-associated (Ia) antigens. *J. Immunol.*, **115**, 1173
18. Jones, E. A., Goodfellow, P. N., Bodmer, J. G. and Bodmer, W. F. (1975). Serological identification of HLA-linked human 'Ia-type' antigens. *Nature (Lond.)*, **256**, 650
19. Ting, A., Mickey, M. R. and Terasaki, P. I. (1976). B-lymphocyte alloantigens in Caucasians. *J. Exp. Med.*, **143**, 981
20. Plate, J. M. D. and McKenzie, I. F. C. (1973). B cell stimulation of allogeneic T cell proliferation in mixed lymphocyte cultures. *Nature New Biology*, **245**, 247
21. Lohrmann, P. H., Novikovs, L. and Graw, R. G. Jr. (1974). Cellular interactions in the proliferative response of human T and B lymphocytes to phytomitogens and allogeneic lymphocytes. *J. Exp. Med.*, **139**, 1553
22. Opelz, G., Kiuchi, M. and Takasugi, M. (1975). Reactivity of lymphocyte subpopulations in human mixed lymphocyte culture. *J. Immunogenet.*, **2**, 1
23. Winchester, R. J., Ebers, G., Fu, S. M., Espinosa, L., Zabriskie, J. and Kunkel, H. G. (1975). B-cell alloantigen Ag 7a in multiple sclerosis. *Lancet*, **ii**, 814
24. Terasaki, P. I., Park, M. S., Opelz, G. and Ting, A. (1976). Multiple sclerosis and high incidence of a B lymphocyte antigen. *Science*, **193**, 1245
25. Compston *et al.* (1976).
26. Dausset, J., Hors, J., Busson, M., Festenstein, H., Oliver, R. T. D., Paris, A. M. I. and Sachs, J. A. (1974). Serologically defined HL-A antigens and long-term survival of cadaver kidney transplants. *N. Engl. J. Med.*, **290**, 979
27. Scandiatransplant Report (1975). HL-A matching and kidney-graft survival. *Lancet*, **i**, 240
28. Opelz, G., Mickey, M. R. and Terasaki, P. I. (1974). HL-A and kidney transplants: Reexamination. *Transplantation*, **17**, 371
29. van Rood, J. J., van Leuwen, A., Persijn, G. G., Lansbergen, Q., Goulmy, E., Termijtelen, A. and Bradley, B. A. (1977). HLA compatibility in clinical transplantation. *Transplant. Proc.*, **9**, 459
30. Belzer, F. O., Perkins, H. A., Fortmann, J. L., Kountz, S. L., Salvatierra, O., Cochrum, K. D. and Payne, R. (1974). Is HL-A typing of clinical significance in cadaver renal transplantation? *Lancet*, **i**, 774
31. Opelz, G. and Terasaki, P. I. (1977a). Effect of blood-group on relation between HLA match and outcome of cadaver kidney transplants. *Lancet*, **i**, 220
32. Opelz, G. and Terasaki, P. I. (1977b). Influence of sex on histocompatibility matching in renal transplantation (Submitted for publication)

33. Opelz, G., Sengar, D. P. S., Mickey, M. R. and Terasaki, P. I. (1973a). Effect of blood transfusions on subsequent kidney transplants. *Transplant Proc.*, **5**, 253
34. Opelz, G. and Terasaki, P. I. (1974a). Poor kidney transplant survival in recipients with frozen blood transfusions or no transfusions. *Lancet*, **ii**, 696
35. Festenstein, H., Sachs, J. A., Paris, A. M. I., Pegrum, G. D. and Moorhead, J. F. (1976). Influence of HLA matching and blood-transfusion on outcome of 502 London Transplant Group renal-graft recipients. *Lancet*, **i**, 157
36. van Hooff, J. P., Kalff, M. W., van Poelgeest, A. E., Persijn, G. G. and van Rood, J. J. (1976). Blood transfusions and kidney transplantation. *Transplantation*, **22**, 306
37. Opelz, G. and Terasaki, P. I. (1976a). Prolongation effect of blood transfusions on kidney graft survival. *Transplantation*, **22**, 380
38. Fuller, T. C., Delmonico, F. L., Cosimi, A. B., Huggins, C. E., King, M. and Russell, P. S. (1977). Effects of various types of RBC transfusions on HLA alloimmunization and renal allograft survival. *Transplant. Proc.*, **9**, 117
39. Opelz, G. and Terasaki, P. I. (1974b). National utilization of cadaver kidneys for transplantation. *J. Am. Med. Assoc.*, **228**, 1260
40. Shaldon, S., Patyna, W. D. and Kaltwasser, P. (1971). The use of testosterone in bilateral nephrectomized dialysis patients. *Trans. Am. Soc. Art. Int. Organs*, **17**, 104
41. Terasaki, P. I., Mickey, M. R. and Kreisler, M. (1971). Presensitization and kidney transplant failures. *Postgrad. Med. J.*, **47**, 89
42. van Hooff, J. P., Schippers, H. M. A., van der Steen, G. J. and van Rood, J. J. (1972). Efficacy of HL-A matching in Eurotransplant. *Lancet*, **ii**, 1385
43. Ferrara, G. B., Tosi, R. M., Longo, A., Azzolina, G. and Carminati, G. (1975). Low immunogenicity of the third HLA series. *Transplantation*, **20**, 340
44. Cochrum, K. C., Perkins, H. A., Payne, R. O., Kountz, S. L. and Belzer, F. O. (1973). The correlation of MLC with graft survival. *Transplant. Proc.*, **5**, 391
45. Opelz, G. and Terasaki, P. I. (1977c). Significance of mixed leukocyte culture testing in cadaver kidney transplantation. *Transplantation*, **23**, 375
46. Bach, F. H., Jarrett-Toth, E., Benike, C. J., Sheehy, M. J., Sondel, P. M. and Bach, M. L. (1976). Three HLA-D region antigens defined by primed LD typing. *J. Exp. Med.*, **144**, 549
47. Rubinstein, P., Falk, C., Martin, M. and Suciu-Foca, N. (1977). Complete typing of the HLA region in families. III. Analysis of responses in the primed lymphocyte test (PLT). *Transplant Proc.* (In press)
48. Kissmeyer-Nielsen, F., Olsen, S., Petersen, V. P. and Fjeldborg, O. (1966). Hyperacute rejection of kidney allografts associated with preexisting humoral antibodies against donor cells. *Lancet*, **i**, 662
49. Patel, R. and Terasaki, P. I. (1970). Significance of the positive cross-match test in kidney transplantation. *N. Engl. J. Med.*, **280**, 735
50. Belzer, F. O., Salvatierra, O., Cochrum, K. C. and Perkins, H. A. (1975). Good kidney graft survival in hyperimmunized patients. *Transplant. Proc.*, **7**, Suppl. 1, 71
51. Thomas, F., Mendez-Picon, G., Thomas, J. and Lee, H. M. (1977). Quantitation of pretransplantation immune responsiveness by *in vitro* T-cell testing. *Transplant. Proc.*, **9**, 49
52. Jones, A. R., Vaughan, R. W., Bewick, M. and Batchelor, R. (1976). Transformation of lymphocytes from patients awaiting cadaver renal transplants. *Lancet*, **ii**, 529
53. Opelz, G., Mickey, M. R. and Terasaki, P. I. (1972a). Identification of unresponsive kidney transplant recipients. *Lancet*, **i**, 868
54. Opelz, G., Mickey, M. R. and Terasaki, P. I. (1972b). Prolonged survival of second human kidney transplants. *Science*, **178**, 617
55. Opelz, G. and Terasaki, P. I. (1976b). Recipient selection for renal retransplantation. *Transplantation*, **21**, 483

56. Morris, P. J., Mickey, M. R., Singal, D. P. and Terasaki, P. I. (1969). Serotyping for homotransplantation. XXII. Specificity of cytotoxic antibodies after renal transplantation. *Br. Med. J.*, **1**, 758
57. Opelz, G., Mickey, M. R. and Terasaki, P. I. (1973b). Blood transfusions and unresponsiveness to HL-A. *Transplantation*, **16**, 649
58. Heideman, M. and Claes, G. (1977). Influence of clinically determined immunologic reactivity on renal transplantation. *Transplant. Proc.*, **9**, 77
59. Halasz, N. A., Orloff, M. J. and Hirose, F. (1964). Increased survival of renal homografts in dogs after injection of graft donor blood. *Transplantation*, **2**, 453
60. van Es, A. A., Marguet, R. L., van Rood, J. J., Kalff, M. W. and Balner, H. (1977). Blood-transfusions induce prolonged kidney allograft survival in rhesus monkeys. *Lancet*, **i**, 506
61. Newton, W. T. and Anderson, C. B. (1973). Planned preimmunization of renal allograft recipients. *Surgery*, **74**, 430
62. Suarez-Ch., R. and Jonasson, O. (1972). Isoimmunization of potential kidney transplant recipients: General frequency and some associated factors. *Transplant. Proc.*, **4**, 577
63. Manzler, A. D. and Nathan, P. (1974). Lymphocytotoxins in a chronic hemodialysis population. *Tissue Antigens*, **4**, 527
64. Opelz, G. and Terasaki, P. I. (1977d). HLA matching and cadaver kidney transplant survival in North America: Influence of center variation and presensitization. *Transplantation* (In press)
65. Opelz, G. and Terasaki, P. I. (1977e). Decreased transplant survival rate of shared and nonshared machine preserved cadaver kidneys. *Transplant. Proc.* (In press)
66. Opelz, G. and Terasaki, P. I. (1977f). Studies on the strength of HLA antigens in related donor kidney transplants. *Transplantation* (In press)
67. Cerilli, J., Holliday, J., Williams, M., Fesparman, D. and Koolemans-Beynen, A. (1977). Immunological evaluation of renal allograft recipients. *Transplant. Proc.* (In press)
68. Yust, I., Wunderlich, J., Mann, D. L., Rogentine, G. N., Leventhal, B., Yankee, R. and Graw, R. (1974). Human lymphocyte-dependent antibody mediated cytotoxicity and direct lymphocyte cytotoxicity against non-HL-A antigens. *Nature (Lond.)*, **249**, 263

8
HLA Complex—Associations with Disease

NICHOLAS R. StC. SINCLAIR and CALVIN R. STILLER

Departments of Bacteriology and Immunology and Medicine,
The University of Western Ontario, London, Ontario, Canada

INTRODUCTION

Throughout the vertebrate series, one particular segment of the chromosome carries the genes for a group of glycoproteins which have the general property of being able to attach to various membrane structures. The genes which contain the genetic information for these membrane proteins are housed within a relatively small portion of the chromosomes, probably in the order of one-tenth of a percent of the total genome. Despite this small genomic representation, the gene products of this particular region play important roles in transplantation rejection, in various cell–cell interactions and, the subject of this review, susceptibility or resistance to various diseases. The region was first recognized because of its production of glycoproteins important in transplant rejection reactions, and because serological techniques were developed to type these antigens, termed histocompatibility antigens, this region in the various species of vertebrates has become known as the major histocompatibility complex (MHC). The adjective *major* was added because this region, above all others, gave the strongest reactions, both in terms of transplantation rejection and in terms of various *in vitro* phenomena which are considered to be correlates of these strong rejection reactions or considered to define antigens directly involved in these transplantation rejections. It was only once the MHC became sufficiently described in terms of its fine genetic structure and in terms of the antigens attributable to this region, that two major biological activities, unrelated to the artificiality of transplantation, became known. The two biological correlates of this region are polymorphism with respect to immune responsiveness and the role that these antigens play in cell–cell interactions.

The purpose of this review is to present observations concerning MHC-associated diseases and to interpret these associations in terms of the two major biological properties of the MHC, that is, its importance in immune responsiveness and in cell–cell interactions. A short description of the MHC and the methods used to delineate its structure will be given. This will be followed by a general classification of MHC-associated diseases and a more detailed look at some of these associations. The review will end with a description of the MHC involvement in immune responsiveness and in cell–cell interactions and an attempt to relate MHC-disease associations to the biological functions of the MHC which are only now being elucidated.

A number of reviews on the MHC associations with disease have appeared over the past two years[1–9]; these provide either more documentation or different points of view from the ones put forward here and, thus, are recommended as further readings into the subject.

DESCRIPTION OF THE MAJOR HISTOCOMPATIBILITY COMPLEX (MHC) IN MAN

Within the MHC four definite (and two provisional) loci have been described (Figure 8.1). These loci encode for human leukocyte antigens (HLA)

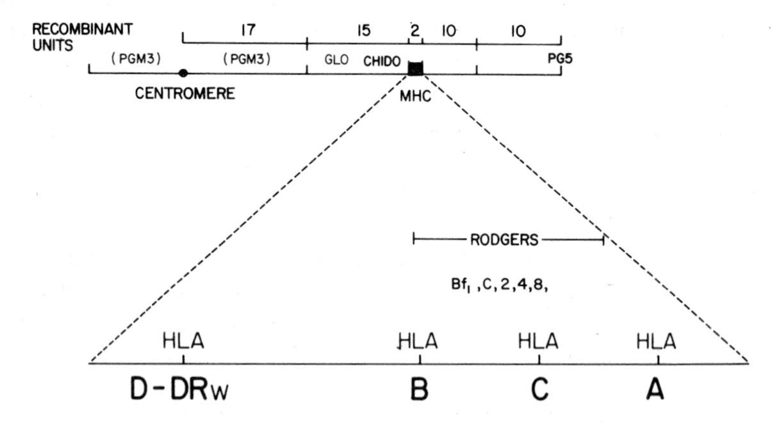

Figure 8.1 The relative positions of MHC and non-MHC loci, as well as the centromere, on the sixth chromosome. The order of the MHC loci are, reading from right to left, HLA-A, C, B and D (DRw). The Rodger's red blood cell group and complement factors BF1, C2, C4 and C8 are closely associated with the MHC. In closer proximity to the chromosomal centromere are phosphoglucomutase-3 (PGM3) and glyoxalase-1 (GLO). The Chido red blood cell locus is located between HLA-D and GLO

A, B, C and D. In addition to this, there are a number of genes that are linked to the MHC. The number of alleles detected at any one of the MHC loci have been increasing with the addition of newly characterized monospecific reagents. The currently known antigens and their gene frequencies in different populations are shown in Table 8.1. Although these loci are at varying recombinant unit distances from each other, linkage disequilibrium exists between particular alleles. Preferential gametic associations between genes at the A and B loci, B and C loci, and B and D loci, have been described and, as will be seen later, some of these haplotypes may have defined association with disease. It is on the basis of linkage with other known chromosomal and genetic markers that the position of the MHC on the sixth chromosome was established, particularly through the use of cell hybridization experiments and correlations with chromosomal markers. Since there are at least four loci, the detection of eight different alleles per individual is possible (assuming heterozygosity). To add to the complexity of this system, B-cell specific antigens have been detected and are thought to be similar to the Ia-antigen system in the mouse. These antigens appear to be coded for by a locus close to or identical with the HLA-D locus which has been termed DRw. However, some Ia-antigens are clearly outside the HLA-D region being in the HLA-A end of the MHC or unlinked to the MHC altogether. A further possibility that an antigen system, defined by the cell-mediated lymphocytotoxicity assay, may be contained within the MHC has been suggested.

Methods used to detect products of the MHC

Serological methods

Historically, the methods used to detect products of the A, B and C regions of the MHC have been serological methods. Sera obtained from either polytransfused patients or multiparous women have been used to determine specificities. The best source is multiparous women who have borne children from the same father, or recipients of repeated planned immunizations from one donor, differing by a single antigen. It is not, however, possible to predict with any degree of certainty the specificity of an antisera until tested.

The most common method used in tissue typing the human today and the method used to describe the A, B, C and DRw profiles, is that of complement-dependent cytotoxicity (CDC). Peripheral blood lymphocytes, obtained by the use of ficol-hypaque separation techniques, are incubated with the specific antisera, a source of rabbit complement, and a supravital dye. After the appropriate incubation period, the number of cells that have taken up this dye are then counted, and the degree of cytotoxicity graded. Similar specificities can be picked up by using agglutination or complement fixation techniques, but these are more laborious and not suitable for routine work.

An *in vitro* assay which measures the amount of antibody-dependent cell-mediated cytotoxicity (ADCC) detects not only A, B and C specificities but other specificities in addition to those detected by the CDC assay. ADCC

Table 8.1 MHC loci gene frequencies (VII Histocompatibility Workshop—Oxford)

MHC antigens	*European Caucasians*	*N. American Caucasians*	*American blacks*	*African blacks*	*Japanese*	*American Indians*
A1	15.8	16.1	8.14	3.92	1.23	2.48
A2	27.0	28.0	16.3	9.41	25.3	45.3
A3	12.6	14.1	7.00	6.37	0.735	0.562
AW23 (A9)	2.41	1.87	10.6	10.8	A9 37.2	A9 23.2
AW24	8.85	7.34	5.14	2.45		
AW25 (A10)	2.04	2.64	0.388	3.50	A10 12.7	A10 0.562
AW26	3.95	3.40	2.33	4.49		
A11	5.06	5.10	2.77	—	6.73	—
A28	4.39	4.18	5.77	8.90	—	2.81
A29	5.83	3.57	2.33	6.37	0.245	0.562
AW30	3.95	2.89	13.0	22.1	0.490	1.12
AW31	2.27	4.53	2.77	4.24	8.71	19.9
AW32	2.94	3.74	1.94	1.50	0.490	1.12
AW33	0.658	1.19	5.09	0.980	1.96	0.562
AW43	—	—	—	4.00	—	—
Blank	2.21	1.32	16.5	11.0	4.24	1.79
B5	5.89	5.86	4.86	3.02	20.9	14.0
B7	10.4	10.5	12.6	7.28	7.06	0.562
B8	9.17	10.4	5.50	7.11	0.253	1.74
B12	16.6	13.8	14.0	12.7	6.46	1.69
B13	3.19	2.59	0.388	1.47	0.758	—
B14	2.40	5.07	4.65	3.56	0.505	—
B18	6.20	3.10	3.60	1.96	—	0.562
B27	4.63	5.60	0.775	—	0.253	6.18
BW15	4.85	5.86	4.72	3.02	9.28	13.7
BW38 (BW16)	1.96	2.47	0.388	BW16 1.49	1.79	BW16 14.5
BW39	3.49	1.38	0.388		4.66	
BW17	5.73	4.91	11.2	16.1	0.573	—
BW21	2.18	3.79	4.39	1.47	1.52	—
BW22	3.64	2.29	3.93	—	6.51	0.562

Table 8.1—*continued*

BW35	9.86	8.63	12.5	7.19	9.38	22.1
BW37	1.12	1.72	1.18	—	0.780	—
BW40	8.11	9.17	3.88	2.01	21.8	16.6
Blank	3.56	2.78	11.0	17.9	7.64	7.81
CW1	4.76	3.71	1.86	—	11.1	10.1
CW2	5.40	6.02	9.22	11.4	1.42	4.63
CW3	9.45	11.4	8.80	5.58	26.3	16.6
CW4	12.6	10.2	12.9	14.4	4.32	23.4
CW5	8.44	5.25	1.39	0.997	1.18	1.13
Blank	59.3	63.4	65.8	67.6	55.6	44.2
DW1	7.90	6.82	*	*	*	*
DW2	9.53	11.7	*	*	*	*
DW3	9.53	8.98	*	*	*	*
DW4	5.11	5.17	*	*	*	*
DW5	9.00	6.10	*	*	*	*
DW6	11.5	8.86	*	*	*	*
D107	5.76	9.83	*	*	*	*
D108	2.54	1.57	*	*	*	*
Blank	39.1	40.9	*	*	*	*
DRw1	6.2	5.2	7.3	—	4.5	—
DRw2	11.2	13.9	13.8	8.7	16.5	8.4
DRw3	8.9	11.8	12.4	11.7	—	9.1
DRw4	10.5	15.9	11.4	4.1	10.3	21.5
DRw4 × 7	7.8	16.5	7.2	3.5	14.4	—
DRw5	15.1	11.9	15.4	7.4	5.4	6.0
DRw6	8.6	10.6	19.1	9.9	6.7	5.9
DRw7	15.5	12.4	12.0	6.6	—	3.7
WIa8	5.6	4.2	7.5	7.2	7.2	12.9
Blank	21.1	13.5	5.3	45.0	45.3	32.5

* No data

utilizes antisera, heat-inactivated to remove any complement, and a third-party source of lymphocytes which act as the effector cell in the ADCC reaction. The assay is a chromium release assay and can be shown to detect HLA-A, B, C and D antigens.

Detection of B-cell antibodies can be carried out using the complement-dependent cytotoxic assay as described above with B-cell enriched targets and longer incubation. This assay may prove to be more reproducible than the mixed lymphocyte reaction in typing for HLA-D. The DRw or those Ia-like antigens coded for the HLA-D end of the MHC are more frequently found on B lymphocytes, although they also occur on the surface of T cells, and it is now possible by this technique to detect several well-defined specificities. Labelling of cells by an immunofluorescent technique also detects B-cell antigens and the ADCC reaction is thought by some workers to also be of use.

Cell proliferation techniques

HLA-D gene products have been detected by the mixed lymphocyte culture (MLC) technique. This is an assay in which the lymphocytes to be typed are incubated with mitomycin-treated cells that are homozygous for the HLA-D antigen. After 5 days in culture, the amount of tritiated thymidine uptake by the unknown cells is measured and a failure to take up more thymidine than the control culture indicates that the unknown cell possesses the HLA-D antigen present on the homozygous typing cell (HTC). This is a difficult assay to read and interpret but several well-known and confirmed specificities of the HLA-D region have been determined using this method. An assay which was thought to detect the same antigen specificities, but which in fact may detect a wider range of specificities, is that of the primed lymphocyte typing technique (PLT). The PLT utilizes the response of lymphocytes in a secondary culture, previously primed in MLC with either homozygous typing cells or cells from a sibling or a parent known to differ by a single haplotype. These two assays appear to complement each other in that there is considerable overlap; moreover, the assignment of HLA-D antigens is best made on the basis of the results of both HTC and PLT assays.

Detection of MHC and non-MHC antigens using cell-mediated lymphocytotoxicity (CML)

Some of the HLA-A, B, C or D antigens, which are recognized by either serological or cell-proliferative assays, may also be recognized through the use of cytotoxic cells directed against these particular antigens. However, the object of CML typing assays is to detect antigens which would not otherwise be detected or defined as groups by serological or cell-proliferative techniques. Therefore, inherent in the methodology are steps which either prospectively or retrospectively exclude reactivities against standard HLA antigens. The cytotoxic cells presently employed have been generated in *in vitro* mixed leukocyte cultures. These cytotoxic cells, which kill the specific stimulator cell, destroy a panel of cells derived from individuals unrelated to the donor of the stimulator cells. One may begin the analysis for CML typing by excluding cytotoxicity which could be explained on the basis of shared MHC antigens between the stimulator cell and the target panel cells. An attempt to exclude shared cross-reactive antigens between the stimulator and target cells could also be undertaken, however, since exclusion is based on the assumption rather than proof that reactions are due to shared antigens exclusion of cytotoxicity based upon the sharing of cross-reactive antigens may be somewhat suspect. One may then take the cytotoxicities remaining and attempt to show correlations with the presence of HLA-A, B, C or D antigens detected serologically. Removal of these significantly associated reactions between the CML typings and the usual HLA antigens again serves to decrease the possibility that one is picking up standard HLA antigens by a somewhat different method. The specificities detected by CML typing cells may be grouped together in clusters or constellations of reactivities against a panel of cells. At present, there are three clusters and each of these clusters shows preferential associations with various serologically defined MHC antigens. There is as yet no clear demonstration of negative associations, as one would expect from allelic series. Cells from HLA-A and B identical but unrelated individuals can be used as responder and stimulator cells in a generation of CML typing cells so that the reactions observed do not relate directly to HLA-A and B antigens. A curious observation has been made by our laboratory in that these CML typing cells which will be cytotoxic to a panel of lymphocytes will not kill the specific stimulator cell or any other targets which share the same HLA-A and B antigens with responder and stimulator cells. It would appear that, in these cases, cytotoxicity is not explicable on the basis of the standard HLA-A and B antigens but may be prevented by these antigens when they are expressed as a group on the surface of the target cell. The targets for CML cytotoxicity may be coded for by areas of the MHC which are at least partially different from those responsible for the standard HLA antigens. Another possibility would be that the targets for such CML activity are encoded by genetic regions not associated with the MHC. Both genetic derivations of CML target antigens may operate at the same time. Indeed, we have evidence from family studies that some CML targets are inherited with the MHC whereas other CML targets are inherited independently of the MHC.

MHC antigen definition and disease associations

The procedures used to detect MHC antigens may influence the analysis of associations between MHC antigens and disease states. The general approach is to find a number of strong reagents which detect certain MHC antigens; this procedure is referred to as clustering. Having found a series of reagents, either sera or cells, one then establishes criteria for the assignment of the MHC antigen detected by these clustered reagents. This may range from being highly restrictive, in which all reagents have to register positive for the antigen, to a fairly loose criteria where only a small number need be positive for the assignment of the antigen. The reason for clustering, which is the definition of a number of reagents which designate a given MHC antigen, relates to the fact that any given reagent must recognize only a portion of the antigen in question and that the combined use of a number of related ('clustered') reagents may define the antigen with greater precision. Since any given reagent has a certain number of 'false positives' or 'false negatives', the multiple determination of the presence or absence of a certain MHC antigen may help lessen the possibility of laboratory error.

The presumption involved in clustering of reagents which define MHC antigens is that they react with these antigens in a somewhat simplistic way. All the reagents within one cluster would be expected to recognize common determinants on the MHC antigens which they identify. However, some of the reagents within one cluster may recognize different, and possibly non-crossreactive, components of a given MHC antigen.

It has become clear that there is no single region in the MHC complex which defines disease resistance or susceptibility. With any given disease, the predominant site for disease association may be restricted to either the A, B, C or D locus. It may be reasonable to assume that further localization of disease associations within the MHC may involve areas smaller than a single HLA locus. That is, it is quite possible that the association of haemochromatosis with A3 may relate to either the left- or the right-hand side of the A3 locus.

Some sera, which are clustered as defining a particular locus, such as A3, may react with structures coded for by either the left- or the right-hand side of the A3 locus. Therefore, if disease associations can be relegated not only to a particular HLA antigen at a particular MHC locus, but, furthermore, restricted to a subregion of this particular HLA antigen, it may be more appropriate to assign the presence or absence of reactions to individual sera which are capable of defining a cluster rather than to an overall assignment of the antigen which the cluster defines.

The problem with this approach is that one has a vast number of sera whose reactions must be compared in a disease and a control population. A useful method to point up the few sera giving very significant positive or negative associations with a disease state is to construct a frequency histogram in which the numbers of comparisons with certain χ^2 values (in increments of two) are given. This can be presented as a table and will show at a glance the number of comparisons which are different from the majority by either occurring in an isolated population separate from the bulk of the comparisons or in a long 'tail' which have χ^2 values giving a significant p-value despite the large number of observations made.

If disease associations are approached from this viewpoint, it may be possible to show that certain reagents defining a given MHC will show a more significant association with a particular disease than with other reagents defining the same MHC antigen. This approach may bring to light evidence that a particular disease state is associated more closely with a portion of a given MHC antigen rather than the presence of the total antigen *per se*. In other words, disease associations may be relegated to 'splits' (sub-specificities) within a given antigen before such 'splits' have been defined by more common means.

Structure and cell-surface behaviour of MHC antigens

MHC antigens (Figure 8.2) may be isolated from cell membranes by one of two classes of procedures. The first, enzyme digestion, allows for the isolation of a dimeric HLA-A or B product made up of β_2-microglobulin and a glycopeptide chain with a molecular weight of 34 000. The β_2-microglobulin is constant in its structure which is comparable to that isolated from urine. The heavy chain demonstrates heterogeneity and possesses four half cysteine bridges. Furthermore, there is a degree of distant homology with immunoglobulin heavy chains, particularly delta-chains. However, the distribution of the cysteines within the primary structure is unlike that of immunoglobulins. When HLA-A or B antigens are isolated using detergent methods, the

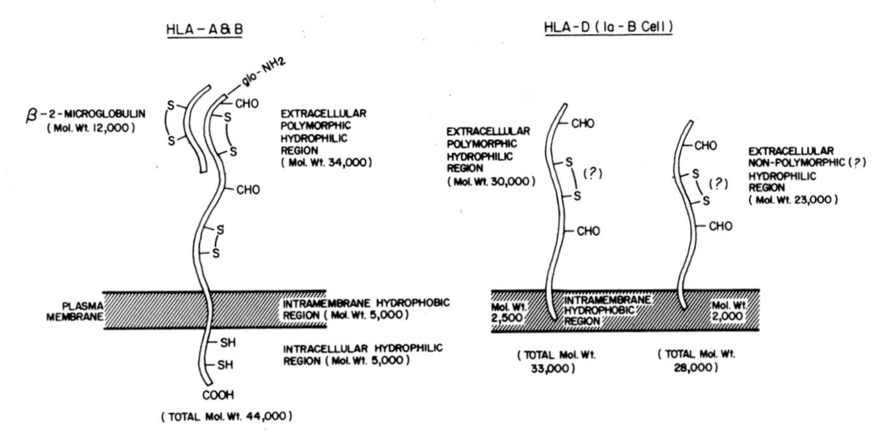

Figure 8.2 Schematic structure of MHC antigens. The HLA-A and B antigens are slightly larger due to an increased length over the Ia antigens of the extracellular and intramembranous portions and the addition of an intracellular hydrophilic region. Also, the HLA antigens A and B associate noncovalently with β-2-microglobulin, whereas the Ia antigen system does not. Ia antigens fall into two different sizes, the larger one being coded for by the MHC and showing polymorphism, whereas the smaller Ia antigen is coded for by genes outside the MHC. The DRw antigens are likely to be found amongst the larger, MHC-encoded Ia antigens

heavy chain has a molecular weight of 44 000 and this molecule may be reduced in size through a 39 000 intermediate to 34 000 by enzymatic digestion with papain. The portions of the molecule removed by papain digestion are, firstly a hydrophilic then a hydrophobic region; the latter represents the attachment site of the HLA-A or B antigens to the cell membrane, while the former may be an intracellular component. Two easily reduced half cysteines exist within the portions of the molecule removed on papain digestion. Therefore, the basic structure of the HLA antigens appears to embody a heavy chain which has a hydrophobic membrane attachment site; this heavy chain is in turn complexed to a light chain (β_2-microglobulin). Attempts to determine whether this heavy–light chain complex is further complexed into oligomers, such as in the immunoglobulin series, have given inconclusive results.

Apart from the enzyme-digested heavy chains which have HLA-A or B antigenicity and attached β_2-microglobulin (with molecular weights of 34 000 and 12 000, respectively), there are a series of molecules with different molecular weights (23 000 and 30 000) which can be purified by gel filtration and used to immunize rabbits. The antibodies produced react with B cells (but not with T cells) and a subpopulation of null cells which possess Fc receptors and are active in ADCC reactions. Furthermore, the antibody against the 23 000 and 30 000 proteins will block the ADCC reaction. These molecules do not appear to be associated with β_2-microglobulin. Because of their cellular distribution and lack of association with β_2-microglobulin, they are thought to be analogous to the Ia antigens of the mouse. In addition there is evidence for population heterogeneity with respect to these isolated antigens. Deoxycholate solubilized molecules have molecular weights of 28 000 and 33 000 and appear to be combined in a dimeric structure. The larger moiety is polymorphic and this polymorphism may be MHC coded. The additional portion of Ia antigen found on deoxycholate isolation, compared to that of enzymatic digestion, represents a hydrophobic membrane attachment site. Therefore, a number of similarities as well as differences exist with respect to the overall structure and attachment of HLA-A and B antigen versus those of the Ia-like (DRw) antigens which are coded for by the HLA-D region of the MHC.

Besides a description of these isolated MHC antigens, an analysis of their behaviour on cell surface membranes is important for the eventual understanding of their biological role. Three major approaches for the study of cell surface topography of MHC antigens have been utilized to determine their natural distribution (by reducing to a minimum redistributions due to the detection agents), their behaviour following cross-linkage, and the influence of their movement on the cell surface on the distribution of other cell surface entities. One may study the natural distribution of MHC antigens, without the intervention of aggregating phenomena, such as capping or patching, by using prefixed cells in which the migration of cell surface components has been reduced or by the use of monovalent antibodies to detect cell surface components. Under these conditions, the MHC antigens appear to be distributed diffusely throughout the cell surface with small clusters of antigen occurring at isolated intervals. Although care must be taken to make sure that small clusters are not artifacts of the detection system, most evidence would suggest that these small clusters are non-artifactual. It is likely that interactions (clusters) involving cell surface entities serve some biological function. Following exposure of MHC antigens on the cell surface to various divalent antibodies, preferably of more than one specificity, these antigens become redistributed into aggregates referred to as patches or caps. Unlike the capping of other molecules, such as surface immunoglobulin or concanavalin-A receptors, there is a requirement for cross-linking, the patching and capping process is slow, and very little of the material becomes endocytosed. Like the capping process induced by anti-immunoglobulin or concanavalin-A, energy is required and, also, colchicine enhances the process. There is no need for cell motility, as with immunoglobulin capping, but not like the concanavalin-A capping. Surface immunoglobulin distributes into one organized cap, whereas MHC antigens may coalesce into more than one cap. It is thought that the phenomenon of aggregation into a single cap is an organized process involving microfilamentous as well as microtubular elements. The less organized multi-capping process exhibited by the MHC antigens may indicate that it is an autonomous system, not being subject to a total cell response which affects other surface entities. One may further analyse the effect of aggregation of one MHC antigen on the distribution of other cell surface entities, a process referred to as co-capping. By studying the co-capping phenomena, one may determine the structural linkage of one cell surface entity to another. MHC antigens of the HLA-A and B type are not structurally linked to each other or to surface immunoglobulins but are linked to β_2-microglobulin in the sense that they will co-cap with this protein. The HLA-A and B antigens are not linked to the Ia (B-cell) antigen in that no co-capping phenomena have been observed between these two MHC antigens. Furthermore, Ia antigens and β_2-microglobulin do not co-cap. Ia antigens, which have some functional relationship to Fc receptors, nevertheless co-cap separately from them. It should not be deduced that various cell surface entities are totally independent and non-interacting. Cell surface entities may associate at certain states and under certain influences. As an example, the binding of monovalent ligands to surface immunoglobulin will induce an association between surface immunoglobulin and Fc receptors. Dynamic and specific forms of interaction may take place between various cell surface entities. These interactions take place in the fluid cell surface membrane and are most likely guided by various submembrane structures such as microfilaments and microtubules.

Although there is a great deal of interest concerning the role that MHC antigens on the surface of cells play in the normal functioning and interaction of cells, as well as in their role as transplantation antigens, it should be pointed out that the MHC components are found in other parts of the cell and probably play important roles in the structural integrity and functional activity involving various intercellular processes. Because of their highly conserved structure in evolution, their presence in substantial amounts on cells, and their demonstrable importance in various immunological and non-immunological processes, it is very likely that these products of the MHC will be shown to play central roles in the functioning of cells, in their organization into a multicellular organism, and possibly in the interactions which occur between organisms within both interbreeding and non-interbreeding populations.

OBSERVED DISEASE ASSOCIATIONS WITH MHC

Introduction and methodology

Just as other genetic markers have associations with diseases described (for example the association of blood groups A with stomach cancer and O with duodenal ulcer), so HLA genes have been described in association with disease. The exact reasons for these associations remain unclear but some theories as to their association will be discussed. Most of the studies have been carried out in a random fashion in which populations with a particular disease are typed within the limits of the reagents of the particular laboratory doing the study and the incidence of a particular antigen determined. This has led to many questionable associations along with a number of very significant ones that have stood the test of additional studies. In interpreting these studies it is important to examine the statistical analysis applied to the data. The usual approach is to calculate the χ^2 for the 2×2 comparison between the presence or absence of a given antigen and a given disease. From the χ^2 value, a p-value may be calculated. If the studies are ones in which large numbers of transplantation antigens are typed and then associations investigated, the p-value for any allele must be corrected for by multiplying it by the number of antigens tested for.

Determining the incidence of antigens in a disease group does not by itself give an indication of the degree of risk to which an individual in the population is exposed by simply possessing that antigen. However, knowing the incidence of the disease in the population being studied and then the observed differences in the HLA antigen expression, the relative risk (RR) can be calculated using the following formula:

$$\mathrm{RR} = \frac{\mathrm{PD}(1-\mathrm{PC})}{\mathrm{PC}(1-\mathrm{PD})} = \frac{\mathrm{DAg}+ \times \mathrm{CAg}-}{\mathrm{CAg}+ \times \mathrm{DAg}-}$$

where PD is the frequency of the antigen in patients; PC is the frequency of antigen in the controls; DAg+ is the percent or number of individuals with the disease and possessing the antigen; CAg− is the percent or number of individuals without the disease and not possessing the antigen; CAg+ are controls with the antigen in question; and DAg− indicates the disease group without the MHC antigen. The personal risk (PR) to an individual with the antigen in question can be determined using the following formula:

$$PR = \frac{PD \times F}{PC}$$

where F is the frequency of the disease in the population.

Classification of MHC and disease associations

One can discern different categories of associations between the HLA complex and disease states (Table 8.2). The *first* is a series of disease associations with either HLA-A, B, C or D. A particular HLA antigen is present in a greater frequency in patients afflicted with these diseases. In most studies in which there is a disease-associated HLA antigen, there appears to be no requirement for homozygosity in order to have a disease association. Therefore, these associations appear to be expressed dominantly but with varying degrees of penetrance. In no case is the penetrance complete; the presence of the particular HLA antigen is not associated with the consistent expression of a disease state. Even in the most striking case, that of ankylosing spondylitis, HLA-B27 is present in approximately 8% of the population, while the disease ankylosing spondylitis has a frequency of less than 0.1% of the population. The observations suggest that a single representation of the gene is sufficient for the existence of susceptibility to the disease state which, however, depends on other factors for complete expression. Initially, there appeared to be an increasing gradient with respect to disease association beginning with HLA-A through HLA-C to HLA-B and even stronger with the HLA-D and perhaps strongest in some cases with certain (DRw) B-cell (Ia-like) antigens. However, it is now clear that, even if such a gradient does exist, each HLA locus has its own strong disease association such as A3 and haemochromatosis, B27 and ankylosing spondylitis, CW6 and psoriasis and DW4-DRw4 and adult-onset rheumatoid arthritis; in each case the 'disease gene' appears to be in or near the locus indicated. There appears to be a greater and greater manifestation of immunological abnormalities as one approaches the HLA-D end in the association between these MHC antigens and disease. The lack of a requirement for homozygosity was thought to rule against the possibility that a defect in immune response is associated with the presence of this particular HLA antigen. From studies in mice, the lack of a response is recessive and, therefore, homozygosity would be required if such a lack in an immune response was the basis for the emergence of these disease states. However, some decreased immune responses in humans have been associated with a single representation of a given MHC antigen, suggesting that non-responsiveness may, in some cases, be dominant. Also

Table 8.2 HLA and disease association

	Antigen (frequency)	*Frequency in population*	*Risk factor*
1. Single gene association			
HLA-A			
Haemochromatosis	A3 (72%)	29%	6
Recurrent herpes labialis	A1 (56%)	25%	4
Pemphigus	A10 (40%)	15%	4
Dust allergies	AW33 (20%)	2%	12
HLA-B			
Ankylosing spondylitis	B27 (93%)	8%	150
Reiter's syndrome	B27 (76%)	8%	36
Anterior uveitis	B27 (55%)	8%	14
Juvenile arthritis	B27 (31%)	8%	5
Behcet's disease	B5 (71%)	13%	16
Subacute thyroiditis	BW35 (80%)	10%	36
	BW17 (29%)	7%	5
Systemic lupus erythematosus	B8 (30%)	23%	2
Myasthenia	B8 (58%)	23%	4
Addison's disease	B8 (50%)	23%	4
Grave's disease	B8 (45%)	23%	3
Coeliac disease	B8 (72%)	23%	8
Dermatitis herpetiformis	B8 (70%)	23%	8
Chronic active hepatitis	B8 (64%)	23%	6
Multiple sclerosis	B7 (45%)	18%	4
Haemochromatosis	B14 (31%)	7%	6
Acute myelogenous leukaemia—remission	B12 (44%)	20%	3
Thyroid disease in Japanese	BW35		
Paralytic poliomyelitis	BW16 (25%)	15%	2
HLA-C			
Psoriasis	T7 (75%)	25%	9
HLA-D			
Multiple sclerosis	DW2 (65%)	24%	6
Chronic active hepatitis	DW3 (66%)	17%	9
Juvenile-onset diabetes	DW3 (36%)	17%	4
	DW4 (38%)	13%	4
Myasthenia gravis	DRw3 (30%)	17%	2
Coeliac disease	DRw3 (96%)	27%	65
Sjogren's disease	DW3 (38%)	17%	3
Thyrotoxicosis (Grave's)	DW3 (53%)	17%	6
Adult-onset rheumatoid arthritis	DW4-DRw4 (62%)	18%	7
Cirrhosis	DRw1		
Diseases in Japanese—thyroid	DHO		4
—juvenile-onset diabetes	DYT		4
Dermatitis herpetiformis	DW3 (80%)	19%	17
2. Two gene association			
Psoriatic arthritis with sacroiliitis	B27 (27%)	6%	6
	BW38 (27%)	3%	12
Psoriasis vulgaris	BW17 (26%)	7%	5
	B13 (19%)	·5%	5
Juvenile diabetes mellitus	B8 (54%)	23%	4
	BW15 (36%)	12%	4

Table 8.2—*continued*

3. MHC haplotype association	
A. Family-restricted haplotypes	
Haemochromatosis	
Ragweed allergy	
Juvenile diabetes mellitus	HLA-D identity in siblings with the disease
B. Haplotypes in populations	
Haemochromatosis	A3-B14
Juvenile-onset diabetes	A1-B8 B8-DW3
Crohn's disease and myasthenia gravis	A1-B8-DW3
Autoimmune disease in Japanese	BW35-DHO BW22J-DYT
Multiple sclerosis	B7-DW2
Systemic lupus erythematosus—severe	A1-B8
—mild	A2-B7
4. Genetic recombination (MHC) and disease association	
Harelip	
Spina bifida	
Juvenile diabetes mellitus	
5. Distortion of linkage disequilibria in disease	
Systemic lupus erythematosus—mild disease	A2-B7
Juvenile-onset diabetes mellitus	A1-B8 B8-DW3
6. Increase or decrease in MHC antigen representation	
Increase —leukaemic lymphoblasts	
—infectious mononucleosis cells	
Decrease—severe combined immunodeficiency disease with adenosine deaminase deficiency	

likely is the association of an abnormal and possibly heightened response with these particular HLA antigens. The other possibility is that these antigens, when expressed on various cell membranes, serve as receptor sites for certain micro-organisms which may interact with and damage the target tissues in these MHC-associated diseases.

A *second* category of genetic association with disease is exemplified by juvenile diabetes. In this case, there appears to be an increase in relative risk in the presence of two HLA-B antigens, such as HLA-B8 and HLA-BW15. This form of heterozygosity at the HLA-B locus in juvenile-onset diabetes, an example of an interaction between two HLA antigens at one locus to induce a heightened disease sensitivity, may be repeated with respect to the occurrence of DW3 and DW4 in this disease.

A *third* category of genetic characteristics is that which shows an increased incidence of the disease in individuals inheriting a particular haplotype within a given family. The implicated haplotype may vary from family to family with respect to the HLA antigens present on that given haplotype. The original demonstration of this phenomenon was that of an increased expression of sensitivity to ragweed allergen but the inheritance of this particular sensitivity within other families has been disputed. However, the original family studies which demonstrated this inheritance were larger, and even if discordant segregation was noted in a number of instances, the linked inheritance seems high enough to suggest a genetic association attributable to linkage on the chromosome carrying the MHC.

A *fourth* group displays an association between increased incidence of crossover events within families and the presence of craniopharyngeal abnormalities, such as harelip. A genetic instability, which may be more widespread than within the MHC but which may be picked up most readily by recombination, deletion and duplication events within the MHC, may be involved in the production of these particular disease states.

A *fifth* type of association between the behaviour of MHC antigens in a disease state concerns the distortion of normal linkage disequilibrium. A number of examples of linkage disequilibrium which appear to be maintained despite the sufficient length of time necessary to allow for randomization include that noted between A1 and B8, A2 and B12 and A3 and B7. Linkage disequilibria also exist between B12 and DW1, B8 and DW3 and B7 and DW2. Linkage disequilibrium disappears within a defined period of generations, depending upon the frequency of recombination between the two genetically linked loci. When linkage disequilibria are still evident despite a sufficient number of generations to allow for an equilibrium to be reached, the maintenance of such a disequilibrium is thought to depend upon some selective advantage for the associated inheritance or expression of alleles present at the two distinct loci. To exemplify an even stronger linkage disequilibrium than that found in the normal population, linkage disequilibria between A1 and B8 and between B8 and DW3 are increased significantly amongst individuals with juvenile-onset diabetes and, indeed, amongst their parents. A preliminary result would suggest that, in mild cases of systemic lupus erythematosus, there is an increase in the A2-B7 haplotype, a combination of genes which does not demonstrate a linkage disequilibrium within the normal population.

A *sixth* group of alterations in the expression of MHC antigens in disease concerns increases or decreases in the various antigens coded for by the MHC. There would appear to be an increase in antigen representation on various leukaemic lymphoblasts and on infectious mononucleosis blasts, particularly with respect to DRw antigens. With respect to chronic lymphocytic leukaemia cells, reactions against these antigens can be blocked by absorption with normal B cells, suggesting that the increases occur in representation of normal DRw antigens. In infectious mononucleosis, there appears to be an increase in DRw-antigen representation on cells which rosette with sheep erythrocytes and have been interpreted to be T cells. The suggestion is that DRw antigens appear on T cells in this disease state or that a minor population of T cells with Ia antigens proliferates preferentially in this disease. Another possibility would be that B cells develop receptors for sheep erythrocytes, the cell surface receptor counterpart of antisheep erythrocyte antibody found in this disease. A further example of an increase in MHC antigens has been noted in ankylosing spondylitis and in Reiter's disease where more anti-HLA-B27 antibody became bound to cell surfaces taken during the active disease as compared to cells taken during remission. In severe combined immunodeficiency disease, the representation of DRw antigens appears to be normal in children possessing normal levels of adenosine deaminase but is decreased in children whose level of adenosine deaminase is low.

It can be seen that alterations in the genetic constitution of the MHC or in the expression of MHC antigens in disease may display many different patterns of associations. This would suggest that there will be no single and simple explanation for the association of certain MHC antigens or phenomena associated with the MHC complex with certain disease states. Rather, the relationship between the MHC and its products and the normal functioning of the multicellular organism as well as its dysfunction may be multifaceted such that each MHC association with disease may require a different explanation.

It has been pointed out previously by other authors that the concept of a 'disease gene' in association with the MHC may be an incorrect view, or at least a distorted view, of the association between the MHC and certain disease states. It may be better to think of the MHC as a very important genetic locus which codes for cell surface structures important in various cell–cell interactions. Certain of these antigens, coded for by genes at one of the four HLA loci, may provide selective advantages which prevent devastating events from occurring, such as massive mortality due to epidemics, but that the presence of these antigens, although protective for a number of untoward events, may predispose to a limited number of somewhat rarer diseases. As an example, the common occurrence of the B8-DW3 haplotype in autoimmune disease may indicate that the immune system in individuals possessing these antigens may be more active in warding off various potentially lethal organisms, but, at the same time, make their bearers more prone to various autoimmune phenomena. In other words, the disease association may be a minor inconvenience (at least in terms of percent incidence) of a gene that confers a protective advantage. Such examples are known from previous studies, a classic case being the resistance to malaria conferred by the inheritance of the sickle cell trait.

Specific MHC antigen associations with diseases

Having given an outline of the types of association which exist between antigens coded for by genes in the MHC and various disease states, specific diseases will be analysed with respect to the presence of certain MHC antigens. Such a presentation is intended to provide specific examples for the preceding generalizations and to point out further complexities which cannot be explained at the present time. In September 1977, the Seventh International Histocompatibility Workshop, held in Oxford, dealt with the association of certain MHC antigens with various disease states. Much of what is to follow is based heavily on the Proceedings of that Workshop[10], as well as on previous reports.

Familial idiopathic haemochromatosis

HLA-A3 occurs more frequently in patients with familial idiopathic haemochromatosis and, although not as consistent, HLA-B14 and B7 have been shown to be increased in various studies. There were no consistent changes in the representation of DRw antigens with this disease. The incidence of DW2 has been reported to be doubled in one study. Families, in which haemochromatosis is found, seem to fall into two general categories; those in which the incidence of A3 in various haplotypes is rather high and those in which the A3 representation is low or absent. In those families in which there are multiple representations of A3-containing haplotypes, there appears to be a reasonable correlation of the disease and/or of iron metabolic abnormalities with the inheritance of A3-containing haplotypes. Many of these haplotypes are A3-B7. The DRw antigens associated with these haplotypes are variable and do not designate the disease-associated A3-B7 haplotypes. In families in which there is a high representation of the above haplotypes, there is a marked increase in iron metabolic abnormalities amongst family members with the same MHC ántigens as those present in the proband. Such a result would suggest that there is a genetic locus located near or in the HLA-A region which is important in this disease and that the alleles present at this loci are recessive in character.

Other studies have suggested that there are two disease potentiating haplotypes associated with haemochromatosis. One involved an A3-containing haplotype and appeared to predispose to abnormal deposition of iron in peripheral tissues such as liver, pancreas or heart. Another haplotype, the antigens of which can vary from family to family, has been defined which dictates the rapidity with which iron is absorbed from the gut. When family members inherit both the A3 antigen and the haplotype which dictates iron uptake, there is an increased likelihood that idiopathic haemochromatosis will occur. These MHC-associated alterations or defects in iron metabolism are instructive because there is little or no reason to suggest any immunopathological mechanisms associated with these abnormalities. Since the MHC antigens play an important role in cell surface components, it is not surprising that certain transport mechanisms would be shown to be associated with the inheritance of given MHC antigens. Furthermore, occult immunopathological mechanisms may be involved in decreasing the barriers to either iron absorption or of iron peripheralization.

In other families, in which there are multiple representations of haemochromatosis and/or iron metabolic abnormalities but in which the A3-B7 haplotype is rare or absent, there appears to be no association between the inheritance of various MHC haplotypes and the presence of the disease. This would suggest that in this latter form of familial idiopathic haemochromatosis, the disease possesses a genetic influence inherited independently of the MHC or indeed is overlaid by strong environmental influences such that the genetic influences are obscured.

Although there is an increase in A3 (relative risk 8.5), B14 (relative risk 6) and B7 (relative risk 2.3) there appears to be no distortion in the linkage disequilibrium observed in patients with idiopathic haemochromatosis with respect to the A3-B14 or the A3-B7 haplotypes. The presence of either of these two haplotypes brings with it a relative risk of approximately 18.

Ankylosing spondylitis

By far the most striking MHC disease association has been that noted with respect to B27 in ankylosing spondylitis. Approximately 90% of individuals with ankylosing spondylitis have the B27 antigen, whereas only 7–9% of control populations possess this antigen. The relative risk (RR), that is, the chances of having the disease given the fact that one possesses the antigen B27, is in the order of 150-fold.

In those individuals who do not possess B27, there is possibly an increase in A2. There is no correlation with any of the DRw antigens, except for a possible decrease in DRw7. Both mild and severe cases of ankylosing spondylitis show an increase in incidence of B27. The severe cases of spondylitis associated with psoriasis, ulcerative colitis, non-specific urethritis and conjunctivitis, or certain forms of dysentry, and Crohn's disease have a significant association with B27. Mild forms of psoriasis and Crohn's disease with spondylitis show a weaker association with B27. The problem may be that clinical assessment of spondylitis in psoriasis and Crohn's disease is more difficult than of that which occurs in ankylosing spondylitis. The mild forms of non-ankylosing spondylitis afflictions may have other (than B27) genetic influences whereas the mild ankylosing spondylitis conditions do not.

In the minority group of patients with ankylosing spondylitis who do not possess B27, increases in some HLA-C and HLA-D antigens have also been reported. Family studies have documented the familial transmission of ankylosing spondylitis primarily with the inheritance of the B27-containing haplotype, but also with the non-B27-containing haplotype present in the proband.

There is a preponderance of males with ankylosing spondylitis. Moreover, a family has been identified in which the father had ankylosing spondylitis but lacked B27, whereas the mother had B27 but no ankylosing spondylitis; all male children with B27 developed ankylosing spondylitis. However, the male preponderance with respect to ankylosing spondylitis was not observed amongst B27 positive family members with the disease or amongst population of 'normal' B27 positive individuals who were then investigated for the disease. This suggests that the disease showed no real sex difference in incidence but that males perceived the problem and sought attention more readily. Thus, the study of MHC association with disease may alter some of the firmly held opinions concerning the overall character of the disease.

Psoriasis

Numbers of HLA-B antigens (B13, BW37, BW16 and BW17) have been shown to be increased in patients with psoriasis vulgaris. B7 is found in lesser amounts as a compensatory phenomena amongst this patient group. Also increased are antigens A1 and AW19, products of linkage disequilibria. Slightly decreased levels of DRw2 and DRw6 have also been noted. However, the major finding has been that HLA-C antisera designated as CW6 showed a strong correlation with psoriasis vulgaris, this association being the overriding one. CW6 is in strong linkage disequilibrium with B13, BW17 and BW37. Therefore, a rather complex association between this disease state and the MHC has been simplified by the designation of a strong association with an HLA-C locus antigen apparently explaining the multiple associations with the various HLA-B antigens. The HLA-CW6 occurred in 32% of a Canadian Caucasian population designated as normal compared to 67% of psoriatics. A moot point concerns whether or not a considerable portion of a control population would have, if thoroughly examined, any of the stigmata which are characteristic of psoriasis. Patients with psoriasis are designated so because the dermatological lesions have reached the level where they are recognized by either the physician or the patient. Many individuals in the 'control' group may be shown to have limited lesions which bear the morphological characteristics of psoriasis. Therefore, the present association given between the presence of CW6 and psoriasis must be considered a minimum estimate of significance. Further studies on this association should include a thorough examination of the control population for limited lesions which have the characteristics attributable to psoriasis vulgaris. Some family studies suggest that the inheritance of the MHC genes and the expression of this disease or of arthritis are strongly associated. There were no significant alterations in the representation of DRw antigens in patients with psoriasis, although there have been some suggestions that either early onset or prolonged duration may be associated with certain DW or DRw antigens. The association of CW6 has been observed in both Japanese and Caucasian populations. A similar constancy in association of a particular MHC antigen with a given disease amongst various racial groups is noted with B5 and Behcet's disease, otherwise such a constancy is rare. The pustular form of psoriasis, as distinct from psoriasis vulgaris, does not show any MHC associations.

Chronic active hepatitis

In the patients not possessing the hepatitis B antigen (UK and Australian study), there is an increased incidence of B8 and DRw3, while there is a decrease in the BW35 antigen. On the other hand, individuals possessing the hepatitis B antigen appear to have a decreased representation of B8 and an increase in BW35. In another study carried out in the United States, patients with chronic active hepatitis who are hepatitis B antigen negative demonstrated a small increase in both B8 and BW35. In cases in which there is an increase in B8, there is also a concomitant increase in A1 which is probably explained by linkage disequilibrium. An increase of A3 and B8 as well as a phenotypic association of A3 with BW35 has been noted in chronic active hepatitis. The DRw antigen is increased in patients with a biopsy diagnosis of cirrhosis.

In addition, there appears to be an increase in DRw3 and B8 in individuals expressing either antinuclear factor or smooth muscle antibody. The associations with the production of smooth muscle antibodies are stronger than that seen with the production of antinuclear factor.

Multiple sclerosis

In Caucasian populations, there is a significant increase in B7 and DRw2 in association with multiple sclerosis. A number of negative correlations have also been reported, resulting from compensatory phenomena due to the increased incidence of B7 and DRw2. HLA-A3 has been reported on some occasions to be increased but such increases, when significant, are explicable on the basis of linkage disequilibrium between A3 and the B7-DRw2 complex. In a preliminary study of a Japanese population, the above associations did not hold; however, increases in BW22, DRw6 and DRw8 were noted. These increases were not as marked as those reported for the Caucasian population. The much weaker association in the Japanese population between MHC antigens and multiple sclerosis may indicate that no susceptibility genes are associated with the MHC in the Japanese, that MHC antigens associated with multiple sclerosis in the Japanese population have not yet been defined (a likely possibility since the blank in DRw antigen designations is 45%) or that the disease-causing genes have lost their association with the MHC. Studies carried out on Arab populations indicate that multiple sclerosis and DRw4 and DRw4 × 7 may be associated. These latter results show that a disease which has similar characteristics in a number of populations may show associations with different MHC antigens.

A number of reports had suggested that there was a higher correlation between DRw2 and multiple sclerosis than between DW2 and this particular disease. However, more recent studies indicate that, although there is a higher percentage of DRw2 than DW2 in patients with multiple sclerosis, there is also an increase in DRw2 over DW2 within a normal population, this leaving the difference between the two populations with the same risk and the same statistical significance.

Apart from the strong association demonstrated between multiple sclerosis and the presence of DW2, there may be an even stronger correlation with an antigen common to both DW2 and DW6-containing cells, which is detected through primed lymphocyte typing and is found in three-quarters of the patients with multiple sclerosis. This 'common antigen' may, in the final analysis, be derived from a separate locus which is in strong linkage disequilibrium with both DW2 and DW6.

Juvenile-onset diabetes

Whereas there are demonstrated associations between juvenile-onset diabetes and the presence of various MHC antigens, there is no such MHC association with maturity-onset diabetes. A number of studies on juvenile-onset diabetes have reported increases in B8, BW15, BW18 and CW3, as well as the increased representation of certain B locus combinations, such as B8-B40 (relative risk 6.9) and B8-B15 (relative risk 5.4). Even more striking increases have been noted for DW3 and DW4 as well as for the B-cell antigens DRw3, DRw4 and DRw4 × 7. When anti-islet cell antibody occurs, there appears to be an increase in a number of HLA-B combinations, such as B8-B40, B8-B18, B8-BW40 and B8-B15. The presence or absence of anti-islet cell antibodies does not appear to influence the association of DRw3, 4 and 4 × 7 with juvenile-onset diabetes. It may be possible to divide patients into two groups based upon fundal changes; those with fundal changes do not appear to have a significant DRw correlation, whereas those without fundal changes have a three-fold increase in the DRw4-DW4 group as well as a two-fold increase in DRw3. Equivalent to that seen with various HLA-B antigens, there appears to be an increased risk when both DW3 and DW4 are present. A similar finding has been noted with respect to the DRw3 and DRw4 antigens. In general, most authors would suggest that, since DRw3 is in linkage disequilibrium with B8 whereas DRw4 shows linkage disequilibrium with BW15, most of the associations in juvenile-onset diabetes are with the HLA-D locus while HLA-B associations represent linkage disequilibrium. This is, however, not a universally shared opinion. Family studies have indicated that DRw4 rather than BW15 houses a genetic factor associated with juvenile-onset diabetes; similar family studies with respect to B8 and DRw3 have been reported recently.

Apart from the increase in the A1-B8 and the B8-DW3 haplotypes in juvenile-onset diabetes and in their parents, there is also an increase in the linkage disequilibrium of these two gene combinations.

Family studies on juvenile-onset diabetes suggest that affected siblings are often MHC identical and that the disease tends to develop in about half of the siblings who are MHC identical to the affected child, suggesting that non-MHC factors also play a role in the emergence of this disease. In selected families in which one parent contributed the DW4 antigen while the other parent contributed the DW3 antigen, all diabetic children possess both the DW3 and the DW4 antigen. In other families, the DW4 haplotype was replaced by other HLA-D-containing haplotypes. A number of recombinant families have been studied in which it could be ascertained that the susceptibility to the development of juvenile-onset diabetes segregated with the HLA-D segment.

Other racial groups show somewhat different MHC associations with juvenile-onset diabetes. In the Japanese population there was an increased occurrence in both DRw3 and DRw4 × 7. However, the increased occurrence of DRw3 did not relate to all the clustered antisera defining this particular antigen, suggesting that only a portion of the DRw3 antigen was increased in juvenile-onset diabetes in the Japanese population. The MHC associations in a South African negroid population with both juvenile-onset diabetes and maturity-onset diabetes were similar; this is unlike the MHC associations with these two forms of diabetes in either the Caucasian or the Japanese population where MHC antigen representation in the maturity-onset diabetes remains normal.

Rheumatoid arthritis

Rheumatoid arthritis can be divided broadly into two types, juvenile-onset and adult-onset. Both show erosive joint lesions. In the adult type, rheumatoid factor and subcutaneous nodules are found frequently but are rare in the juvenile-onset type. On the other hand, fever, skin rash and lymphadenopathy are frequent in the juvenile type but rare in the adult type. In females with adult-onset rheumatoid arthritis, there is a highly significant increase in DW4, DRw4, DRw4 × 7 and BW15. Amongst the males, increases have been noted in DRw4, DRw4 × 7 and BW40, but the increase in DRw4 × 7 was due to the increase in the DRw4 antigen. The relative risk for individuals possessing DW4 or DRw4 is approximately 6.

The female adult-onset rheumatoid arthritics can be divided into those under and over the age of 41; the younger group possesses a significant increase in both DRw4 and DRw4 × 7, whereas the older group does not. Rheumatoid arthritis represents one disease in which there is no consistent HLA-A, B or C antigen associations but there is a strong association with a HLA-D antigen. Increases in DW4 range from three- to seven-fold. There also appears to be an association between the presence of rheumatoid factor and DW4, although DW4 is not associated with the presence of rheumatoid factor in the absence of clinical arthritis. The juvenile-onset rheumatoid arthritics do not demonstrate the same increase in the DW4–DRw4 complex but there is an increase in a specificity designated TMO (which is found in 1% of controls but in 21% of those with the disease); this antigen appears to be associated with the DW107 antigen but is not the same as DRw7.

Myasthenia gravis

There is an overall increase in A1, B8 and DRw3, suggesting the incrimination of a whole haplotype in the genesis of myasthenia gravis. However, before the whole haplotype can be incriminated, it must be shown that each locus is associated in a primary fashion with disease and not secondarily through normal linkage disequilibrium. In other words the linkage disequilibrium must be shown to intensify in this disease compared to controls, as happens in juvenile-onset diabetes. In individuals lacking B8, there is an increase in BW25 and CW4. Such associations are not seen in the patients with thymoma as distinct from other thymic abnormalities. The presence of these antigens does not seem to correlate with thymic disease, other autoantibodies or reduced serum IgM or isohaemagglutinin titres. The increased incidence of DW3 has been accompanied by a decreased incidence of DW2 in a Caucasian population. Although HLA-B8 and DW3 are increased in Caucasians, there seems to be a stronger association in the Japanese population with BW35. Furthermore, the DRw2 antigen group is increased significantly in the Japanese population with myasthenia gravis.

Coeliac disease

Just as with myasthenia gravis, there appears to be an increase in the A1, B8 and DRw3 haplotype, with an increase in the strength of disease association as one approaches the HLA-D end of the MHC. This suggests a primary disease association with the HLA-DW3 antigen and secondary associations through linkage disequilibria with both A1 and B8. The incidence of DW3 amongst patients with coeliac disease does not appear to be as high as that seen with DRw3. Since in this particular study there were large numbers of intermediate stimulations in the homozygous typing procedure for DW-typing, extra antigens may be present in the homozygous typing cells which can be recognized by lymphocytes taken from individuals with this disease. There has been a report of a B-cell antibody raised against individuals with coeliac disease which was not MHC associated.

Systemic lupus erythematosus

Patients with SLE and A1-B8 appear to have more severe renal complications than those who have A2-B7. Family studies indicate these groupings are haplotypes. These results suggest that various haplotypes may predispose to the character rather than the presence of the disease. The A2-B7 haplotype is unusual in controls but yet is fairly common amongst the SLE patient group indicating a distortion in linkage disequilibrium within this disease category.

Another demonstration of distortion of linkage disequilibrium occurs in haplotypes carrying the C2 deficiency gene. This deficiency is associated with an A10-B18-DW2 haplotype, an uncommon association in the general population.

Sjogren's disease

In this disease there is an increased incidence of DW3. Furthermore, a number of B-cell antisera which determine different DRw antigens within a normal population react with cells from patients with Sjogren's disease with greater frequency. There have been reports of increases in B8, DW3, DRw3, DRw5 and DRw6 in Sjogren's disease. There is some similarity amongst the disease associations with respect to Sjogren's disease and systemic lupus erythematosus.

Malignant diseases

Although the initial associations of an HLA antigen with disease involved patients with malignancies, these associations have been rather limited with respect to the broad range of malignant diseases and have shown relative risks in the order of 1.3 to at most 3.5. Such results have been considered by many to be disappointing, especially in view of the rather rich associations between the MHC and malignant diseases in mice. Nevertheless, three varieties of malignant disease appear to show some limited increases. Hodgkin's disease is associated with increases in B5, BW35, B18 and BW15. There may be increases also in A1 and B8. Some documented increases in certain antigens with disease duration have been noted. Also, certain antigens appear to be associated with either decreased or increased lengths of remission.

An interesting observation has been made with respect to nasopharyngeal carcinoma in the Chinese. The initial observation was an increase in the blank at the HLA-B locus, that is, an increase in an undefined B antigen. A new B antigen, Singapore 2 (Sin 2, BW46), has been identified and this antigen in concert with A2 appears to be increased in patients with nasopharyngeal carcinoma.

In the overall study of patients with acute myelogenous leukaemia (AML) there have been slight and non-statistically significant increases in A2, and patients with A1-B8 or A2-B12 haplotypes appear to survive longer (although such differences did not reach the level of statistical significance). The incidence of HLA-B12 also increases throughout the disease course. Three particular haplotypes (A1-B8; A2-B12; and A3-B15) are associated with approximately 50% remission rates whereas other haplotypes give a 28% remission rate. There appears to be an increased representation of Ia antigen on the surface of AML blasts; these positive reactions, detected with the various DRw sera, are totally absorbable with normal B cells indicating that these increases involve heightened antigen representations of normal differentiation antigens. With chronic lymphocytic leukaemia there is an increased representation of DRw antigens on the surface of the leukaemic cells compared to those detectable on normal control B cells.

Autoimmune endocrinopathies—racial differences

Amongst Caucasian populations, autoimmune diseases are associated most commonly with the B8-DW3 haplotype; this is replaced with the BW35-DHO haplotype in the Japanese population. It is of interest that these two pairs of antigens in the two populations show a similar frequency and degree of linkage disequilibrium. Despite the fact that HLA-DHO in the Japanese population appears to be equivalent to DW3 in Caucasian populations with respect to overall incidence, linkage disequilibrium and disease associations, the DHO antigen is defined by DRw2, rather than DRw3, sera. In Caucasian populations, juvenile-onset diabetes shows a strong association with the B8-DW3 haplotype, similar to other forms of autoimmune diseases, whereas in the Japanese population, another HLA-D antigen, DYT, is common in this particular disease group. The HLA-DYT antigen is associated with B-cell antigens defined by sera within the DRw4, 7 and 4×7 clusters. In Caucasian populations, the DW4 antigen is also increased in diseases with autoimmune characteristics, such as rheumatoid arthritis and juvenile-onset diabetes.

An interesting crossreactivity has been demonstrated with respect to B-cell antibodies and various antithyroid, thyroglobulin and microsomal antibodies which appear in Grave's and Hashimoto's diseases.

POSSIBLE EXPLANATIONS FOR THE ASSOCIATION BETWEEN MHC AND DISEASES

As can be seen from the foregoing, the association between the MHC and various disease states is by no means trivial. Relative risks of over 100 have been recorded and it is evident that a number of instances in which the relative risk exceeds five are common. These important associations would suggest that there are a number of direct connections between the expression of certain MHC antigens and the susceptibility to given disease states. There are three important biological consequences which show associations with the MHC. These are the association between MHC and immune responsiveness, the importance of the MHC in various types of cell–cell interactions,

Table 8.3 Genetically associated (determined?) immune responsiveness in man

Antigen	*Exposure*	*Measurement*	*Genetics*
Australia antigen	endemic	presence of antigen	BW35
Mycobacteriumleprae	endemic	disease incidence	HLA linked (family study), ?DW2-WIa2 low responders
Tetanus toxoid	immunization	blast transformation	BW35-DHO-low responders (Japanese)
Streptococcal antigen (SK-SD)	ubiquitous	lymphocyte proliferation and skin test	B5 associated
Rubella virus	immunization	antibody titre	BW17, A28
Vaccinia	immunization	lymphocyte proliferation	CW3—low responders
Influenza	immunization	antibody titre	BW60 associated
Diphtheria toxin	immunization	antibody titre	non-HLA linked
Measles	ubiquitous	antibody titre	HLA linked—MS patients with A3-B7-high responders
Typhoid and/or yellow fever	epidemic	disease mortality	B7 low responders
Mycobacterium tuberculosis	endemic	history of tuberculosis	B8—positive history (susceptibles or survivors?)
Herpes simplex	endemic	lymphocyte proliferation	DW2 in MS patients low responders
Ragweed	seasonal	skin test	A2 (B12) B7 and crossreacting antigens
Rye grass	seasonal	skin test	B8
Glutin	general	antibody, lymphocyte proliferation and skin test	DW3 associated
Avian proteins	incidental	precipitating antibodies	DW6 associated
Phytohaemagglutinin	none	lymphocyte proliferation	B8 in males

and the genetic and structural relationship between MHC antigens and a series of fetal antigens which appear to dictate morphogenesis. A brief description of these three biological consequences attributable to the MHC will be dealt with.

MHC and immune responsiveness

There are a number of studies which show a relationship between various MHC antigens and their ability to respond to various microbial and non-microbial antigens. Table 8.3 gives a list of antigens towards which some of these MHC-associated immune responses are directed. This table is an expanded version of that presented by van Rood at the Third International Congress of Immunology, July 1977. The presence of certain MHC antigens may be associated with either high or low responses to various antigens. These results appear to be different from murine studies in which low responsiveness is a recessive trait. In some instances, the measurement was the presence or absence of disease and, again, certain MHC antigens may be associated with the presence of the disease in question. There have not yet been published any data demonstrating that certain MHC antigens are found in increased numbers amongst individuals showing resistance to various forms of infection. One would have predicted that resistance to disease would be detectable in individuals carrying certain MHC antigens since immunological responsiveness is, in many instances, a dominant trait. Certain MHC antigens seem to define low responders, such as B7 and DW2. Other antigens would appear to define high responders such as B8 and DW3. It is of interest that the B8-DW3 complex is associated with many autoimmune diseases; possibly, the high responsiveness and the propensity to develop autoimmune disease may be correlated. However, there are instances in which genetic low responders have appeared to be susceptible to autoimmune phenomenon such as the BW35-DHO haplotype in the Japanese. The generally low responder B7-DW2 haplotype is found in increased incidence in multiple sclerosis; this may suggest that certain low responder MHC antigens may be associated with autoimmune disease or that multiple sclerosis is essentially a disease of immunodeficiency.

High responders and MHC

B8 has been associated with increases in various immunological diseases and was analysed with respect to responsiveness to PHA in young and old individuals. No differences were found amongst the young age group (20–50 years of age) whereas in the old age group (70–100 years of age) the males possessed a high response to PHA and had a higher representation of B8 whereas the females possessed a low response to PHA and had a lower incidence of B8 in that population. A comparison of severe versus mild systemic lupus erythematosus shows that the severe group had a high representation of the A1-B8 haplotype whereas the mild cases had a high representation of the A2-B7 haplotype. These results taken together may indicate that the B8 antigen marks a high responder gene.

An interesting example of the association between immune responsiveness and the presence of a particular MHC antigen concerns the presence of B8 in increased numbers amongst individuals who have rye grass allergies but in whom there is no marked overall increase in IgE serum levels. These individuals do not have widely ranging atopies. On the other hand, individuals with multiple allergies, including rye grass, and increased levels of IgE do not show an increase incidence in the B8 antigen. The latter would suggest that these forms of allergies are under non-MHC control. Furthermore, widespread increases in immune responses of the IgE type may fall under polygenic control such as is the case for immune responses against complex antigens in mice.

Low responders and MHC

A number of examples of low responsiveness associated with certain MHC antigens have come to light recently. In one instance, the *in vivo* administration of tetanus toxoid induces the ability of lymphocytes obtained from these individuals at a later time to respond with lymphocyte proliferation on *in vitro* exposure to tetanus toxoid. A Japanese population may be divided into those whose lymphocytes can be induced to a state of responsiveness by tetanus toxoid immunization and a smaller percent of the population who cannot. HLA-BW35 is increased in the low responders and, in this Japanese population, the BW35 antigen is in strong linkage disequilibrium with HLA-DHO (an HLA-D antigen). The BW35-DHO haplotype is associated in the Japanese population with an increased incidence of autoimmune disease.

A similar situation exists amongst a Caucasian population on vaccination with vaccinia virus. In this case, the Caucasian population demonstrated an increased amount of CW3 in the low responders compared to the high responders. The same authors have noted that leprosy (tuberculoid form) is found amongst siblings which have inherited the same MHC haplotypes in greater frequency than would be expected.

An interesting study on the role of B7 in epidemics has been described in which a family of Dutch immigrants to Surinam were devastated by a typhoid (mortality 50%) and yellow fever (mortality 20%) epidemics. The incidence of HLA-B7 was 0.01 compared to 0.14 in a control population picked because of its correspondence to the founding stock. These would suggest that immune responses to typhoid and/or yellow fever are decreased in individuals with HLA-B7.

An increased incidence of HLA-B8 individuals in Newfoundland has been found among individuals who have a history of tuberculosis. Whereas 56% of those with a positive history have B8, only 20% of a group with no history of tuberculosis have B8. Whether this represents increased susceptibility to tuberculosis or an increased survival rate, once having contracted the disease, is not known.

In patients with multiple sclerosis, the presence of antibodies to measles antigen is found in individuals who have a higher incidence of B7 and those multiple sclerosis patients with DW2 have decreased lymphoblastic responses to herpes simplex. Normal individuals have neither of these MHC associations with respect to these immune reactivities.

MHC and cell interaction

There are many examples of MHC restrictions with respect to the expression of cytotoxicity or with respect to cell–cell co-operation. All of these restrictions are explained on the basis of modifications on or closely associated with the MHC. These modifications induce a form of recognition which involves both the alteration as well as the MHC antigen structure. Examples of MHC restricted cell–cell interactions range from the ability of macrophages and T cells to collaborate, provided that they share common H-2I (mouse) or HLA-D (man) antigens, to the ability of cytotoxic cells to kill target cells bearing various antigens (virus-induced, or minor histocompatibility antigens) provided that the cytotoxic and target cells share serologically defined antigens (H-2K and H-2D in mouse and HLA-A or B in man).

The ability of cells altered by infectious agents to serve as targets for cytotoxic T cells depends upon the sharing of at least one H-2K or H-2D region antigen between the murine target and the cytotoxic cell. This is so even when the virus antigens are fully expressed on completely allogeneic cells. Therefore, this restriction is not based upon the lack of a receptor for virus or lack of expression of viral antigens. The noted MHC restriction with regard to cytotoxic attack is thought to be due to either a requirement for dual recognition of both the infectious agent antigen and some portion of the MHC or that the MHC becomes altered in some way through the appearance of the viral antigen and that the attacking cell recognizes this alteration. Perhaps some combination of these two processes is the basis for MHC restriction in cytotoxic attack against altered cells. Similarly, the MHC restriction in cellular co-operation within an immune response may indicate dual and/or altered self recognition when one cell presents the antigen to another cell. Since the expression of cytotoxicity and various forms of collaboration within the immune system involve the recognition of MHC antigens, there could easily be an effect of various MHC antigens on either form of cell–cell interaction. That is, certain MHC antigens, be they from the HLA-A, B, C or D locus, may be either better or worse in mediating effector–target cell interactions or specific cell–cell co-operation between cellular components of the immune response. Certainly, such MHC-dependent modulation of cell–cell interactions would have a distinctive bearing on the outcome of a number of disease states in which environmental antigens of either an infectious or non-infectious nature play a role.

We have recently described a form of cell-mediated cytotoxicity in which there was no MHC restriction, that is, a requirement for a syngeneic relationship between cytotoxic and target cells. In this system, the antigen system recognized appears to be a backbone structure, only a portion of which is coded for by the MHC. This backbone structure is not recognized when interacting cell types have in common all the antigens of the HLA-A and B loci. It may be that the MHC not only provides a background upon which entities capable of inducing cell–cell interaction may be displayed, but also, the MHC may serve as a barrier which shields other cell surface elements from interaction with nearby cells. In other words, the cell surface economy is served in some ways by cell–cell interaction; however, other cell–cell interactions may be detrimental to cellular activities. The MHC may operate to control both 'cell-interaction' and 'cell-isolation'.

MHC and receptors for infectious agents and antigens

Although experiments carried out in animal models on the MHC restriction phenomena on the ability of cells to serve as adequate targets have suggested that the restriction is not due to the inability of the virus to penetrate the target cell and to express itself on the cell-surface membrane, examples of polymorphism within a population for receptors for infectious agents have been noted. These include the requirement for the Duffy antigen to allow easy access of the malarial parasite into erythrocytes. Other examples of MHC disease associations may relate to the possibility that the MHC antigens serve as receptors for various infectious or allergenic antigens or that the MHC products act as attachment sites for antigen- or microbial-receptors coded for by another part of the genome.

MHC and the complement system

Although little reference has been made to the various genes responsible for a number of complement components of both the classical and the alternate pathway, it has been clear from a number of studies that genes of either a structural or regulatory nature are housed within the MHC. Deficiencies in some of these complement components are associated with forms of human disease, but the correlation between these human diseases and MHC inheritance or association has not yet been clearly defined. More work is required to determine whether or not MHC disease associations operate through disordered complement metabolism.

MHC and molecular mimicry

A number of studies have been carried out to determine whether or not the antigen coded for by the MHC and various environmental antigens (bacterial or viruses) are crossreactive to any great degree. Examples of such cross-reactivity have been noted by serological analyses. Furthermore, a number of examples of transplantation rejection, consequent to exposure to various micro-organisms, have been reported and suggest that antigens carried by the micro-organisms can sensitize recipients to antigens present on allo-grafted tissue. If such molecular mimicry does exist, it may be that individuals possessing MHC antigens which crossreact with various infectious agent antigens may be more susceptible to those infectious agents if resistance to them depends upon an adequate immune response. Molecular mimicry may not only be the basis of some inabilities to respond to certain environmental antigens, but such mimicry, if it mimics allogeneic antigens, may predispose to heightened immune responses.

MHC and T system in embryological development

The murine MHC is located in close genetic association with a locus (T) which codes for proteins more primitive than and highly analogous to the MHC antigens. These fetal antigens are found during early developmental life and disappear with the appearance of the adult-type MHC antigens. This genetic structure was originally recognized because a large number of developmental defects were mapped to this area of the chromosome. These defects ranged from a slightly shortened tail to failure to develop beyond a certain embryological stage. Various forms of vertebral abnormalities, reminiscent of spina bifida in humans, have been attributed to this and nearby loci. Therefore, it would seem that the MHC is in close genetic association with and preceded by the activation of a system which codes for protein required for cell–cell interactions necessary for embryological development. Although separated on the chromosome by a considerable distance, there are very few recombination events between the MHC and T locus and linkage disequilibria between alleles at these two loci are evident, presumably because recombinants are selected against. It is of interest that abnormally high recombinations in the MHC in humans is associated with a number of fetal maldevelopments. Therefore, the MHC may represent an ontological advance over a more primitive system important for cell–cell interaction. The analogy does not stop at this point, however, since the proteins coded for by this primitive system resemble very much and show homologies to the HLA-A and B antigens. The system even shows the tandem duplication characteristic of the MHC.

CONCLUSIONS

The fact that the MHC has such important biological consequences such as the control of immune responsiveness, cell–cell interactions, complement levels and embryological morphogenesis, must be considered important in the eventual understanding of the relationship between the presence of certain MHC antigens in a number of disease states. Clearly, no final explanation can be given but a number of provisional conclusions concerning the explanation of MHC associated diseases may be made. It is unlikely that any single explanation will suffice for all known MHC disease associations. There appears to be no single 'disease gene' within the MHC. The range of diseases which show MHC association is rather large and they cannot be thought of as possessing any single common characteristic. Although most of the associations demonstrated between the presence of certain MHC antigens and disease states are positive associations, this in no way suggests that there would be a consistent explanation for such associations. Probably certain MHC disease associations are consequent to hyperactive immune responses, whereas in other cases the association appears to exist because of hypoactive immune responses. In some cases, the MHC disease associations have served to point out the common ground between two disease states previously thought of as separate, while, in other cases, the MHC disease associations have led to a separation into two entities in a particular disease state thought of previously as homogeneous. A system which not only controls immune responsiveness and cell–cell interactions in the generation or expression of immune responses, but also appears to be involved in many other forms of cell–cell interaction may influence the economy of the cell, organism, and, indeed, of populations, such that certain untoward events, such as diseases, would be either more or less likely.

Even if MHC disease associations exist, this should not be construed as suggesting that MHC antigens are instrumental in the induction of the disease state. The disease state may be the product of some noxious agent while the disease association may simply reflect either the likelihood of an event such as infection or the likelihood of untoward reactions to infection; that is, mechanisms helpful in getting rid of infection may, when prolonged, lead to a disease.

The peculiar propensity for associations between MHC antigens and certain diseases seems particularly noticeable when the diseases come from a group of illnesses which are characterized by being subacute or chronic, often involving unknown aetiology, and displaying forms of disordered immune response or disordered inflammatory processes. The reasons for associations of such diseases with MHC inheritance is not understood. Perhaps the preponderance of such reported associations may simply be technical in the sense that diseases of known aetiology are ones which tend to be investigated with respect to the constellation of MHC antigens. Examples of the influence of MHC antigen groups on acute infectious diseases are known, indicating that the MHC also plays a role in the outcome of diseases of known causation.

Whatever the explanation for the association between various diseases and the MHC, it would seem reasonably certain that forms of medical intervention may be envisaged which are based on the knowledge of the MHC system and its disease associations. Genetic counselling based upon the use of typing for HLA antigens to determine the likelihood of siblings developing a disease present within a family is the most obvious form of medical intervention. Furthermore, it is quite possible that spermatozoa selection, based on the exclusion of sperm possessing HLA antigens associated with a given disease state within a family, can be envisaged as a workable form of medical intervention. This seems to be a distinct possibility since MHC antigens are represented in their haplotypic expression in a population of sperm. It may be possible, therefore, to select for haplotypes within a disease-bearing family in which MHC haplotypes not expressed by the proband will be favoured. Whether or not such a procedure would be beneficial in the long run remains to be seen; however, it would appear possible to remove from a population haplotypes associated with susceptibility to certain diseases. As a form of immunological engineering such approaches would seem to hold the most promise. However, animal models for MHC disease associations similar to those in man are required before one could apply such a procedure to clinical disease.

Apart from the possibility of altering the inheritance of certain MHC-associated 'disease genes', more research is required in the direction of attempting to determine precise reasons for the association between certain MHC antigens and susceptibility to certain disease states. Part of the investigations which will help elucidate mechanisms is the continued search for such associations within the population. However, once most of the categories for disease association have been established, a state of the art which we are fast approaching, various incisive animal experiments will be required to elucidate more fully the mechanisms behind MHC disease associations. Such work will require novel and precise models for the investigation of such associations; this leaves the field open to those in immunobiology and experimental medicine who have both the knowledge of immunogenetics as well as an understanding of the clinical diseases to be investigated. Model building, that is, the finding of experimental models for clinical diseases associated with the MHC, is in its infancy and will itself be the subject of approaches referred to as 'immunological engineering'. One can, therefore, look forward to a development in this particular field beyond the descriptive, even though such descriptions will continue to be of value. As the field of MHC disease associations expands into intuitive and reductive models, the inventiveness of the scientific mind will keep this field an intellectually interesting and a clinically profitable field of research endeavour.

ACKNOWLEDGEMENTS

N. R. StC. Sinclair is presently a Research Professor of the Medical Research Council of Canada. Grant support for work carried out during the writing of this review has come from the Medical Research Council of Canada, the National Cancer Institute of Canada, the Canadian Arthritis and Rheumatism Society, the Kidney Foundation of Canada, and The Richard and Jean Ivey Fund.

The authors are indebted to Rosemary Marianik for her excellent secretarial work throughout the preparation of this manuscript.

References

1. Dausset, J. (1976). Le complexe HLA. IV. Les associations entre HLA et maladies. *La Nouv. Presse Med.*, **5**, 1477
2. Bach, F. H. and van Rood, J. J. The major histocompatibility complex—genetics and biology. *N. Engl. J. Med.*, **295**, 927
3. Dausset, J. (1977). La physiologie et la pathologie du complexe HLA. *Ann. Immunol.*, **128C**, 363
4. Svejgaard, A., Platz, P., Ryder, L. P., Nielsen, L. S. and Thomsen, M. (1975). HL-A and disease associations—a survey. *Transplant. Rev.*, **22**, 3
5. Dausset, J. and Hors, J. (1975). Some contributions of the HL-A complex to the genetics of human disease. *Transplant. Rev.*, **22**, 44
6. van Rood, J. J., van Hooff, J. P. and Keuning, J. J. (1975). Disease predisposition, immune responsiveness and the fine structure of the HL-A supergene. *Transplant. Rev.*, **22**, 75
7. Dausset, J. (1977). HLA complex in human biology in the light of associations with disease. *Transplant. Proc.*, **9**, 523
8. Dupont, B. and Svejgaard, A. (1977). HLA and disease. *Transplant. Proc.*, **9**, 1271
9. Dausset, J. and Svejgaard, A. (1977). *HLA and Disease* (Copenhagen: Munksgaard)
10. Kissmeyer-Nielsen, F., Bodmer, W., Thorsby, E. and Walford, R. L. (1977). Abstracts for the Seventh Histocompatibility Workshop. *Tissue Antigens*, **10**, No. 3

9
Immunological Manipulations in Renal Allotransplantation

RONALD D. GUTTMANN
Transplant Service, Royal Victoria Hospital and McGill University, Montreal, Quebec, Canada

---

INTRODUCTION

The treatment of patients with end-stage renal disease has evolved into an important branch of medical therapeutics. At the present time there are more than 30 000 patients on chronic haemodialysis, the majority of whom may be awaiting renal transplantation, and since 1962 over 30 000 renal transplants have been carried out around the world. In spite of numerous predictions that this therapeutic effort would be a dismal failure, many patients today owe the significant prolongation of their lives to the important development of means of caring for patients with chronic renal failure and with kidney transplants by refinements in haemodialysis and the use of immunosuppressive medications. Society is demanding more and more that facilities be available for the treatment of chronic renal failure by both the artificial kidney and transplantation, thus the numbers of patients who enter this treatment phase are growing. This is producing large overall economic pressures bolstered by the fact that it is widely accepted that if a kidney transplant is successful the patient is afforded the best type of restoration to a normal quality of life in all aspects. These factors as well as the intellectual challenge should be the major driving forces in various attempts to understand the basic immunological and clinical problems underlying transplantation.

It should be recognized that many of the developments in clinical transplantation have come through important empirical steps that would not have been possible without the contributions of many dedicated scientists and clinicians and transplant programmes around the world sensing the need for the treatment of patients before research laboratories provided answers to problems of specific immunosuppression which will be dealt with in other chapters of this book. Furthermore, it should be stressed that in spite of the lack of specific information in many of the areas that deal with the manipulation of the immune response in man, in particular the use of immunosuppressive drugs in transplantation patients, the efforts in this area have been of heuristic value in that these drugs are being used to treat many other types of immunological diseases with many of the general therapeutic principles having been learned in the clinical transplantation setting.

Finally, it has been the broad interest in the question of tissue typing and histocompatibility immunogenetics for transplantation applicability with the ultimate goal of finding a well-matched kidney for every recipient that has opened up new vistas in the understanding of cell surface antigens and the genetics of the immune response, knowledge which is applicable to a wide variety of other disease mechanisms representing problems for human populations. Thus, in spite of the general problems of defining the real usefulness of tissue typing as it applies to cadaveric clinical transplantation, the important contributions of histocompatibility transplantation research are spread to a multitude of other important biomedical problems and this area is likely to be of value in the understanding of the genetic predisposition, aetiology and pathogenesis of those diseases that are related to the function of the major histocompatibility complex.

It is the purpose of this chapter to outline the general principles involved in the problems of allograft rejection and to then examine some of the clinical approaches that can be taken to modify this process as well as to give some insight into the major non-immunological but very important clinical problems of patients.

ALLOGRAFT REJECTION

The rejection of a renal allograft is a process of a high order of complexity which follows the sensitization of the recipient by the cell surface or histocompatibility antigens of the donor. Sensitization causes activation of several biological systems of immunity whose effector mechanisms collectively, in various quantities and with a number of different types of interactions result in tissue destruction. Examples of these effector mechanisms are direct activation of lymphocytes into killer cells, lymphokine secretion, antibody formation and fixation, complement system activation, coagulation, platelet aggregation, neutrophil, and macrophage mediated tissue destruction. Thus, the pathological features that are seen in rejection are a reflection of the involvement to various degrees of each of these types of effector systems depending on both quantitative and qualitative factors. These reaction steps, and the type of pathogenetic mechanisms which may occur, are initially a function of the degree of genetic disparity between donor and recipient (factors of immunogenicity and immune responsiveness) and are modulated by quantitative factors of previous recipient sensitization as well as other modifying factors which occur after a transplant when individuals are receiving treatments designed to suppress their immune response.

Effector mechanisms are activated following sensitization of the recipient by the cell surface transplantation antigens of the donor. There are four mechanisms which have been considered to be possibly responsible for sensitization by allografts. The first of these involves the release of so-called 'passenger leukocytes'[1-3] which are probably a heterogeneous group of cell types including T and B lymphocytes and macrophages[4] which are contained within the interstitium of the grafted tissue and are passively transferred and released from the graft after allotransplantation. In addition, a second mechanism of sensitization may occur which is a function of recipient lymphocyte circulating through the graft and activated by antigen contact, a process termed 'peripheral sensitization'[5]. Whether or not these lymphocytes actually leave the graft after antigen contact to 'instruct' other cells in the process of recognition and generation of effector mechanisms is not certain. Further, the contribution of this type of sensitization in the sequence of immunological events is not known; however, it is likely that the interaction of these circulating host lymphocytes within the graft may result in cells which proliferate locally[3] and conceivably cause some component of tissue damage. Another mechanism of sensitization is related to the fact that during the surgical process of transplantation there is interruption of blood flow, and ischaemic damage to some degree is encountered in all organ allografting situations. Damaged cells may release antigenic surface components in particulate form into the circulation and thus there may be some contribution to sensitization by this mechanism[6]. Finally, it is conceivable that ischaemia or cell turnover with resultant cell membrane antigen release may cause soluble surface antigens to be released into the circulation which may additionally immunize the recipient. The presence of soluble histocompatibility antigens in the plasma is most likely due to lymphocyte turnover as a normal physiological event. Whether or not an organ such as the kidney can release soluble histocompatibility antigens is not established and whether or not such soluble antigens would induce a suppressed immune response rather than a heightened immune response is also not clear.

PASSENGER LEUKOCYTES

The most compelling evidence for the predominant mechanism of sensitization is that relating to the release of passenger leukocytes. This does not necessarily exclude the participation of other cell types in sensitization, and it is believed that once sensitization has occurred other graft structures are immunologically specific targets in rejection by virtue of their possession of cell surface histocompatibility antigens. The evidence for passenger leukocytes is based on two significant experimental observations that were independently described. Steinmuller[1] was able to show that mice rendered immunologically tolerant by foreign strain lymphoid cell injection, when subsequently used as donors of skin to genetically identical or syngeneic normal animals, caused sensitization to occur to the strain which had induced tolerance while the syngeneic skin grafts survived permanently. At the same time, Elkins and Guttmann[2] using a local graft-versus-host reaction of the rat kidney were able to demonstrate that the immunologically specific stimulus of the cellular proliferative reaction which resulted in renal parenchymal damage was related to a circulating cell having access to the kidney at the time the reaction was carried out rather than a cell of the renal parenchyma. These haematopoietic cells were thus postulated to serve as immunogenic stimuli for the inoculated cell in the local graft-versus-host reaction and it was thus concluded that renal tissue was damaged secondarily as an innocent bystander. These local graft-versus-host reaction experiments led to the postulate that 'passenger leukocytes', i.e. the non-essential haematopoietic and non-parenchymal cells in the kidney should be considered as important immunogenic stimuli in rejection[2]. Subsequently, further studies were carried out in the inbred rat renal allograft model which demonstrated that there were drug sensitive cells of bone marrow origin serving as a major immunogenic stimulus for the rejection of kidney allografts which could be demonstrated in different ways[3]. These experiments demonstrated that if bone marrow chimaeric rats were produced and kidneys of these rats were transplanted into genetically identical recipients, then cell infiltrates typical of acute cellular rejection were generated. In this type of situation, the donated kidneys possessed foreign haematopoietic cells even though the renal parenchyma was genetically identical to the recipient and these foreign cells in the kidney served as the immunogenic stimulus for the generation of infiltrates. Thus, it was concluded from these types of studies that cellular infiltrates of rejection, in part, represent an interaction between recipient lymphocytes that may proliferate as a response to foreign haematopoietic cells in the genetically identical donor organ. Further experiments showed that by using bone marrow chimaeric rats as kidney donors of a genetically foreign or allogeneic strain but with a syngeneic haematopoietic system induced prior to transplantation, the vigorous rate of allograft rejection would not be evoked. In this experimental situation the donor kidney parenchyma was foreign and the haematopoietic cells in the kidneys at the time of transplantation were compatible with the recipient and rejection was significantly delayed. Thus, haematopoietic cell disparity was clearly shown to be an important factor in the genesis of acute rejection.

If such haematopoietic cells or 'passenger leukocytes' were important cells in the pathogenesis of rejection and served as the sensitizing stimulus, the question was posed whether or not they could be eliminated from the grafted organ prior to transplantation. In this regard, experiments were undertaken in an attempt to pretreat the donor of kidneys in an experimental situation to evaluate whether or not allograft immunogenicity could be reduced by this potentially clinically useful type of approach. It was possible to demonstrate that pretreatment of donor with cytotoxic drugs could render these kidneys less immunogenic in that the rate of rejection was markedly altered[7]. This finding was compatible with a previous observation showing that kidneys transplanted after donor pretreatment with antithymocyte serum also had a slight effect on retarding the rate of rejection[8] and perfusion of canine kidneys with antilymphocyte globulin has been shown to alter survival[9]. These donor pretreatment findings have been extending by a number of investigators[10–14] and the concept that passenger leukocytes are important mediators in allograft rejection is well established[15]. Additional evidence has been obtained using an experimental model of allotransplantation which has shown that the sensitizing haematopoietic cells may be either T or B lymphocytes[4] and other experimental systems[16] have demonstrated that these cells are important in the afferent arc, i.e. the sensitization phase, which is probably a role of greater significance for them then as graft targets for host effector mechanisms. This type of conclusion is also based on the observation that donor pretreatment with cytotoxic drugs is not effective in reducing immunogenicity when the recipients have been pre-immunized (Guttmann, unpublished).

Experimental studies have attempted to determine how donor pretreatment with cytotoxic drugs actually may work in reducing the immunogenicity of organ allograft. These studies have been carried out assuming that the cytotoxic drug effect on peripheral circulating lymphocytes may be similar to the effect on tissue 'passenger leukocytes' in the organ allograft; thus *in vitro* tests have been applied to an analysis of the mechanism of drug action in this type of system[17]. Lymphocyte culture studies were done to look at the effect of donor pretreatment on this function. It could be demonstrated that following pretreatment with cyclophosphamide there was a dose–response decrease in proliferation triggered by mitogen stimulation using phytohaemagglutinin as well as a decreased response in the mixed leukocyte interaction (MLI). These diminished responses in the MLI were found in both two-way as well as one-way systems even though only one population of lymphocytes came from pretreated donors. Thus, the pretreatment affected both cellular responsiveness as well as the stimulatory ability of these lymphocytes. It was further demonstrated that the decreased ability to react in the MLI was a time-dependent phenomenon and that the reduction in the stimulatory ability or responsive ability after drug pretreatment was not solely due to cell death in culture but in part due to specific surface alterations of lymphocytes after pretreatment which may affect their ability to immunize or their ability to circulate in the physiological pattern in the recipient. These *in vitro* studies showed that lymphocytes harvested within 2 h after pretreatment showed only a slight decrease of response but longer periods of time up to 4 h yielded significant depressions of lymphocyte responses. This indicates that there is a minimum optimal time following donor pretreatment to produce lymphocyte dysfunction which should be considered and this correlates well with the *in vivo* results obtained. These types of responses of lymphocytes may remain depressed as long as 72 h after pretreatment. Further studies demonstrated that the serologically detectable antigens on the cell surface were affected by donor pretreatment suggesting that they are present in less concentration on lymphocytes that have been injured by the pretreatment drugs. Other functions relating to cell membrane extensibility or mobility of molecules through the lipid portion of the plasma membrane were relatively unaffected by pretreatment.

Thus, *in vitro* evidence suggest that pretreatment with cyclophosphamide alters those protein synthetic functions which result in cell membrane transplantation antigen and receptor expression while the lipid membrane functions of the cells were not significantly altered. It is conceivable, although unlikely, that pretreatment of donors with these drugs may affect expression of transplant antigens on other graft cells such as the parenchymal cell or the endothelial cell. However, in the absence of direct evidence for this hypothesis and the compelling evidence that these high drug doses do affect lymphocytes, alteration of haematopoietic cells is the favoured possibility as providing the best explanation for how graft immunogenicity may be altered. The effect that is seen with cytotoxic drug pretreatment is probably different from that obtained by *in vitro* incubation of cells with enzymes[18] or perfusion of organs[19] with mitogens where macromolecular complexes may be formed and released into the circulation.

To extend the principle of donor pretreatment to larger animals used for outbred organ grafting experiments, it has been found in the dog that such pretreatment is able to promote prolonged graft survival[11–13]. However it was found that the dog is extremely sensitive to renal damage by cytotoxic drugs in the presence of ischaemia which manifest itself in the form of cortical necrosis[12]. It was found that preservation manoeuvres such as pulsatile perfusion, or prolonged cold storage of organs in the presence of donor pretreated organs resulted in a very high incidence of cortical damage. These problems could be experimentally overcome by using the plasma containing the metabolites of the cytotoxic drugs in a pulsatile perfusion system using normal kidneys. This provides further evidence that preservation need not necessarily be excluded with pretreatment protocols and furthermore suggests that such pretreatment approaches may be used in future with organs from live donors once they have been removed and can be manipulated on pulsatile perfusion equipment with active perfusates.

THE PATHOPHYSIOLOGY OF ACUTE REJECTION

After sensitization has occurred and effector mechanisms are activated there are predictable sequences of pathological events leading to tissue injury. It should be stressed that the relative immunogenicity of the organ and the responsiveness of the recipient, are both such complex functions that the nature of the pathology seen may be variable; nonetheless the sequence of events has been demonstrated experimentally in a variety of ways. Normally, in non-presensitized recipients acute renal allograft rejection manifests itself with a progressive accumulation of large mononuclear cells in capillaries, in perivascular distribution, and then with generalized interstitial invasion by rapidly proliferating cells which differentiate into three distinct cell types[20]. Early in the rejection process these large mononuclear cells have been identified as part of the T lymphocyte lineage[21] and later on they reflect the wider spectrum of functional cell types which may include B lymphocytes, macrophages, plasma cells, mast cells and fibroblasts[22]. Cellular rejection is associated with progressive ischaemia. This ischaemia may be profoundly manifest as disturbances of blood flow and blood flow distribution[23,24], and in addition to vascular endothelial damage, perivascular infiltrates are present around large vessels which are involved in controlling blood flow to the organ. The progressive endothelial injury in acute renal allograft rejection may be associated with significant deposition of fibrin, platelet aggregates in glomerular capillaries and in the late stage the disease events are associated with tubular cell damage and necrosis[8,25–29].

Once sensitization has occurred in a recipient and the organ is transplanted, the secondary response in the presensitized individual causes pathological events of a totally different nature. In this type of response, if the level of preformed circulating antibodies is high, hyperacute rejection may occur. Hyperacute rejection is defined as rejection which may occur within minutes or hours with complete graft dysfunction[30]. On the other hand, if presensitization has occurred and the current levels of circulating antibodies are not extremely high the recipient will respond with an amnestic response largely dominated by antibody formation and what is operationally defined as accelerated rejection will occur. This may require 3 to 7 days for full expression with its characteristic pathology dominated by haemorrhagic necrosis of the tissue.

In hyperacute rejection, the sequence of humoral and pathogenetic events has been sequenced in experimental cardiac allograft studies using the inbred rat model[31–33]. The first event to occur in hyperacute rejection is the fixation of immunoglobulin G on vessel and parenchymal cell wall with the subsequent activation of the complement system and deposition of complement components. This leads to the rapid aggregation of platelets in the microvasculature of the organ with actual obstruction to blood flow and organ cell death due to progressive hypoxia. Concurrently there is invasion of the tissue with polymorphonuclear leukocytes which release their granules containing hydrolytic enzymes and tissue necrosis proceeds. A further event in the pathogenesis of hyperacute rejection is the degranulation of mast cells which may be present in the allografted tissue. In accelerated rejection which occurs at a slower rate, the principle feature is haemorrhage into the interstitium of the tissue with ultimate necrosis. These events are thought to be related to endothelial cell rupture which follows antibody and complement deposition and platelet aggregation occurring at a slower rate than that seen in hyperacute rejection.

It is possible to show experimentally that during the pathogenetic events of hyperacute rejection, antibody deposition alone on endothelium and parenchymal cell membrane is not sufficient in itself to cause tissue damage since the participation of an active complement system is essential[33]. Secondly, it is possible to demonstrate that hyperacute rejection can occur in the absence of polymorphonuclear leukocytes[34]; thus it has been possible to demonstrate that the platelet aggregation and obstruction of the microvasculature has a key role in the progressive hypoxia in cell death in hyperacute rejection[33]. Thus it is antibody binding with complement components and a subsequent interaction of platelets related to the activation of the complement system that represents the central focus of tissue damage in hyperacute allograft rejection.

CLINICAL TRANSPLANTATION

Selection of patients

Most patients under 55 years of age who present with chronic renal failure are potential candidates for renal allotransplantation. At the present time, patients are identified into high- and low-risk categories[35] with high-risk patients being considered those individuals over 45 years of age and extremely young children as well as those patients who have serious systemic diseases some of which may be transmitted to the allograft.

It should be pointed out, however, that renal allotransplantation and the treatment of renal failure on the artificial kidney are complementary therapeutic modalities and for most patients dialytic therapy is carried out before transplant and after a transplant fails which is before the next transplant. There have been no attempts in our programme to deliberately select out very high-risk patients; on the other hand, experience is showing that for patients over 55 years of age, transplantation offers little more than a similar quality of life prolongation than obtained by treatment with the artificial kidney. Since there is a problem of scarce resources such as cadaveric kidneys, it is felt that these should be reserved for those patients who have a reasonable expectation of life. At the present time, there is no compelling reason to exclude patients from transplantation who have systemic diseases such as juvenile diabetes with nephropathy, systemic lupus erythematosus, and cystinosis, because even if it can be shown that recurrence of disease in the transplant may occur to some degree these patients may in fact have a considerable life prolongation following transplantation.

Tissue typing for renal transplantation

The role of histocompatibility typing in clinical transplantation is well established for live related donors and remains a controversial issue in transplantation for cadaveric renal allografts. The principles of tissue typing and the future expectations for this field are outlined in another chapter of this book. In living related donor selection, tissue typing is useful once it has been established that a family member is willing to donate an organ, the sole acceptable motivating criterion being that of an altruistic response to help a terminally ill loved one. At this point, it is judicious to attempt to find an HLA-MLC identical sibling if possible or a haplotype matched parent or sibling to be considered as a donor. The lymphocyte cross-match test should be negative and it has been our policy to attend to renal transplantation as early as possible when living donors are available to avoid entering the patient into a dialysis phase which in most cases is unnecessary.

In the case of cadaveric allotransplantation, histocompatibility matching and clinical results have not convincingly demonstrated a correlation and thus extraordinary efforts to obtain good matches by long-term preservation and shipment techniques do not seem justified. Prospective cadaveric donors and transplant recipients should be HLA typed and this information becomes important if the first transplant fails and a second transplant is required. It is thus possible to avoid shared antigenic specificities between the first and second or third donors when given to a patient as a subsequent transplant. The tissue typing lymphocyte cross-match, however, is essential. It must be established without doubt that the cross-match is negative and that there are no preformed cytotoxic antibodies in the patient that react with donor lymphocytes prior to the transplant. This test has been standardized[36] with a 1 h incubation time following the addition of complement to the patient's serum and donor lymphocytes. However, prolonged incubations of 3 h, in our experience, have brought out an additional 15% of positive tests which were negative at 1 h and these are considered a warning that a particular donor should not be used or that one may run the risk of hyperacute rejection. Recently it has been suggested that a positive cross-match against B lymphocytes rather than T lymphocytes may not be necessarily indicative of a poor prognosis[37]; but these results are preliminary and should be viewed with caution at the present time.

The mixed lymphocyte culture reaction[38,39] can be done in the cadaveric–donor–recipient combination as a rapid test or retrospective test and can certainly be done in the live related donor situation. Mixed lymphocyte culture non-reactivity between two related individuals represents evidence for genetic identity at the LD sublocus of the major histocompatibility complex and the results of renal transplantation between family members so matched has been excellent. It is, however, controversial with respect to what a weak MLC reaction means compared to a strong MLC reaction in other than MLC non-reactive live donor transplant situations, particularly in the situation of cadaveric donor transplants. It has been suggested that low MLC reactivity to a particular donor may be associated with a better result[40], but it is not known whether such low reactivity represents general anergy on the part of the patient or truly a better matched organ. Whether the MLC test should be used selectively for patients who are awaiting cadaveric renal transplant is similarly not known. In fact, it can be shown in experimental models that a good MLC reaction, and thus a good proliferative response, is essential for generating the phenomenon of prolonged survival by active immunological enhancement[41]. This may occur perhaps through the generation of suppressor lymphocytes.

The arguments for or against tissue typing and matching and various selection tests in cadaveric renal transplantation are of more than passing academic interest since they may provide a selection mechanism whereby certain patients will receive allografts sooner than other patients while waiting on the artificial kidney. It is thus incumbent upon those scientists, who claim to have important selection tests, to establish with the most vigorous methodologies that indeed these selection tests are clinically important. Confirmation of these results should be obtained as quickly as possible because of the selection bias effect that such claims have. Until such immunological tests for selection are substantiated, it has been our practice to use medical priority considerations and length of waiting time for a cadaveric kidney as the important criteria for selection to receive transplants.

Pretransplant management

An important issue in the problem of the pretransplant period has been the question of whether patients should undergo bilateral nephrectomy or not prior to transplantation. This manoeuvre should be undertaken when patients have had renal diseases which have been associated with infection to remove a possible source of post-transplant infection. In certain cases where hypertension is unmanageable, it is clearly justifiable to remove kidneys pretransplant. Whether or not this should become a routine procedure is controversial. It is our experience that patients who have not undergone pretransplant bilateral nephrectomy may have a higher incidence of post-transplant hypertension in the first transplant year; however this hypertension is manageable by drugs and long-term follow-up of 5 years has revealed that this group of patients have blood pressures that are not different from the group that underwent bilateral nephrectomy prior to transplantation for other reasons. In the absence of other evidence, routine nephrectomy would seem to be poor practice in general because of the morbidity and mortality risks; the anephric patient on haemodialysis has a more difficult time coping with additional fluid restriction and volume problems as well as the problem of maintaining adequate haemoglobin due to the removal of an important erythropoietin secreting organ. Thus, at the present time there would seem to be no standard routine policy of nephrectomy that is deemed advisable based on current information.

The helpful or harmful role of blood transfusions pretransplant has been controversial, but recent evidence[42,43] seems to suggest that those patients who received blood transfusions prior to renal allotransplantation may fare better than those patients who did not, an observation made clinically many years ago[44]. This type of data adds some confusion to the issue of whether or not dialysis units should adopt a deliberate transfusion policy in the course of treating patients with chronic renal failure. This is an important point because transfusing a population of patients with chronic renal failure may prejudice the chances and possibly lengthen the waiting time of certain patients, who respond to these transfusions with the development of lymphocytotoxic antibody, if receiving a renal transplant. In this regard this question must be viewed as extremely serious and carefully obtained data must be accumulated to determine whether or not this phenomenon is really true or is exaggerated due to the fact that a special patient population (i.e. those who have not become sensitized by repeated transfusions) has been selected out for transplantation. The most compelling reason for not having a routine transfusion policy in dialysis units is the fact that transfusions are the mode of transmission of serum hepatitis which poses a dangerous risk to haemodialysis and transplant personnel and patients. Transfusions must be given to patients when there are medical indications while they are awaiting renal transplantation but an extremely cautious view should be taken for a routine policy prior to transplant. Whether or not transfusions actually induce specific enhancing antibodies or antibodies to Ia region antigens, which allow a better overall result is as yet not clear.

DONOR PRETREATMENT

The rationale for the clinical use of donor pretreatment to reduce allograft immunogenicity has been largely based on rat experiments and the supporting evidence for the approach has been confirmed by a number of laboratories cited above. The drug experiments in the rat which demonstrated that 5 h was a sufficient minimal time for donor pretreatment indicated that a clinical approach would be possible. With the acceptability of the use of heart-beating brain-death cadaveric donors, the simplicity of the protocol and the demonstration of events similar to those seen in experimental models can suggest viable clinical approaches. The pretreatment role in cadaveric renal transplantation is one of an important adjunct. The transplant surgery itself, subsequent surgical complications, possible recurrent renal disease, and the management of rejection with immunosuppressive drugs and the side-effects of these drugs in long-term management are equally important aspects of the total process of patient care and treatment whose long-term goal is providing patients with an adequately functioning cadaveric allograft and a low morbidity state. Thus, in considering the problems in clinical renal allotransplantation, all of the aforementioned problems must be discussed for an adequate appreciation of how a patient population and individual patients are cared for.

Clinical donor pretreatment is carried out in the following way[45–47]. The transplant team undertakes the care of the heart beating mechanically ventilated cadaver donor after the diagnosis of irreversible brain damage has been made by two neurospecialists, and consent for renal transplantation has been obtained from the next of kin. At this time blood is drawn for tissue typing and lymphocyte function studies. The donor pretreatment is given in the form of intravenous cyclophosphamide followed by intravenous methylprednisolone. Initially 5 g of methylprednisolone and 3 g of cyclophosphamide were infused intravenously into the donor over a 5–10 min period; subsequently cyclophosphamide was increased to 5 g along with 5 g of methylprednisolone, and a subsequent series of 7 g of cyclophosphamide was used with 1 g of methylprednisolone and, most recently, 7 g of cyclophosphamide has been used with 4 g of methylprednisolone. Because the *in vitro* human lymphocyte function studies that were done initially did not completely bring lymphocyte responsiveness down to background levels[48], the protocols were altered with that goal in mind. After the drugs have been given, the transplantation team manages the donor by monitoring the blood pressure of the cadaver, using dopamine or isoproterenol if necessary, and promotes diuresis with adequate electrolyte fluid replacement and occasionally large doses of furosemide. In general, the kidneys that have been transplanted in our programme have had minimal warm ischaemia times, are generally flushed with Ringer's lactate solution at 4 °C and are usually transplanted within 6 to 8 h. We have not used this protocol with pulsatile perfusion techniques although this has been carried out by other groups. The cadaver is maintained for a minimum of 4–5 h after drug pretreatment and in some cases, due to the logistics of organizing the transplant and waiting for cross-match results and calling in appropriate recipients, we have delayed harvesting kidneys as long as 12 h following pretreatment. It can be shown in the pretreated cadaver donor that if blood is obtained prior to the pretreatment, 1 h following pretreatment and at a later time before the kidneys are harvested and lymphocytes are isolated, a result similar to that seen in the experimental model is obtained[48]. The drug effect on these lymphocytes in terms of their ability to respond to phytohaemagglutinin

(PHA) and in two-way MLI has been observed. These studies have demonstrated that there is a time-dependent decrease in lymphocyte responsiveness to PHA and in the two-way MLI indicating that both simulating and responding abilities have been affected by drug pretreatment in man. These curves have further suggested that the time after pretreatment is a crucial variable and 4–5 h seems to be the minimum amount of time to achieve a significant effect on lymphocyte function *in vitro* after pretreatment. These function studies provide good evidence that the drug effect over a short period of time on lymphocytes is adequate, such that these *in vitro* tests may be useful to develop more optimal protocols for pretreatment.

There are a number of possible theoretical reasons why donor pretreatment may not be effective because of the problems encountered in the management of the unstable cadaver donor. If the donor is hypotensive and acidotic it is highly unlikely that the drug will be activated in sufficient quantity or be able to get into the graft tissues at sufficiently high concentration to be taken up by haematopoietic cells. Also if high doses of steroids interfere with the optimal activation of cyclophosphamide by the hepatic microsomes, alterations in the protocol may have to be undertaken and we are awaiting proof of this point. In this case, it would be wise to first infuse cyclophosphamide and delay prednisolone for several hours[47]. If the pretreatment interval is too short, the pretreatment will not be effective and it should be stressed that it is not adequate to simply infuse the drugs and harvest the kidneys immediately or leave the donor in a relatively unphysiological state. Since donor pretreated kidneys can still stimulate a rejection episode, if the post-transplant immunosuppressive regimen is inadequate or if the patients are treated late for rejection or if follow-up is not frequent enough these kidneys may be lost for other reasons. Donor pretreatment is a useful adjunctive measurement which has been confirmed by others and can assist the complex problem of transplantation. As such, its chief value is that it is a manoeuvre that is not harmful to the patient but is a pretransplant manipulation.

Post-transplant management

Once a transplant has been carried out the major clinical problems that are to be faced are those of rejection and the complications of drug therapy. While tissue typing and matching in the live related donor situation is an important selection tool and while donor pretreatment can reduce cadaver graft immunogenicity, once a transplant is done one must contend with and manipulate the major clinical problems mentioned above.

There are a variety of post-transplant immunosuppressive protocols used by many centres with azathioprine and prednisone as the cornerstones of long-term therapy. Many centres routinely use antilymphocyte globulin in addition to the chemical approach, and at our centre cyclophosphamide infusions are combined with high dose methylprednisolone in the treatment of rejection[49,50]. The use of antilymphocyte serum in our programme has been confined to those cases of severe rejection which seem not to be responding to the high dose drug infusions.

The chemical immunosuppressive regimen at the Royal Victoria Hospital is as follows: azathioprine is given at a dose of 1.5 to 2 mg/kg per day with the large majority of patients receiving an arbitrary 125 mg daily and a lesser number 100 mg daily with the white blood count remaining above 5000/mm^3. Prednisone is given in an initial dose of 100 mg/day reducing by 10 mg every 4th to 5th day until 50 mg is reached. Prednisone is reduced by 5 mg each week until a level of 25 mg is reached and is maintained until 5 months post-transplant, reduced then to 20 mg/day at 8 months and to 15 mg/day at 1 year. No patient receives more than 15 mg of prednisone daily after the first transplant year. In the case of steroid induced complications or serious infections we do not hesitate to immediately place patients on 30 mg of prednisone on alternate days and cease therapy with azathioprine if clinically appropriate. This is done at any point during the early or late post-transplant period where our clinical judgements suggest that an infectious process is going on and the patient is at significant risk. Since May 1972 recipients have received routine infusions of 750 mg methylprednisolone and 400 mg cyclophosphamide on post-transplant days 0, 2, or 3, 7, 14, and 21. The approach towards the treatment of acute rejection, which may be characterized by fever, rise in serum creatinine, with or without oliguria, is to administer an intravenous infusion of 750 mg methylprednisolone followed by 400 mg cyclophosphamide intravenously over a 1-hour time period for each drug. On the day of this type of infusion we do not use routine azathioprine or prednisone. Cyclophosphamide is included as a part of the infusion if the WBC is greater than 2500/mm^3. The rationale for high dose cyclophosphamide infusions derives from experimental studies using the rat renal transplant model showing its effectiveness in prolonging renal allograft survival when given in single high periodic doses[51]. After such a high dose drug infusion for the treatment of acute rejection, patients are placed on 200 or 100 mg oral prednisone on the following day depending on whether the serum creatinine has risen or fallen. The infusion may be repeated on the following day, often a third time 2 days later until we observe that either (1) oliguria has reversed or the creatinine has begun to decrease or (2) closed renal biopsy shows that the inflammatory infiltrate is cleared or is predominantly composed of pyknotic cells as evidence of cell death. Percutaneous renal biopsy can be an extremely useful indicator for distinguishing between the type of rejection, i.e. cellular or accelerated as shown in Figure 9.1, as well as a useful indicator for the cessation of immunosuppressive therapy when a lack of inflammatory infiltrate is apparent even though the patients may have a considerable amount of renal failure. The closed biopsy is useful in the early post-transplant period where one is dealing with a primarily non-functioning kidney to establish whether or not acute tubular necrosis is present. In this setting, occasionally one finds evidence for rejection which must be treated with immunosuppressive drugs, and occasionally one finds acute pyelonephritis to be vigorously treated with antibiotics. In the late post-transplant months, closed renal biopsy can help in the diagnosis of chronic rejection with features of interstitial fibrosis and glomerular sclerosis which is untreatable, pyelonephritis, recurrent disease, and the

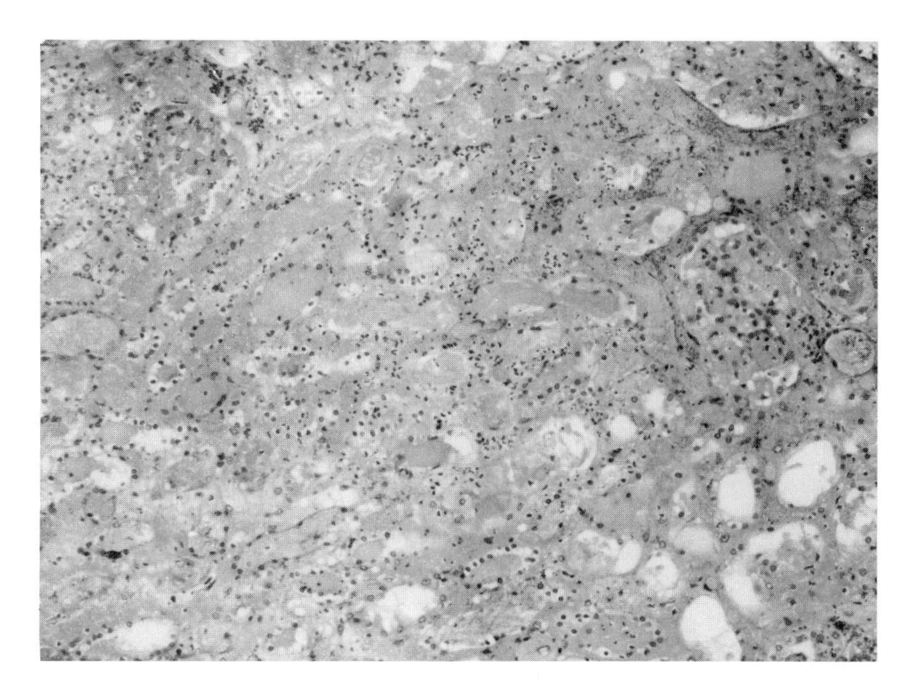

Figure 9.1 Accelerated rejection of a cadaveric renal allograft. Deteriorating function and a histological picture incompatible with reversibility indicated that transplant nephrectomy should be carried out ($\times 110$). (Courtesy of Dr J. Knaack)

interesting and as yet poorly understood mild renal failure episodes associated with viral infections. Immunosuppressive infusions are not used in these instances. Closed renal biopsy has been indispensable in patient management provided that a specific answerable question is asked such as the type of rejection, other renal lesions mimicking rejection, or adequacy of therapy based on cell infiltrates. While it is recognized that many vascular and tubular lesions can be prominent during rejection, these pathological changes *per se* may not warrant high dose chemotherapy and many of these parenchymal changes are spontaneously reversible. After rejection episodes have responded to high dose chemotherapy, prednisone is rapidly tapered back to the original schedule described above by 50 mg increments from

200 to 100 mg and then by 10 mg increments every other day from 100 mg downward until the normal protocol dose of prednisone dose is reached. Local X-ray to the kidney during an acute rejection has been used as an adjunctive measure. It is confined to 150–200 rads for three consecutive days during the first rejection episode and only when no improvement in renal function occurs following drug infusions and where biopsy evidence shows an immature mononuclear cell infiltrate.

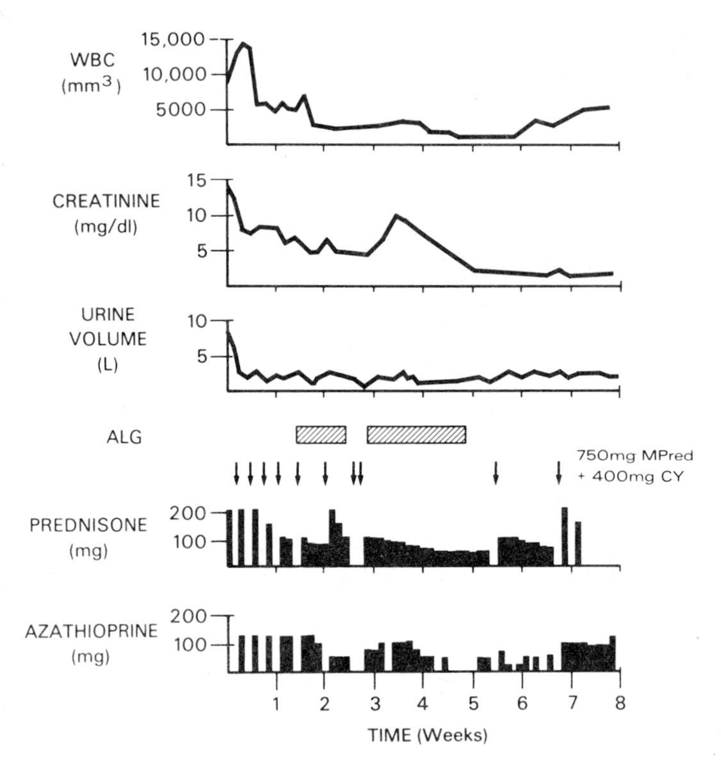

Figure 9.2 The course of a patient who had two very severe rejection episodes marked by fever, oliguria and decreasing renal function. The first episode responded to a short course of ALG and infusions of cyclophosphamide and methylprednisolone temporarily, however a second course of ALG was given as the signs of rejection reappeared.

While antilymphocyte globulin has received widespread use its role in renal allotransplantation still remains controversial[52]. One of the major considerations in the use of antilymphocyte globulin (ALG), which is generally made in horses or rabbits immunized with human lymphoblast or thymocytes or thymocyte membranes, is that when it is used with azathioprine and prednisone, the immunosuppressive effect seen is an effect of the entire drug regimen and not just the ALG alone. There has been a wide gamut of toxicities associated with regimens that incorporate antilymphocyte globulin including fever, serum sickness, anaphylaxis, platelet aggregation reactions, and it may not be without significant morbidity and mortality. Nonetheless, as with every drug, experience allows one to learn to use it in a particular regimen along with the other chemical agents in

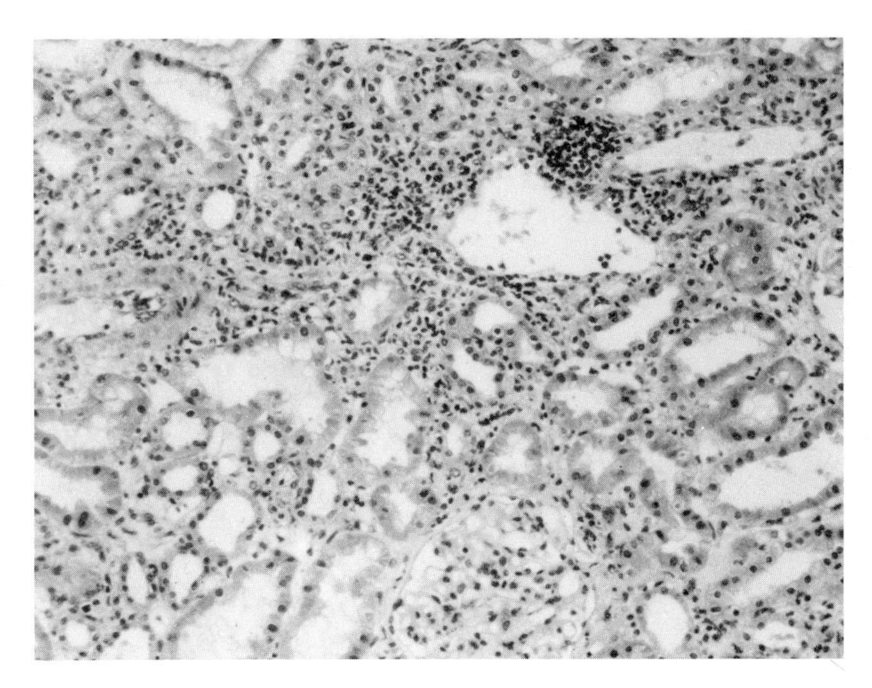

Figure 9.3 Early acute cellular rejection prior to the institution of infusion chemotherapy and ALG as detailed in Figure 9.2 ($\times$ 160). (Courtesy of Dr J. Knaack)

a potentially beneficial way. A significant problem with ALG is that its immunosuppressive potency varies from batch to batch and no standard test or battery of tests have convincingly been shown to measure this immunosuppressive potency of the preparations destined for human use. We have confined our use of antilymphocyte globulin to patients who are undergoing very early acute rejections within the first 2 weeks post-transplant and who do not seem to be responding to high dose drug infusions. In these instances renal biopsy shows massive cellular infiltrates and renal failure is worsening. When a minimum of two drug infusions of cyclophosphamide and methylprednisolone fail to induce a response we have added ALG in concentrations from 7.5 mg/kg/day to 30 mg/kg/day for 5–10 day courses and have seen dramatic reversal of oliguria and renal failure, and a decrease in the febrile response of rejection in about half of the patients. The case that is illustrated in Figures 9.2–9.4 indicates how following the termination of a short course of ALG a second rejection episode ensued, which was reversed by the next course of ALG given to the patient. Thus, ALG can be used as an adjunct and can be restricted to those patients who are not responding well to standard chemical treatment.

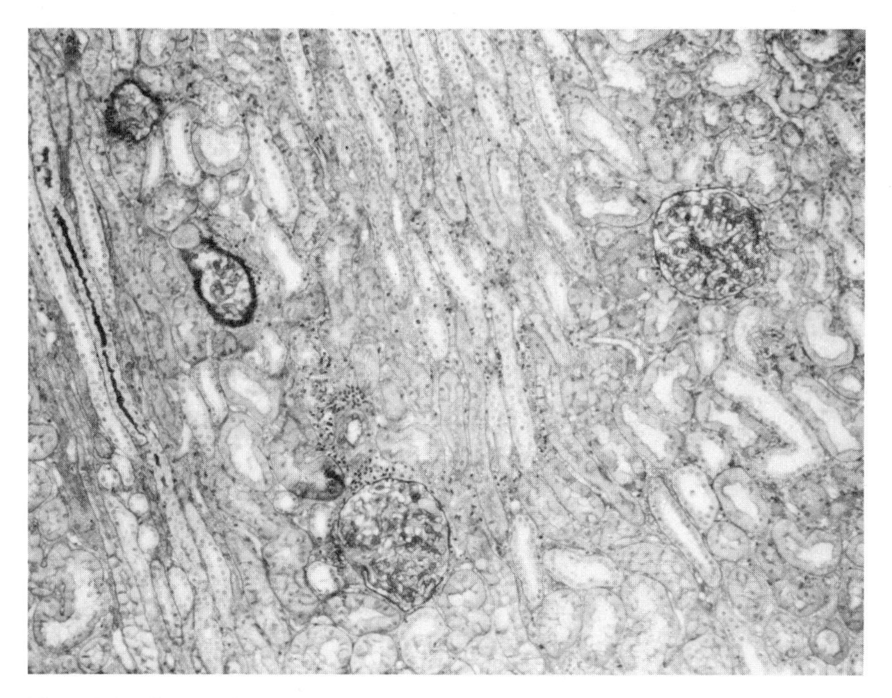

Figure 9.4 Clearing of the infiltrates of rejection following infusion chemotherapy and ALG to treat acute rejection (×110). (Courtesy of Dr J. Knaack)

An additional important step in patient management has been related to efforts to reduce long-term immunosuppressive drug morbidity and mortality. We have had cause to withdraw immunosuppressive therapy on a temporary basis in the face of severe viral, fungal, or bacterial infections. In most cases azathioprine is withdrawn completely and prednisone is reduced to 30 mg on alternate days. This type of drug regimen is followed until we are certain that the patient has recovered from the infection both in terms of objective clinical data including the absence of fever as well as subjective evidence provided by the patient. We have noted that prior to complete clearing of fever, the patient will undergo alternate day fevers associated with viral infections (particularly cytomegalovirus and coxsackie viruses) with the fever swings correlated with whether or not prednisone had been given on the particular day. These alternate day fevers then subside and generally patients are clearly improved clinically and after a short follow-up period immunosuppressive drugs can be reinstituted. At this time we would generally reinstitute 25 mg/day of azathioprine with additional 25 mg increments over a 1–4 week period and continue on alternate day steroids in some cases some for many months. Some patients are returned to the original prednisone dose according to the schedule of the routine protocol. It has been impressive that few acute rejections during these periods occur as a consequence of this type of post-transplant drug therapy withdrawal during the course of infectious diseases and it has not been obvious that the infections encountered have triggered acute rejection with the possible exceptions of Gram-negative bacterial infections. On the contrary, many infection associated instances of renal failure which have been documented by biopsy are due to non-specific glomerular and tubular lesions which are not associated with known experimental forms of rejection and may be related to the infectious agent itself, either in the form of immune complex disease or other types of nephrotoxicity. Renal function generally improves following the clearing of infection, in spite of withholding immunosuppressive drugs.

One of the most difficult problems in renal transplantation is seen in patients who have recently had rapidly progressive forms of glomerulonephritis and show recurrent disease after transplantation, illustrated in Figure 9.5. It is as yet impossible to predict which patients may develop

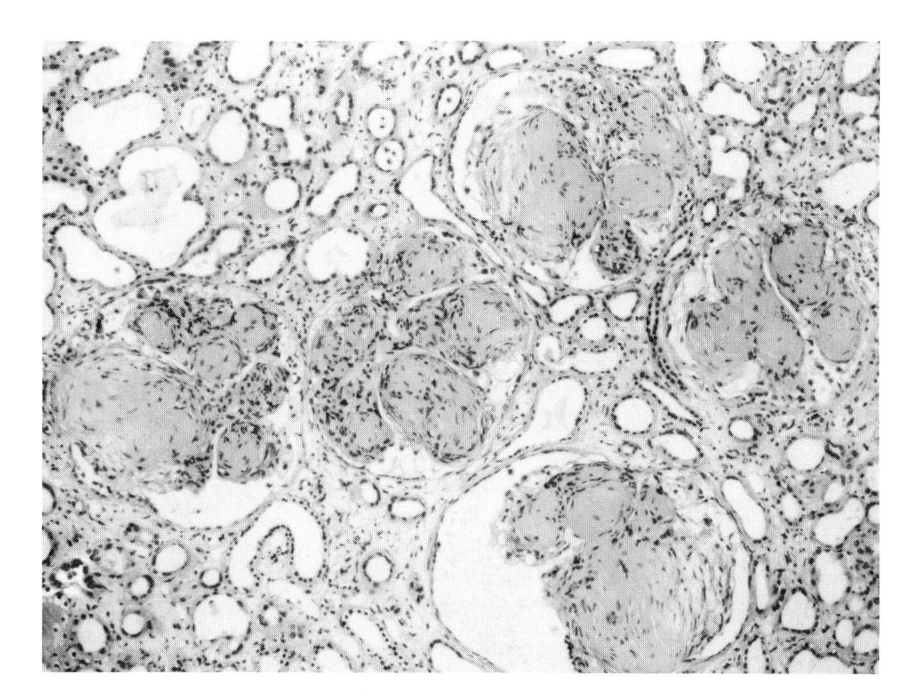

Figure 9.5 Recurrent glomerulonephritis in a cadaver renal allograft $4\frac{1}{2}$ years post-transplant. The lesions are identical to those of the patient's original disease and were documented to develop very slowly during the life of the graft ($\times$ 160). (Courtesy of Dr J. Knaack)

recurrent disease although it has been considered prudent not to carry out renal transplants in those patients who still have evidence of activity of their original disease but rather wait for a quiescent period. Nonetheless, recurrent disease may develop histologically and cause some functional abnormalities after transplantation. It has been our experience that treating these recurrent diseases with high dose methylprednisolone and cyclophosphamide infusions, as we would treat acute rejection, has been useful and has in most instances allowed survival of the allograft with the recurrent disease progressing either very slowly or regressing. In these cases, the immunosuppressive drug infusions have been started very early for this treatment purpose owing to the early diagnosis of recurrent lesions on biopsy. The proportion of patients that develop recurrent disease are small in our experience.

Another important transplant complication which must be attended to and which can mimic acute rejection is renal arterial stenosis, which may have an incidence of approximately 10% post-transplant. This can cause severe and unmanageable blood pressure problems in patients and can induce renal failure. Many of these patients can be managed with drug therapy, but when this becomes difficult corrective surgery is advisable. It is essential when patients have severe unexplained hypertension post-transplant, that renal arteriography is carried out and that biopsy confirms that the likely cause of the lesion is related to the vascular problem. Only in this way can the potential for surgical cure be properly assessed.

In vitro immunological monitoring tests to manage patients

Renal transplant patients can be characterized with a variety of *in vitro* tests. While theoretically this opens possibilities for monitoring, it must be kept in mind that post-renal transplant patients are well monitored in terms of clinical signs and daily renal functional measurements in the form of serum creatinine which is a relatively inexpensive chemical test requiring a very small amount of blood. Nonetheless, the search for specific immunological tests, helpful to the clinician, is useful and may be helpful in understanding and characterizing the patient's status before, during and after rejection. It remains to be established that long-term monitoring of every patient with an allograft has major clinical usefulness.

The best established test in terms of its utility in the diagnosis of rejection is the leukocyte migration inhibition test as illustrated in Figure 9.6[53,54]. In this test, blood from the recipient is obtained, lymphocytes are isolated and put in capillary tubes and migrate into tissue culture medium which contains a subcellular fraction of donor spleen cells as antigen. If sensitized cells are in the blood at the time, the normal migration of the patient's leukocytes are inhibited and this has been correlated with an impending rejection. Unfortunately, migration of blood leukocytes is not normal once the patient has been treated with large amounts of steroids and thus this test is not helpful in detecting a continuing rejection. Following the reversal of rejection it is often found that the cells of patients will migrate more than normal and that the serum may contain blocking factors as illustrated in Figure 9.7.

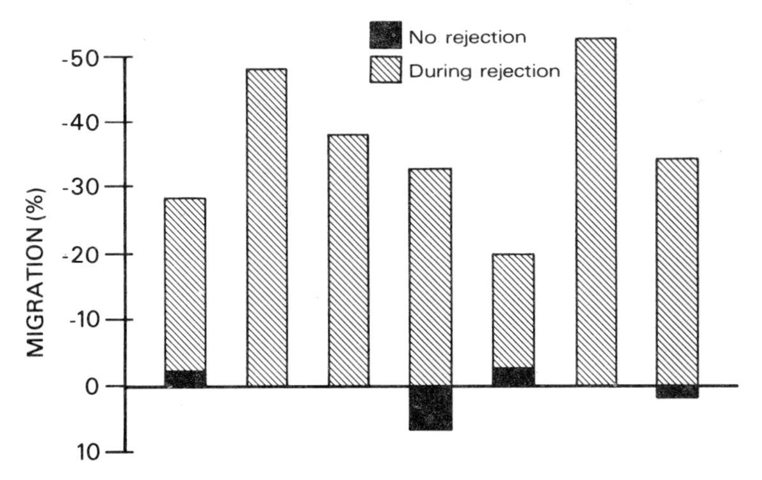

Figure 9.6 Leukocyte migration inhibition studied in seven patients during a renal allograft rejection episode and four times during quiescence. A significant alteration in the normal pattern of migration was seen during rejection. (Courtesy of Dr R. Falk)

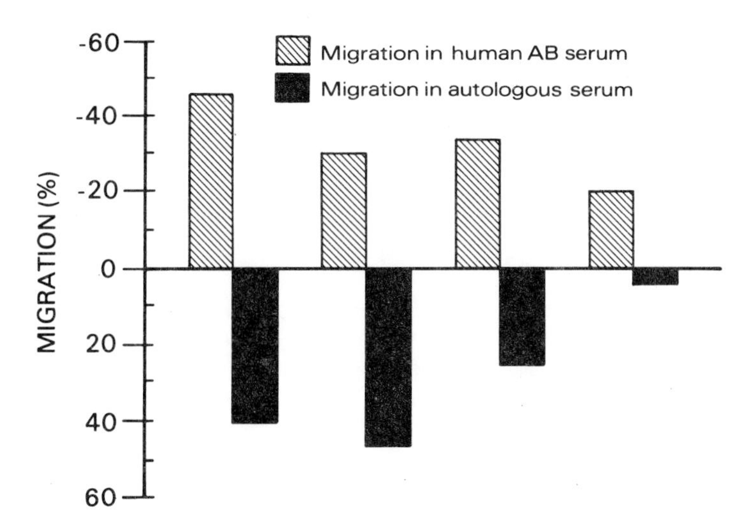

Figure 9.7 Leukocyte migration inhibition studied in four patients during their course. They all showed strong cell-mediated immunity to donor antigens; however this was blocked in the presence of their own serum indicating a modulating effect by humoral components. (Courtesy of Dr R. Falk)

Another test that has been found to correlate with an acute rejection is the test of cell-mediated lymphocytolysis where one detects killer T cells in the circulation of patients during rejection[55]. This test requires a large blood sample from the patient and the availability of specific donor target cells to be labelled with chromium 51 as a marker of injury. As a daily routine test it is not yet established as a practical tool.

Other immunological tests have been used to monitor rejection such as spontaneous blast transformation, the post-transplant MLC reaction, and lymphocyte dependent antibody assay which await confirmation as tests which may be clinically useful. While they are descriptive and may characterize a particular state of the patient during an immune response to an allograft, they have yet to be shown helpful in either selecting a particular donor recipient combination with a good prognosis or being useful as clinical tests in manipulating therapy.

The population of patients and results of renal transplantation

The results of renal transplantation particularly when combined with an adequate dialysis programme where patients may be shifted from one programme to the other have been excellent in recent years. In spite of the fact that in our own programme we accept equal numbers of high- and low-risk patients for transplantation it is possible to reduce overall mortality to $<5\%$ in the first post-transplant year and to less than 3% per year subsequently.

Generally patients over 55 years of age are discouraged from transplantation, however there are exceptions to this in our experience. In the recipient population, pretransplant bilateral nephrectomy is only undertaken for patients that have polycystic kidney disease, pyelonephritis, other problems of infection of the urinogenitary tract, and is not done routinely for patients with glomerulonephritis. Pretransplant thymectomy or splenectomy is not routinely carried out. In terms of the populations of patients that have received cadaveric transplants in our programme, approximately two-thirds have had cytotoxic antibody on routine antibody screening against a random pool and thus we deal predominantly with a sensitized group of patients. In terms of tissue typing and matching, since we do not have a large recipient pool of patients that await transplant, our matches tend to be poor. In fact, over 80% of the transplants carried out in the patients who receive pretreated kidneys had one or no antigens matched. We have placed no significance on the pretransplant MLC reaction between lymphocytes of the cadaveric donor and the recipient although through drug pretreatment we find that the final MLC done between pretreated donor and recipient is low. Thus the use of standard HLA typing is an important point not in the current transplant but to avoid shared antigens if the patient requires a second or third transplant. Thus, HLA typing has not been an important variable when it has been possible to use donor pretreatment to reduce allograft immunogenicity. Whether this is related to the pretreatment alteration of passenger leukocyte HLA-D region antigens or LD antigens or not remains speculative. However, no matter what the role of histocompatibility typing ultimately may be in renal transplantation, at the moment what is important is the adequacy of donor pretreatment with an effective post-transplant allograft treatment regimen for rejection incorporating sensible clinical judgement.

Since many of the patients have had multiple transfusions, previous allografts, and previous pregnancies in some of the female patients, a high quality pretransplant cross match test is obviously important and in this regard the 3 h cross-match is essential to attempt to avoid hyperacute rejection.

The 3-year graft survival rate in patients receiving pretreated kidneys has been 71% with no exclusions while a non-pretreated group shows 44% at the same time period. The impressive consequences of the pretreatment protocol have been the lack of severity of acute rejection episodes although in absolute numbers these occur roughly in the same frequency as in kidneys that have come from other non-pretreated donors. It remains to be seen whether or not the addition of ALG to the early drug regimen of treating acute rejection will be able to reverse the 15–20% of early rejections that become irreversible and appear to be an accelerated haemorrhagic rejection by histological criteria. The important consequence of effective donor pretreatment and early reversal of rejection is subsequent long-term excellent renal function in patients and a noticeable tendency towards a short hospital stay following the transplant. Similar results have been obtained at another centre using this approach[47].

In spite of the numerous problems that may occur in patients post-renal transplant, the overall results that have been achieved, with empirical methods that have been derived as more and more experience with immunosuppression has been gained, have been very impressive. It is well known that post-transplant, long-term patients may not be completely immunologically suppressed yet there is no evidence that they reject their allograft and one must question the mechanism of long-term allograft survival. Numerous studies have demonstrated that patients may develop lymphocytotoxic antibody in their serum post-renal allotransplant but there has been no correlation with good long-term allograft survival and this parameter. There has been tremendous interest in the so-called 'blocking factors' which were initially thought to be enhancing antibody, later were thought to be antigen–antibody complexes and recently there has been suggestion that anti-idiotypic antibody may be associated with long-term graft survival. There is no convincing evidence yet, that in the drug treated human recipient of renal allograft that any of these so-called enhancing agents play a clear role in graft prolongation. It is certain that central immunological tolerance, i.e. that form of specific unresponsiveness which is associated with clonal deletion, does not occur in these patients since once immunosuppressive drug therapy is stopped, patients may reject their allografts which is also evidence that graft adaptation by so-called re-endothelialization of the graft with donor cells probably does not take place. One other possible mechanism is that of the continued generation of suppressor lymphocytes due to the generation of these regulatory cells by continual release of donor antigen from the graft. While it is still uncertain whether or not suppressor cells exist in patients with long-surviving allografts, they can be demonstrated easily in *in vitro* systems, and can be shown to have both donor specificity and non-specificity. The non-specific immunosuppression induced by the drug in addition to the above mentioned blocking factors and cellular mechanisms may all be operative to a greater or lesser degree in individual patients and it is a summation and preponderance of these inhibitory effects over the destructive immune response mechanisms that allow long-term graft survival. Other non-specific factors such as late chronic viral infections may contribute to unresponsiveness and those patients who may have had infections with immunosuppressive viruses such as cytomegalovirus may represent other types of mechanisms that add to the total picture of long-term graft survival.

CONCLUSION

In the overall scope of the problem of renal transplantation and the kind of immunological engineering that is done to see patients through the complex problem, there are two important steps or general areas to be considered. One is the reduction of allograft immunogenicity before the graft is in place and the second is the development of adequate methods for the post-transplant immunosuppression, the use of drugs during infectious problems, and the adequate use of drugs during rejection episodes. Every attempt must be made to increase the number of cadaveric donor organs available, and with this the establishment of high-quality centres that can deal with all of the problems of obtaining organs locally without necessarily resorting to logistically complex long-distance shipping operations except for highly selective and specific reasons for a few patients in need of a particular tissue-type organ. Finally, it will be extremely important to derive solid data on the fate of all patients entering the chronic renal failure stage of their illness in terms of their fate on haemodialysis and after transplantation in combined programmes. In spite of renal transplant patients possibly being the most carefully studied subjects in medical history owing in part to pioneering efforts of Dr Joseph E. Murray who was instrumental in establishing the International Transplantation Registry and developing patient flow sheets useful in management and analysis of cases, and the ability for transplant clinicians to publish their observations quickly, there remains a large amount of information that is needed before the treatment problem can be sensibly put into a global perspective for health planners, economists, and the society in general. This data should soon be forthcoming.

References

1. Bach, F. and Hirschhorn, K. (1964). Lymphocyte interaction: A potential histocompatibility test *in vitro*. *Science*, **143**, 813
2. Bain, B., Vas, M. R., and Lowenstein, L. (1964). Genetic studies on the mixed leucocyte reaction. *Science*, **145**, 1315
3. Balch, C. M., Wilson, C. B., Lee, S. and Feldman, J. D. (1973). Thymus-dependent lymphocytes in tissue sections of rejecting rat renal allografts. *J. Exp. Med.*, **138**, 1584
4. Beyer, M. M. and Friedman, E. A. (1975). Prolonged survival of rabbit skin and kidney allografts following donor treatment with cytosine arabinoside. *Transplantation*, **19**, 60
5. Billingham, R. E. (1971). The passenger concept in transplantation immunity. *Cell. Immunol.*, **2**, 1
6. Busch, G. J., Schamberg, J. F., Moretz, R. D., Strom, T. B., Tilney, N. L. and Carpenter, C. B. (1977). Four patterns of human renal allograft rejection: A cytologic and *in vitro* analysis of the infiltrate in 24 irreversibly rejected kidneys. *Transpl. Proc.*, **9**, 37
7. Callender, C. O., Simmons, R. L., Toledo-Pereyra, L. H. *et al.* (1973). Prolongation of kidney allografts perfused by antilymphocyte globulin *in vitro*. *Transplantation*, **16**, 377
8. Chassot, P. G., Beaudoin, J. G. and Guttmann, R. D. (1974). Prolongation of kidney allograft survival in dogs with donor pretreatment. *Surg. Forum*, **25**, 314
9. Cochrum, K. C., Salvatierra, O. and Belzer, R. O. (1974). Correlation between MLC stimulation and graft survival in living related and cadaver transplants. *Ann. Surg.*, **180**, 617
10. Dossetor, J. B., MacKinnon, K. J., Gault, M. H. *et al.* (1967). Cadaver kidney transplants. *Transplantation*, **5**, 844
11. Elkins, W. L. and Guttmann, R. D. (1968). Immunogenicity of circulating host leucocytes. *Science*, **159**, 1250
12. Ettenger, R. B., Terasaki, P. I., Opelz, G. *et al.* (1976). Successful renal allograft across a positive crossmatch for donor B lymphocyte alloantigens. *Lancet*, **ii**, 56
13. Falk, R. E., Guttmann, R. D., Beaudoin, J. G. *et al.* (1972). Leukocyte migration *in vitro* and its relationship to human renal allograft rejection and enhancement. *Transplantation*, **13**, 461
14. Falk, R. E., Guttmann, R. D., Falk, J. A. *et al.* (1972). A study of cell-mediated immunity to transplantation antigens in human renal allograft recipients. *Transpl. Proc.*, **4**, 271
15. Forbes, R. D. C., Kuramochi, T., Guttmann, R. D. *et al.* (1975). A controlled sequential morphologic study of hyperacute cardiac allograft rejection in the rat. *Lab. Invest.*, **33**, 280
16. Forbes, R. D. C., Guttmann, R. D., Kuramochi, T. *et al.* (1976). Non-essential role of neutrophils as mediators of hyperacute cardiac allograft rejection in the rat. *Lab. Invest.*, **34**, 229
17. Forbes, R. D. C., Guttmann, R. D. and Kuramochi, T. (1977a). Controlled studies of the pathogenesis of hyperacute cardiac allograft rejection in actively immunized recipients. *Transpl. Proc.*, **9**, 301
18. Forbes, R. D. C., Guttmann, R. D. and Pinto, M. (1976). Hyperacute rejection of cardiac allograft in a rat strain with a hereditary platelet function defect. *Lab. Invest.*, **37**, 158
19. Freeman, J. S., Chamberlin, E., Reemstma, K. and Steinmuller, D. (1971). Rat heart allograft survival with donor pretreatment. *Circulation* (Suppl. I), **43**, 120
20. Gardner, L. B., Guttmann, R. D. and Merrill, J. P. (1968). Renal transplantation in the inbred rat. IV. Alterations in the micro-vasculature in acute unmodified reaction. *Transplantation*, **6**, 411
21. Guttmann, R. D., Lindquist, R. R. and Parker, R. M. (1967). Renal transplantation in the inbred rat. I. Morphologic immunologic and functional alterations during acute rejection. *Transplantation*, **5**, 668
22. Guttmann, R. D., Lindquist, R. R. and Ockner, S. A. (1969a). Renal transplantation in the inbred rat. IX. Hematopoietic origin of an immunogenic stimulus of rejection. *Transplantation*, **8**, 472

23. Guttmann, R. D. and Lindquist, R. R. (1969b). Renal transplantation of the inbred rat. XI. Reduction of allograft immunogenicity by cytotoxic drug pretreatment of donors. *Transplantation*, **8**, 490
24. Guttmann, R. D., Beaudoin, J. G. and Morehouse, D. D. (1973). Reduction of immunogenicity of human cadaver renal allografts by donor pretreatment. *Transpl. Proc.*, **5**, 663
25. Guttmann, R. D., Beaudoin, J. G., Morehouse, D. D. *et al.* (1973). Immunosuppression and rehabilitation following cadaveric renal transplantation. *Urology*, **1**, 102
26. Guttmann, R. D., Falk, R. E. and Kuramochi, T. (1974a). Thymic influences on cardiac allograft immunogenicity. *Transplantation*, **18**, 93
27. Guttmann, R. D. (1974b). Membrane properties and functional activity of lymphocytes from cyclophosphamide-pretreated rats. *J. Immunol.*, **112**, 1594
28. Guttmann, R. D., Beaudoin, J. G., Morehouse, D. D. *et al.* (1975). Donor pretreatment as an adjunct to cadaver renal transplantation. *Transpl. Proc.*, **7**, 117
29. Guttmann, R. D. (1976). Manipulation of allograft immunogenicity by pretreatment of cadaver donors. *Urol. Clin. N. Am.*, **3**, 475
30. Guttmann, R. D. (1977). *In vitro* correlates of rejection. II. Rat mixed lymphocyte reactivity *in vitro* and cardiac allograft acute rejection, hyperacute or accelerated rejection and prolongation by active immunization. *Transplantation*, **23**, 153
31. Jeffery, J. R., Guttmann, R. D. and Charpentier, B. (1976). *In vitro* monitoring of cadaver kidney donor pretreatment by lymphocyte culture. *Clin. Exp. Med.* (In press)
32. Kawabe, K., Guttmann, R. D., Levin, B. *et al.* (1972). Renal transplantation in the inbred rat. XVIII. Effect of cyclophosphamide on acute rejection and long survival of recipients. *Transplantation*, **13**, 21
33. Kissmeyer-Nielson, F., Olsen, S., Petersen, V. P. *et al.* (1966). Hyperacute rejection of kidney allografts associated with pre-existing humoral antibodies against donor cells. *Lancet*, **ii**, 662
34. Lindquist, R. R., Guttmann, R. D., Merrill, J. P. and Dammin, G. J. (1968). Human renal allografts. Interpretation of morphologic and immunohistochemical observations. *Am. J. Pathol.*, **53**, 851
35. Lindquist, R. R., Guttmann, R. D. and Mahabir, R. N. (1970). Fibrin deposition as a pathogenetic mechanism producing glomerulopathy in long-surviving renal allografts. *Transplantation*, **9**, 65
36. Lindquist, R. R., Guttmann, R. D. and Merrill, J. P. (1971a). Renal transplantation in the inbred rat. VI. Electron microscopic study of the mononuclear cells accumulating in rejecting renal allografts. *Transplantation*, **12**, 1
37. Lindquist, R. R., Guttmann, R. D. and Merrill, J. P. (1971b). Renal transplantation in the inbred rat. VII. Ultrastructure of the glomerulus during acute renal allograft rejection. *Transplantation*, **11**, 1
38. Lindquist, R. R., Chen, F. D. and Guttmann, R. D. (1972). Ultrastructural studies on the proximal renal tubule during *in vitro* and *in vivo* ischemia. In: *Reversibility of Cellular Injury due to Inadequate Perfusion* (T. I. Malinin, R. Zappa, F. Gollan and Q. B. Callahan, eds.), p. 300 (Springfield, Ill.: Chas. C. Thomas)
39. Monaco, A. P., Campion, J. P. and Kapnick, S. J. (1977). Clinical use of antilymphocyte globulin. *Transpl. Proc.*, **9**, 1007
40. Najarian, J. S., May, J. and Cochrum, K. C. (1966). Mechanism of antigen release from canine kidney homotransplants.*Ann. N.Y. Acad. Sci.*, **129**, 76
41. Opelz, G. and Terasaki, P. I. (1977). Enhancement of kidney graft survival by blood transfusions. *Transpl. Proc.*, **9**, 121
42. Porter, K., Dossetor, J. B., Marchioro, T. L. *et al.* (1967). Human renal transplants. I. Glomerular changes. *Lab. Inves.*, **16**, 153
43. Simmons, R. L., Kjellstrand, C. M., Buselmeier, T. J. *et al.* (1971). Renal transplantation in high-risk patients. *Arch. Surg.*, **103**, 290

44. Simmons, R. L., Rios, A., Toledo-Pereyra, L. H. and Steinmuller, D. Modifying the immunogenicity of cell membrane antigens. *Am. J. Clin. Pathol.*, **63**, 714
45. Steinmuller, D. (1967). Immunization with skin isografts taken from tolerant mice. *Science*, **158**, 127
46. Steinmuller, D. and Hart, E. A. (1971). Passenger leucocytes and induction of allograft immunity. *Transpl. Proc.*, **3**, 673
47. Stiller, C. R., St. C. Sinclair, N. R., Abrahams, S. *et al.* (1976). Anti-donor immune responses in prediction of transplant rejection. *N. Engl. J. Med.*, **294**, 978
48. Strober, S. and Gowans, J. L. (1965). The role of lymphocytes in the sensitization of rats to renal homografts. *J. Exp. Med.*, **122**, 347
49. Stuart, F. P., Garrick, T., Holter, A. *et al.* (1971). Delayed rejection of renal allografts in the rat and dog by reduction of passenger leucocytes. *Surgery*, **70**, 128
50. Terasaki, P. I. and McClelland, J. D. (1964). Microdroplet assay of human serum cytotoxins. *Nature*, **204**, 998
51. Toledo-Pereyra, L. H., Ray, P. K., Callender, C. O. *et al.* (1973). Renal allograft prolongation using phytomitogens to mask graft antigens. *Surgery*, **76**, 121
52. van Rood, J. J., van Leeuwen, A., Persijn, G. G. *et al.* (1977). HLA histocompatibility in clinical transplantation. *Transpl. Proc.*, **9**, 459
53. Zincke, H. and Woods, J. E. (1974). Attempted immunological alteration of canine renal allograft donors. *Transplantation*, **18**, 480
54. Zincke, H., Woods, J. E., Roses, J. and Kimbler, R. W. (1976). The use of procarbazine hydrochloride versus cyclophosphamide in donor pretreatment in cadaveric renal transplantation. *Proc. Mayo Clin.*, **51**, 693
55. Zincke, H. and Woods, J. E. (1977). Donor pretreatment in cadaver renal transplantation. *Surg. Gynecol. Obstet.*, **145**, 183

10
Solid Tumour Immunotherapy

D. W. JIRSCH* and R. E. FALK†

* St Michael's Hospital and † Toronto General Hospital, University of Toronto, Toronto, Ontario, Canada

---

Tumour immunotherapy has emerged as a new discipline in the past two decades. Evidence for the possible beneficial effect of immunological manipulation of the tumour patient has developed since the turn of the century when William B. Coley intentionally infected tumours with streptococcal cultures in an attempt to induce regression[1–4]. Though occasional patients had remarkable disease regression and even long remission, most did not respond and the treatment fell into disuse.

Modern tumour immunology has a more certain experimental basis and dates from the demonstration by Foley in 1953 that tumours possessed distinctive antigens which are different from histocompatibility antigens and can be recognized by tumour-bearing hosts[5]. Such tumour-associated antigens are apparently capable of evoking both cellular and humoral immune responses in cancer patients[6]. Frequently the clinical course of disease will correlate well with the immune response to such tumour-associated antigens. Recent evidence suggests that the effectiveness of host immune defences may be limited because growing tumours can evade host protective immune surveillance mechanisms by producing both specific and non-specific immunosuppression. A variety of mechanisms has been postulated: these include the immunosuppressive effect of antigen or tumour-directed antibody, antigen–antibody complexes, suppressor T cells and more specific factors related to the tumour itself[6–8].

IMMUNE RESPONSE TO TUMOURS

Recent observations suggest that the monocyte or macrophage series of cells may play a central role in the immune response to tumours. Other cell types unquestionably involved are the so-called 'B' lymphocytes, which produce antibodies, and the 'T' lymphocytes, which function either in co-operation with B cells in antibody production or as specific cytotoxic effector cells. These killer T cells are effective both by cell to cell contact and through the production of lymphokines. Lymphokines may interact with macrophages to inhibit their migration from the site of antigen or tumour and, as well, they may activate macrophages so that they become specifically cytotoxic (Figure 10.1).

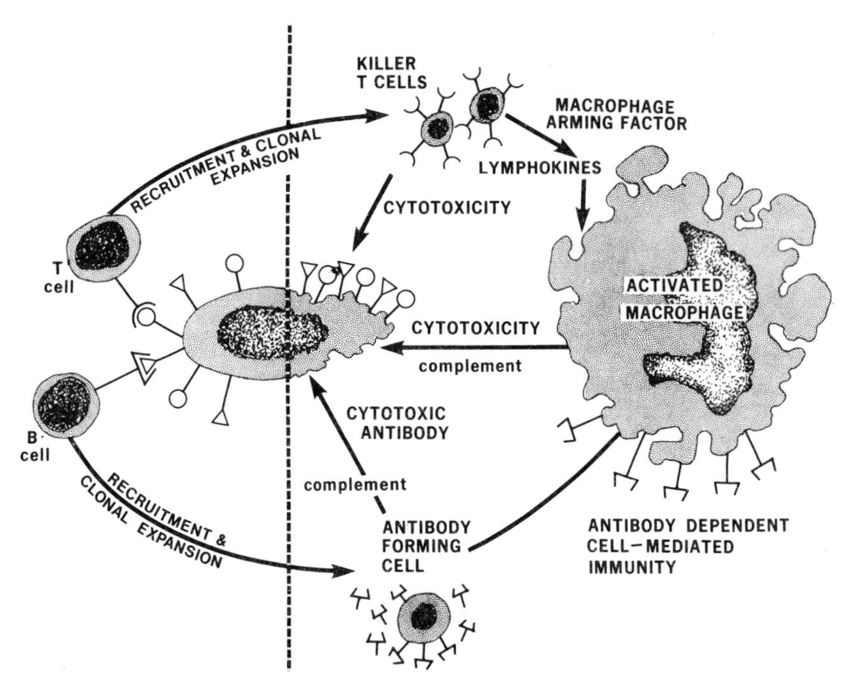

Figure 10.1 Immune destruction of the neoplastic cell. Both T and B cells react to tumour-specific antigens. Activated T cells are cytotoxic; as well they release molecular substances which 'arm' or activate macrophages with consequent tumour cell destruction. Activated B cells produce antibodies which may be tumouricidal in the presence of complement. Since macrophages bear receptors for the Fc component of antibodies, attachment of cytotoxic antibodies to macrophage may effect specific antibody-dependent cell-mediated immunity and tumour cell death

Macrophages appear singularly important in processing tumour antigen, which is thought to be presented either to T or B cells. Presentation to a relevant B cell could result in antibody production, while presentation to a specific T cell could result in the generation of cytotoxic effector cells and lymphokine production. A negative function of T cells has recently been described, termed the suppressor T cell effect[9]. This has been explored in various animal models and has been found to effect a specific inhibition of immunological responsiveness to various antigens. Suppressor T cells appear early after tumour induction and their numbers decrease after tumour excision. The existence of suppressor T cells in clinical tumour circumstances has not, as yet, been demonstrated except in an indirect fashion[10]. Further *in vivo* experimental data indicate that the elimination of T-cell formation, either totally or partially, can increase an effective anti-tumour reaction. The observation that suppressor T cells are extremely radiosensitive suggests several new prospects for more effective immune manipulation in the neoplastic process[11].

A major function of macrophages may involve tumour cell killing by direct cell to cell contact. In order to induce this destruction such macrophages must be activated, a process which may be achieved in several ways. Macrophage activation can be effected by T cells which have been in contact with tumour antigen[12]. This does not require specific cell to cell contact, as T cell supernatants, in appropriate conditions, can produce macrophage activation. This activation is not specific and such activated macrophages will kill any tumour cell but will not kill normal cells. Alternatively, non-specific macrophage activation may be induced by contact with bacterial antigens such as Bacillus Calmette Guerin (BCG) or *Corynebacterium parvum (C. parvum)*. After experimental infection of animals or in cell culture systems which coapt macrophages and bacterial antigens, macrophages become non-specifically activated and will non-specifically kill tumour cells.

Since certain studies have shown that macrophages form 10–50% of the cells of a tumour, one wonders, if these are all activated, why do they not destroy the tumour? Possibly such macrophages are, in fact, activated but are overloaded with tumour antigen to the extent that their activity is paralysed or inept. Indeed, such macrophage paralysis can be shown with non-tumour particles. Macrophages harvested from malignant ascitic fluid have been shown to be fully activated but have little clinical or experimental effect on inhibiting tumour growth in specific circumstances. One way in which they can be stimulated, however, is by the administration of bacterial antigens. These probably act to increase the rate of antigen process by macrophages, hence macrophage activity. Several recent reports have indicated that in clinical neoplasia both circulating monocytes and peritoneal macrophages are more active than cells derived from normal individuals[13,14]. This activity was observed prior to any immunostimulation and did not correlate with improved clinical prognosis. This again suggests that an 'abortive' type of macrophage activation may occur in neoplasia.

In addition to paralysis of macrophage activity, certain other factors may be involved in protecting tumours from immune reactivity. The role of suppressor T cells has previously been mentioned. The antibody products of B cells may also in themselves be immunosuppressive in that combination of anti-tumour antibody with tumour antigen (soluble antigen–antibody complexes) have been shown to be immunosuppressive in a variety of circumstances. These complexes are capable of interfering with the cytotoxic action of effector cells of either T cell or macrophage origin. This 'blocking effect' has been shown to occur both at the effector cell level and at the tumour cell surface, depending on which animal model is used[15–18]. It is likely that both sites of activity are involved. The evidence for the clinical immunosuppressive effect of antigen–antibody complexes in patients is, as yet, indirect but such complexes can be demonstrated in various clinical circumstances associated with growing tumours. Following excision of tumours, it is at times possible to demonstrate antibody excess, which may itself disappear with tumour recurrence.

The complexity of the cellular interactions involved in the immune response to neoplasia is apparent. To further complicate matters, it is often extremely difficult to demonstrate any difference in immunological responsiveness between cancer and non-cancer patients[19]. They tend to show the same heterogeneity of responses until well-advanced tumour disease is present when it is generally possible to demonstrate a decreased immune response to tumour. By this time it is usually too late, from the patient's point of view, to effect tumour eradication. Even this inadequate response usually disappears once there is widespread tumour dissemination.

Despite the complex possibilities of immune responses to tumour-associated antigens, an increasing amount of information indicates that immunological manipulations may, in fact, decrease the recurrence rates of tumours and increase patient survival time under certain conditions. As such, immunotherapy is a welcome addition to the armamentarium of the oncologist. For many tumours, surgical removal is curative. As diagnoses are made earlier, the surgical cure rate should be expected to improve. Despite potentially curative surgery, however, many patients continue to develop recurrent cancer because of the failure of local therapy to completely eradicate every cancer cell. Similarly, radiation may be highly effective as a form of local therapy, but again will not affect systemically disseminated tumour cells. Although chemotherapy is systemic in effect, it is curative only when the disseminated tumour cell load is very small. This failure is easily explicable since chemotherapeutic agents act on the basis of single hit kinetics, and the same drug dose is required to achieve each fractional decrease of the tumour cell burden, whatever the size of the residual tumour cell pool. In comparison, under optimal conditions, the immune response could theoretically kill all remaining tumour cells following immunotherapy. In this context, current efforts are directed toward preventing recurrence of surgically removed tumours or control of non-resectable tumours.

TUMOUR IMMUNOTHERAPY

The potential methods of tumour immunotherapy can be divided into four groups:

1. Non-specific immunotherapy, which involves the administration of bacterial antigens such as BCG or *C. parvum*. These act as potent non-specific stimulators of the reticuloendothelial system but also affect T- and B-cell function.
2. Active specific immunotherapy, which involves the active stimulation of the immune system with tumour vaccines in an attempt to induce specific immunity against tumour antigens.
3. Passive immunotherapy, which involves the administration of tumour-specific antisera.
4. Adoptive immunotherapy, which involves the administration of immune lymphoid cells or subcellular components from another host rendered immune to the specific tumour.

Non-specific immunotherapy

The rationale for non-specific immunotherapy is based on the observation that certain bacterial substances, such as BCG, *C. parvum*, mixed bacterial toxins, certain fractions of the tubercle bacillus (methanol extractable residue (MER)) and certain polynucleotides all have the ability to stimulate immune host responses non-specifically to infectious agents including viruses, fungi and bacteria. The mechanisms for these interactions are largely unknown but the immune response to a wide variety of antigens is seemingly enhanced.

Immunotherapy with BCG

In the first decade of this century, Calmette and Guerin, working at the Pasteur Institute, developed an attenuated strain of *Mycobacterium bovis*, the so-called Bacille Calmette-Guerin (BCG)[20]. This is a virulent bacterium which has been used as immunoprophylaxis against tuberculosis for well over half a century and has been administered to millions of patients without serious adverse effects. The observation that BCG enhanced host resistance to a wide variety of bacterial infections[21,22], coupled with the evidence of tumour-specific antigens, motivated its use in the clinical and laboratory milieu as a possible immunotherapeutic agent. Animal studies demonstrated that BCG administration enhanced resistance to the growth of transplanted tumours[23,24]. Pretreatment with BCG was most effective, and established tumours were generally refractory to systemic BCG immunotherapy[25]. In most experimental tumour cell systems, the clinical efficacy of BCG therapy has required obvious proximity of the tumour cell and BCG[26] as well as an intact immune response. In experimental solid tumour systems it has been demonstrated that BCG, given when the tumour burden is lowered by excision of the primary tumour, decreases the number of metastases which subsequently develop[27,28]. Many of the factors that determine the success or failure of BCG immunotherapy in animal models have been defined[25].

These include the following:

1. The tumour host must be capable of developing an immune response to BCG for immunotherapy to be successful. In most animal tumour models, if the immune response to BCG is blocked, the protective effect is lessened. However, BCG does have an antitumour effect in thymectomized and irradiated animals.
2. Tumour size is a critical factor in limiting the effectiveness of BCG immunotherapy.
3. The host must have the ability to develop an immune response to the tumour antigen or antigens.
4. Successful immunotherapy with BCG may require the injection of an adequate number of viable organisms.
5. BCG and tumour cells must come in contact. Proximity is best achieved by intratumour injection, but systemic BCG therapy is demonstrably effective in laboratory animals.

The activity of the reticuloendothelial system is augmented by BCG, as demonstrated by increased clearance of carbon particles from the circulation[27]. Humoral antibody synthesis to unrelated antigens is also increased by BCG treatment[27].

There is strong evidence to suggest that the effect induced by adjuvant BCG treatment is mediated by macrophages, since tumour suppression is abrogated in silica treated rats[29]. Other studies indicate that a large part of the antitumour effect of intralesional BCG treatment is non-specific and is the result of the induction of a local delayed hypersensitivity reaction within the tumour nodule[25,28–30]. In these instances, tumour cells are killed as innocent bystanders at the site of an intense hypersensitivity reaction evoked by the bacteria. *In vitro* studies have demonstrated, moreover, that macrophages can be activated non-specifically by PPD or BCG, and, once activated, the macrophages can inhibit tumour growth by direct contact.

In addition to the non-specific destruction of neoplastic cells, the large numbers of macrophages attracted by the immune response to BCG may facilitate the processing and presentation of tumour antigens to immunologically relevant or competent lymphocytes within the tumour or in the regional lymph nodes with amplification of tumour-specific immunity. A theoretical consideration in the use of BCG is the observation that PPD is a B-cell mitogen[31]. The possibility that it is functioning as a polyclonal activator for B cells, promoting a thymus-independent antibody response, is now under assessment. It suggests the intriguing possibility of independent B-cell activation even in the face of T-cell suppressive activity.

Complications of BCG immunotherapy

Both local and systemic complications have been encountered with the use of BCG. Systemic reactions depend on the route of administration, the number of previous injections and possibly on the dose of BCG. The intensity of the reaction to intradermal BCG depends mainly on the number of previously administered injections. Initial vaccinations produce small ulcers that evolve over 1 or 2 months and are associated with local lymphadenopathy. Following three or four injections, however, a local reaction appears within 24 h with itching and ulceration; serous discharge forms at the injection site. Once patients are sensitized to tuberculin, intratumoural injection of BCG is almost invariably associated with chills, fever and malaise. Systemic symptoms begin 4 to 6 h post-inoculation and usually subside within 36 to 48 h, although they occasionally last longer. Febrile responses do occur but usually dissipate quickly[25,27]. Severe hypersensitivity reactions and anaphylaxis have been found with repeated intralesional BCG injections. Two patients have died from apparent reactions to intralesional injections of BCG; hypotension and intravascular coagulation followed intralesional administration of BCG for malignant melanoma[32]. Since neoplasms are often very vascular, intralesional injection may force a large number of organisms into the circulation. This mandates use of the smallest effective dose for cutaneous injection, with small numbers of lesions treated at any specific time.

Certain risks of BCG administration are due to the fact that live organisms are inoculated. Persistent BCG infection has been observed in immunosuppressed patients at vaccination sites and in lymph nodes, bone and visceral organs; miliary disease has been found at autopsy in patients given BCG immunotherapy. Since BCG organisms are profoundly susceptible to single antituberculous drug therapy, any evidence of systemic bacillary disease (manifest by malaise and a 'flu-like' syndrome) should be treated immediately with isoniazid. Other systemic responses or reactions reported following BCG injection include erythema nodosum, uveitis, vitiligo, pancytopenia, hepatic dysfunction, hepatosplenomegaly and jaundice with granulomatous hepatitis.

In contrast to intratumoural injection with BCG, the administration of BCG by intradermal, multiple puncture or scarification techniques is usually well tolerated and produces only mild fever and malaise for 1 or 2 days[27,32]. No instances of anaphylactic reaction or marked toxicity have been reported with these methods of administration and the incidence of hepatic dysfunction is low. Patients may, however, develop painful lymphadenopathy near vaccination sites. The fever and malaise that follow scarification respond to aspirin and antihistamines[25]. Alternative routes for use of BCG have included intraperitoneal and intrapleural[33–35]; both produce variable systemic reaction with evidence of local inflammatory reaction. Systemic effects can be diminished by decreasing the dose or by administering isoniazid immediately after inoculation; since the organism is attenuated it is responsive to single agent antituberculous therapy. The oral route has also been used with the subsequent development of hypersensitivity[36–38].

This produces minimal side-effects even with prolonged use and permits administration of massive doses. Since the organism or its breakdown products are absorbed from the gut, the potential immunostimulant is in direct proximity with gastrointestinal malignancy.

A serious potential hazard of BCG administration is immunological enhancement of tumour growth[39]. Enhancement or rapid tumour growth has been thoroughly demonstrated in some experimental animal tumour systems. In these models, BCG was given in large doses prior to or shortly after the transplantation of a tumour. Repeated administration of BCG has also been reported to depress cellular immunity in man and animals as measured by delayed cutaneous hypersensitivity reactions to certain common skin test antigens[40]. There have been anecdotal reports of accelerated tumour growth in patients who have received BCG. For these reasons, caution must be exercised in clinical trials using repeated large doses of BCG. Immune responses should be monitored in such patients to detect any immunosuppressive effect of BCG therapy.

Immunotherapy with *Corynebacterium parvum*

The anaerobic diphtheroid bacterium *C. parvum* has been found to be the most potent bacterial stimulant of the macrophage system currently available. A single injection of killed organisms provokes a prolonged and intense phagocytic response due to activation of the reticuloendothelial system. *C. parvum* also possesses a strong adjuvant property, demonstrable either by substituting it for myobacteria in complete Freund's adjuvant or by injecting it into animals prior to antigen administration. *C. parvum* shares with BCG the capacity to increase resistance to a wide range of experimental animal tumours[41,42]. Unlike BCG, *C. parvum* has the advantage of being effective in the form of a formalin-killed vaccine. In the laboratory, it was first demonstrated that a single intravenous injection of *C. parvum* (8–12 days after subcutaneous tumour transplantation) was effective in delaying the appearance of a subcutaneous mammary carcinoma. Once the tumour was palpable, however, *C. parvum* was ineffective in inhibiting tumour growth. Further studies showed that a single intraperitoneal injection of *C. parvum* 3 days following tumour establishment could inhibit the growth of the same mammary tumour and other unrelated sarcoma tumours as well[43]. Similar tumour models have shown significant, but usually transient, inhibition of tumour growth in response to *C. parvum* administration. Despite demonstrable tumour suppression, even in T-cell deprived mice[44], systemic *C. parvum* therapy effect has been short and few complete regressions have been recorded. Toxicity has been established for both intravenous and intraperitoneal injection routes. Subcutaneous or intradermal injections of *C. parvum* are well tolerated and result in marked splenomegaly, hepatomegaly and stimulation of local lymph nodes. Although local injection of *C. parvum* near tumour sites is experimentally as effective or even more effective than systemic injection, again few complete tumour regressions have been recorded. Direct intratumoural injection of *C. parvum* has resulted in regression of primary tumours and animals cured by such intralesional injection of *C. parvum* have been found to be subsequently highly and specifically immune to tumour rechallenge. Of even greater interest, the combination of systemic immunostimulation (using *C. parvum*) and cytoreductive chemotherapeutic agents, has produced dramatic growth inhibition of established solid tumours and some lasting regressions. Similarly, the combination of *C. parvum* immunostimulation with specific active immunization against tumour with inactivated tumour cells has proven effective[41].

The mechanism of action of *C. parvum* is unclear but direct reticuloendothelial cell activation is probably responsible[43]. Injected animals show massive proliferation of macrophages and lymphocytes in secondary lymphoid organs. Such animals are demonstrably able to clear injected carbon particles more swiftly than untreated controls. *C. parvum* also acts as an adjuvant to certain antigens and can protect against subsequent challenge with pathogenic organisms. Systemic infection with *C. parvum* has been shown capable of depressing T-cell mediated immune responses (spleen and peripheral blood lymphocytes). Since antitumour immunity has long been considered a T-cell mediated response, the finding of T-cell depression by *C. parvum* was considered not a direct effect on T cells but secondary to interaction with macrophages. Further studies have suggested that B-cell function may be enhanced with *C. parvum* injection, but again the relevant mechanism is probably an indirect one mediated via the macrophage[45]. More specifically, it has been demonstrated that the *in vitro* antitumour activity of peritoneal cells from mice treated with *C. parvum* is macrophage mediated. Indeed, many strains of *C. parvum* produce a chemotactic factor that specifically attracts macrophages. The observed *in vitro* antitumour activity of peritoneal cells from T-cell deprived and nude mice treated with *C. parvum* suggests that the participation of T cells is not essential and is consistent with *in vivo* studies[46]. Summarily, the antitumour effect of *C. parvum* probably depends on non-specific macrophage stimulation. *C. parvum* is further capable of boosting specific antitumour responses when it is injected mixed together with tumour cells. The antitumour effect of intralesional injection of *C. parvum* is probably produced both by local and non-specific macrophage activation plus augmented tumour-specific immunity.

Systemic administration of *C. parvum* may thus be advantageous in the instance of disseminated human tumours. This would result in generalized non-specific stimulation of the reticuloendothelial system and, secondly, would provide an opportunity for administered *C. parvum* to come into proximity with tumour deposits, with subsequent production of both local non-specific macrophage activation and an augmented specific immune response.

Non-specific immunotherapy with other agents

The induction of local delayed hypersensitivity reactions is clinically effective therapy for primary epidermal tumours, including, particularly, the intractable skin cancer syndromes. Studies by a number of investigators have shown that the induction of delayed hypersensitivity reactions at tumour sites results in regression and eradication of malignant neoplasms. The immunogens which will elicit immune antitumour reactions are not related to tumour antigens. A wide variety of materials, ranging from simple chemical compounds to complex biological substances, can exert the same antineoplastic effects by triggering the immune system to elicit selective cancer cell destruction[47]. Although the stimulus or trigger for the immune response in this instance is not specific, the final destructive effects are selective against tumour. In this context, while tumours are eradicated by immune challenge reactions, healing can proceed simultaneously at the same site; microscopic examination has verified cancer cell destruction with adjacent normal cell growth and viability. These observations again indicate that certain aspects of the antitumour pathways of cell-mediated immunity are not specific for tumour antigens since tumour regression can be produced with immune challenge by antigens apparently tumour unrelated. In patients with basal and squamous cell carcinomas of skin, for example, it has been demonstrated that the induction of a local delayed hypersensitivity reaction in tumour tissue by DNCB administration and other agents causes selective destruction of cancer cells. The induced local delayed hypersensitivity reaction to DNCB has resulted in the resolution of more than 90% of superficial basal or squamous cell carcinomas[47]. This therapy has also been applied to systemic cancers which involve the skin, such as metastatic surface breast deposits, or melanomas and infiltrates arising from lymphomas, mycosis fungoides and Kaposi's sarcoma. Application of sensitization agents has usually not been limited to the site of clinical disease, but has extended over the anatomic region or site of the neoplasm. Concentrations of the sensitizing agents that have been applied to these areas have been effective below the lowest concentrations to which delayed hypersensitivity reactions could be demonstrated in normal skin[47,48].

A specific agent deserves mention: levamisole is a drug that has been used widely in animals and in man as an antihelminthic. It has recently attracted attention because it seems to stimulate immune responses[43,49]. Its mechanism of action is, again, unknown but it may act on macrophages to stimulate phagocytosis. Anergic patients have shown restored delayed hypersensitivity responses within 48 h of levamisole administration. Experimentally, transplanted sarcoma tissues can be suppressed and the number of metastatic deposits can be reduced in adult mice treated with levamisole. This suggests a stimulatory effect on tumour immunity. Although certain experimental models have not been affected by levamisole administration, clinical usefulness has been claimed in a variety of disorders.

Active immunotherapy

With active immunotherapy, efforts are made to increase patient immunity by (1) altering tumour-specific antigens to render them more antigenic, (2) coupling tumour antigens with carriers, or (3) mixing tumour antigens with adjuvants to stimulate host reticuloendothelial cells. Most attempts at active immunotherapy in man have involved administration of vaccines of whole tumour cells, inactivated and incapable of proliferation. Inactivation can be achieved by irradiation, mitomycin-C treatment, freezing and thawing and heat inactivation. Repeated efforts have been made to increase tumour antigenicity by modifying tumour cells[6]. These attempts have included coupling highly antigenic carrier protein, such as rabbit gammaglobulin, to tumour cell surfaces, modification of tumour-specific antigens by chemical treatment or linking substances, such as concanavalin-A, to the tumour cell surface. Immunological adjuvant agents such as BCG or *C. parvum* have also been used in combination with whole tumour cells or modified tumour antigens to enhance host immune tumour responses. Active immunotherapy has been used most extensively in patients with advanced disease following failure of more conventional treatment modalities. Studies have shown that such autoimmunization procedures can augment patients' immune responses to their own tumour. Recently a human tumour antigen preparation has been mixed with Freund's complete adjuvant (FCA) to produce effective immunity to lung cancer[50]. The purified antigen in this case produced specific delayed hypersensitivity reactions upon rechallenge, and correlated with patient maintenance of a post-surgical disease-free state. Most previous attempts involved the use of whole, irradiated tumour cells plus FCA and did not produce comparable results.

Passive immunotherapy

Since a growing tumour is often associated with the development of both humoral and cell-mediated immune responses directed against the neoplasm, passive immunotherapy is based on the notion that administration of antitumour antiserum may be beneficial. This is debatable since there is experimental evidence suggesting that antitumour antibodies, perhaps in complex with antigen, may be responsible for the resistance of certain tumours to immune destruction. Passive immunotherapy with antitumour sera has a long history[51]. In this form of treatment experimental animals are immunized with components of the patient's tumour. The resulting antitumour antiserum is then administered to the tumour-bearing patient. Attempts at this form of therapy have been reported since the turn of the century and continue to appear, although results have been generally discouraging. The use of antitumour serum is generally associated with significant side-effects since it contains antibodies against normal tissue antigens of the host who, indeed, may react in hypersensitive fashion to the foreign gammaglobulin. This first problem could be minimized with the development of highly purified tumour antigen[52]. An alternative source of antiserum possibly useful for patients with a given tumour would be that derived from patients 'cured' of their own malignancies. Although occasional spectacular results have been reported with this form of passive immunotherapy, its reported benefit has been limited. A recent clinical trial of this approach in malignant melanoma has failed to produce significant benefit.

Adoptive immunotherapy

Cell-mediated immunity, as manifest by delayed hypersensitivity responses, is a form of reactivity that can be adoptively transferred from one individual to another by means of lymphoid cell transfer. The use of transferred lymphoid cells in the treatment of neoplasia is a relatively new development dependent on the demonstration of the important role of cell-mediated immunity in transplant rejection and tumour immunity. Experimentally, transfer of lymphocytes from tumour-immune rodents to syngeneic hosts has permitted transfer of resistance to specific tumour cell challenge. The difficulty in this regard with human tumours is due to rejection and destruction of transferred lymphocytes, secondary to histocompatibility differences between host and donor. This objection has been documented clinically with allogeneic lymphoid cell transfers, which have been largely disappointing; objective improvement has been obtained in only a small number of circumstances. That small success documented may be due to non-specific stimulation of the immune response with allogeneic cells rather than transmitted specific immune capabilities.

The largest series of patients treated by specific adoptive immunotherapy has consisted of patients who have been grafted with a histologically similar malignant tumour within a matched group. Following initial tumour rejections, patients have been transfused with leukocytes derived from individuals who have rejected their tumour grafts. Although some clinical responses have been noted, the results have not been striking. Other sources of lymphocytes have included those obtained from patients cured of their malignancies and autologous lymphocytes grown in tissue culture in the presence of tumour cells with subsequent reinfusion[6]. Autologous thoracic duct lymphocytes have been sensitized *in vitro* by incubating them with mitomycin-C treated tumour cells. Mitomycin-C treatment inhibits tumour cell replication and does not permit further growth when such cells are reinfused into the patient along with the putatively sensitized lymphocytes. Some apparent clinical responses have been reported, but the results are not striking. Autologous lymphocytes have similarly been exposed *in vitro* to phytohaemagglutinin and have been reinfused or injected directly into tumour deposits with some success.

Specific extracts of sensitized lymphoid cells have become the object of recent experimental interest. (A complete discussion of transfer factor is included in Chapters 2 and 3.) In this context, interest in 'immune RNA' was first stimulated by the observation that RNA extracted (a) from lymphoid cells previously exposed *in vitro* to specific antigens, or (b) from lymphoid tissues of animals immunized to specific antigens *in vivo*, could convert normal non-immune lymphoid cells to specific immunological reactivity. Transplantation antigen immunity could be successfully transferred with RNA from the lymphoid tissues of sensitized donors. Subsequent studies have confirmed the ability of immune RNA to transfer antitumour immunity. The antitumour activity of such material may be abrogated by ribonuclease treatment but not by treatment with other enzymes. Transfer of antitumour immunity in tissue culture with immune allogeneic RNA has been demonstrated: lymphocytes of melanoma patients free of disease have been used as RNA source material and have rendered normal allogeneic lymphocytes cytotoxic in tissue culture. RNA from normal lymphocytes did not cause lymphocytes to become cytotoxic to melanoma cells in control studies. Since immune RNA is a small molecule and poor immunogen, it has obvious advantages. Not only are the problems of HLA incompatibility, serum sickness and anaphylaxis circumvented, but successful interspecies transfer of cell-mediated immunity has been accomplished. This has suggested that xenogeneic RNA extracted from animals immunized with tumour could be produced in large quantities to permit patient treatment. A variety of patients with gross or minimal residual tumour (melanoma, hypernephroma, sarcoma, breast carcinoma, cholangiocarcinoma, gastrointestinal carcinoma) have been treated with immune RNA[53]. Small numbers of these patients have shown subjective clinical improvement. Most of the patients have shown increased peripheral blood lymphocyte cytotoxicity for tumour target cells following immune RNA treatment. Sheep immune RNA, as used in these studies, was injected intradermally and was completely free of significant local or systemic toxicity and was very well tolerated. Because of the subjective nature of the trials, it is too early to evaluate therapeutic usefulness with regard to tumour growth and patient survival.

IMMUNOTHERAPY OF SPECIFIC TUMOURS

Sarcomas

Historically it was with sarcomas that the beneficial effect of treatment with bacterial or Coley's toxins, derived from *Erysipelas*-producing streptococci, and from *Bacillus prodigious* (now known as *Serratia marcescens*) was first described. In particular the course of Ewing's sarcoma was favourably influenced by bacterial toxin therapy combined with surgery and/or radiotherapy[54]. Thus far, however, no programme has proved effective in controlled studies for human sarcomas. Individual patient responses have been noted in patients immunized with cultured osteosarcoma cells[55] and in patients immunized with irradiated autologous sarcoma cells mixed with live BCG[56]. Patients with osteogenic sarcomas have been treated by autologous vaccine administration following the amputation of the involved extremity[57,58]. Statistical analysis of these patients did not show significantly different survival compared to a controlled population, but did suggest that those patients vaccinated with lysed tumour cells survived longer than control patients[58]. In another group of osteosarcoma patients immunized with allogeneic tumour cells and BCG following amputation, three of 17 patients survived 3 years, while none of 12 non-immunized patients survived this long[59]. In a larger group of patients who received adjuvant immunotherapy postoperatively, 16 of 27 patients (59%) with soft tissue sarcomas have survived 3 years. In contrast, only six of 32 patients who did not receive immunotherapy survived this long[60]. In another study 11 patients with sarcomas were immunized with X-irradiated, allogeneic, cultured sarcoma cells or with viral oncolysates[61]. Eight of the 11 patients showed intensified immune reactions to the allogeneic cells used for immunization (even in patients with metastases) and expansion of the compartment of lymphocytes that were cytotoxic to cultured sarcoma cells[62,63]. Cultured osteosarcoma cells of one patient were infected with influenza virus and the patient was thereafter immunized with crude membrane preparations of these cells. The patient developed cytotoxic antibodies and lymphocytes to autologous osteosarcoma cells[63]. Similarly, a 4-month-old infant with intra-abdominal malignant teratoma and embryonal rhabdomyosarcoma received chemotherapy followed by a low dose regimen of continuing cytosine arabinoside and intracutaneous BCG. Following treatment, serum factors were found which potentiated lymphocyte-mediated cytotoxicity; prior to treatment serum factors had blocked the lymphocyte-mediated cytotoxicity to autochthonous tumour[64].

Patients with sarcomatous tumours have been immunized with allogeneic frozen and thawed tumour homogenates and then repeatedly cross-transfused with plasma and leukocytes from one another[65,66]. For variable periods of time 13 of 54 patients treated thus have shown a decrease in the size of metastatic lesions. The cross-transplant/cross-transfusion type of immunotherapy was first introduced in the treatment of malignant melanoma[66]; when applied to the treatment of sarcomas, this technique has only occasionally brought about remission. Of four patients with sarcomas who received cross-transplants of tumours and cross-transfusions of leukocytes, two of the three patients with osteogenic sarcomas showed partial remission. HLA-matched sibling lymphocyte transfusion resulted in a notable 6-month complete remission in a patient with ovarian carcinoma[68]. In eight patients with metastatic osteosarcoma, passive immunization with xenogeneic immune serum or active immunization with sarcoma extract failed to alter the clinical course[69].

Since the results with adjuvant chemotherapy in osteogenic sarcoma have been impressive, combination of immunotherapy with these chemotherapy regimens could produce improved results in the future and may lead to an eventual cure of the disease. At present, the 5-year results of various randomized studies are awaited.

Malignant melanomas

The production of antibody to cytoplasmic and membrane components of melanoma cells has been confirmed, but the significance of this event is not known[70–73]. It appears that these antibodies occur in the sera of patients with tumours other than melanoma, and they occur in healthy donors commonly, but the titre of antibodies is significantly higher in patients with melanoma than that found in sera of tumour-free melanoma donors. Melanoma patients have further been shown to have circulating complement-dependent antibodies that will lyse melanoma cells[73]. These may not be found in patients with macroscopic tumour or visceral metastases. The presence of cytolytic antibodies has correlated roughly with survival. As expected, patients with cytolytic antibodies survive longer than those without. A drop in the titre of such antibodies has been observed in patients with disseminated disease. The fate of such antibodies under these circumstances is not known. They may be bound to tumour cells, destroyed by tumour cells or, alternately, they may be destroyed by anti-idiotypic and anti-allotypic antibodies[74,75].

In malignant melanoma the capability of lymph node lymphocytes to immunologically react to autologous melanoma antigen is of paramount importance in tumour spread, in contrast to the primarily haematogenous spread of sarcomas[76–78]. Melanomas as a rule invade regional lymph nodes first, and widespread visceral metastases occur only thereafter, throughout both lymphatic and haematogenous routes. The blastogenic response of lymphocytes from patients with widespread melanoma appears weaker than that of patients with localized tumours[79]. Circulating lymphocytes of patients with melanoma can kill or inhibit the growth of cultured autologous or allogeneic melanoma cells[80–87]. The presence of serum factors blocking lymphocyte-mediated cytotoxicity was found to signify advancing tumours and widespread metastases. In other patients with cytotoxic lymphocytes, no demonstrable blocking serum factors and growing tumours have been found. A fluctuation of blocking factors in serially tested patients has also been documented without clinical correlation[88]. In other studies, non-melanoma bearing individuals have yielded lymphocytes that expressed cytotoxicity to melanoma cells to the same extent and with the same incidence. The number of normal reactors, especially among American blacks, is certainly large[89]. Another well-documented event must be considered. At one time lymphocyte-mediated cytotoxicity did not appear to be related to the clinical stage of disease, but recent lack of lymphocyte-mediated cytotoxicity in advanced clinical disease has been encountered. However, when non-reactor lymphocytes are washed, their capacity to react has been restored[90]; the low molecular weight substance eluted from non-reactor lymphocytes presumably represents solubilized melanoma antigen. If this is so, circulating soluble tumour antigens can incapacitate lymphocytes.

In addition to lymphocyte-mediated cytotoxicity, macrophages are capable of phagocytosing autologous melanoma cells[91]. This may represent one of two possibilities. Experimentally, non-specifically activated macrophages can distinguish between normal and tumour cells and direct their cytotoxic activity toward tumour cells. Alternatively, cytophilic antibody bound to macrophages may mediate specific target cell phagocytosis, an interaction easily demonstrable in man[92].

There are certain features of the disease entity of malignant melanoma which suggest immunological host defence mechanisms. Spontaneous regression of melanomas is well documented[93], as is regression of a primary focus while lymph node metastases persist. The occasional stabilization of advanced disease and long periods of dormancy between removal of a primary focus and appearance of metastatic disease also suggest immune interaction. Similarly, the regression of a halo naevus[94] with its characteristic dense lymphocytic infiltration suggests that these lymphocytes are functional. Indeed, antibodies reactive with malignant melanoma cells do occur in patients with regressed halo naevi. Mechanisms beyond those of immunity probably significantly influence tumour growth rate, but well retained late sensitivity responses to a variety of antigens coincide with a better prognosis for melanoma-bearing patients. In contrast, low titres of antibodies have been found in patients with widespread melanoma. The reactivity of lymphocytes cytotoxic to allogeneic melanoma cells has been found to be related to the stage of the disease[95] but skin reactions to melanoma antigens do not regularly correlate with disease stage. Since there is a known good correlation between lymphocytic infiltration of primary melanoma disease and a good delayed hypersensitivity response[96,97], the premise that persons with melanoma are deficient in circulating T-cell lymphocytes may be invalid.

A wide variety of T-cell and macrophage stimulants have been used in the treatment of malignant melanoma. In this regard, the effectiveness of BCG is probably not restricted to non-specific immunostimulation. Studies suggest that guinea-pig hepatoma and mouse and human melanoma cells all share common cell surface antigens with those of BCG organisms[97–99]. Thus, immunization with BCG may provide some level of tumour-specific protection.

BCG has been used extensively in the treatment of human malignant melanomas[100–112]. Morton *et al.*[100] have utilized intratumour injection of BCG in extensive trials to treat recurrent melanoma. Individual tumour nodules were injected with 0.1 to 0.5 ml of Glaxo strain BCG. Complete regression was reported in 91% of the nodules injected in 36 patients with intracutaneous lesions. In six of the 36 patients, uninjected intracutaneous nodules were also observed to regress. In patients with subcutaneous or visceral disease, however, the response of injected lesions dropped to 31% (eight out of 26) and, furthermore, no regression of uninjected nodules was noted. In the series of Bornstein *et al.*[107], five out of 15 patients treated with intralesional BCG responded well; one patient had a complete remission with regression of both injected and uninjected lesions. Responding patients' sera did not have blocking activity, but sera taken from patients whose tumours grew quickly after BCG injection contained factors which blocked melanoma-directed lymphocyte toxicity. While BCG therapy following surgical excision of tumours improved the survival of patients with metastatic or recurrent melanomas, serial evaluation of cell-mediated immunity was not of prognostic value and the level of immune response did not change with BCG therapy[109].

Zeigler and co-workers[113,114] have reported a four-phase treatment programme for patients with stage 4 melanoma. In phase one, the patient is sensitized with BCG; in phase two, cutaneous and subcutaneous nodules are injected directly with BCG. Autochthonous lymphocytes are activated *in vitro* with neuraminidase-treated tumour cells and readministered to the patient in phase three, while phase four consists of subcutaneous inoculation of irradiated neuraminidase-treated autochthonous tumour cells and BCG. One hundred and forty-two patients were treated over $3\frac{1}{2}$ years[115]; at the time of reporting, 34% had died, 43% were alive with disease and 23% had complete regression and remained free of disease. In contrast, it appears that immunotherapy has little to offer patients with extensive or visceral disease. Guttermann *et al.*[112] have reported on 89 patients with stage 3 melanoma treated with dimethyl-triazeno imidazole carboxamide (DTIC) administered intravenously, combined with BCG (Pasteur strain) given by scarification. Comparisons of DTIC–BCG treated patients with those treated with DTIC alone revealed significant improvement in the DTIC–BCG group when disease was confined to lymph nodes and subcutaneous tissues, and to a lesser extent, in patients with pulmonary involvement. Patients with visceral metastases showed no improvement with DTIC–BCG over DTIC alone. A somewhat different approach employing adjuvant immunostimulation has been utilized with both primary resectable and metastatic melanoma patients. Repeated administration of BCG per os in extremely high doses has been demonstrated to be safe and produce sensitization to tuberculin. In the initial follow-up of patients with primary or resectable melanoma an improvement has been noted in terms of decreased incidence of recurrent disease and thus prolongation of survival[105]. For the future treatment of malignant melanoma it is apparent that intensive investigation of a combination of surgery, chemotherapy and immunostimulation is required.

During immunotherapy of malignant melanomas with BCG, occasionally severe, even fatal, complications have occurred[116–121]. Granulomatous hepatitis responds to isoniazid but anaphylaxis and disseminated intravascular coagulation can be life-threatening[119]. Intralesional injections of BCG elicit these complications; BCG applied through the scarification technique is much safer. A final problem is that enhanced growth of metastatic tumour following immunostimulation has been reported, particularly in patients in which subcutaneous and lymph node metastases were directly injected with BCG[120,121]. In some cases accelerated tumour growth coincided with the appearance or increase of serum lymphocyte-blocking factors.

Sporadic case reports contend that transfusion of blood from patients with regressed or cured melanoma can induce remission in melanoma patients[122,123]. No contemporary trials of passive immunotherapy have been reported. Immune sera derived from patients with malignant melanoma and immunized with autologous tumour cells in Freund's adjuvant could occasionally effect temporary regression with intralesional injection. The cross-transplantation of live tumour cells and later exchange of white blood cells and serum has been reported. Nadler and Moore[66] produced partial regression of melanoma in 16 out of 86 patients and complete regression in two. Their patients, matched for blood and tumour types, were inoculated subcutaneously with live tumour cells from a partner. After five days each pair was cross-transfused with white blood cells daily over a period of 5 to 15 days. Employing a scheme of cross-transplantation of live tumour cells and exchange of white blood cells and serum, Krementz and Samuels reported tumour regression in two out of nine patients[124]. Humphrey[125,126] and his co-workers modified the Nadler and Moore scheme. Tumour cells were homogenized and frozen and thawed three times to make the preparation acellular. Paired patients were immunized with intradermal and subcutaneous inoculation of the cell products and then underwent cross-exchange of white blood cells and serum. The tumour preparation was later refined by centrifugation, taking only the final supernatant fluid after centrifugating at 102 000 *g* for 30 minutes. Treatment with these preparations, followed by exchange of white blood cells and serum has produced an overall objective response in 20 out of 86 patients with melanoma. Although the incidence of delayed hypersensitivity activity was greater with the ultracentrifuged fraction, clinical response was about the same in both groups. The transfer of autologous lymphocytes cultured with melanoma cells or allogeneic sensitized lymphocytes has been reported anecdotally without any major benefit. The use of transfer factor in the treatment of melanoma is reviewed in this volume (Chapters 2 and 3).

Carcinoma of the breast

Immunotherapy for breast cancer is attractive to all who consider the evidence for immune phenomena in relation to the problem. Although putative breast cancer antigens have been isolated, they are only weakly antigenic and it has been difficult to demonstrate or identify useful antigen–antibody interactions in breast cancer[127–132]. Clinically, however, breast carcinoma is one of the tumours in which regional lymph node reactivity to tumour correlates well with prognosis[133–136]. A defensive role of the regional lymph nodes in preventing the spread of breast carcinoma has been postulated. Indeed, the regional lymph node lymphocytes of patients with breast carcinoma are capable of reacting to mitogens and respond to stimulation with breast carcinoma antigen to a greater degree than lymphocytes taken from the circulating blood pool[137,138]. The common occurrence of lymph node metastases notwithstanding, these data support the notion that the regional lymph nodes of patients with breast cancer are immunologically competent and suggest that they may be able to retard tumour spread. Good correlation has been shown between the presence of complement-fixing antibody directed toward solubilized breast carcinoma antigen, lymphocyte infiltration of breast tumours, sinus histiocytosis in regional lymph nodes and clinical prognosis[139]. Thus, complement-fixing breast carcinoma antibody appears to be an important prognostic factor, inasmuch as false-positive reactions are rare and the reaction of the breast carcinoma antigen with antibody depends on participation of the Fab fragment. Cell-mediated reactions to breast carcinoma antigens have been studied *in vitro* by lymphocyte blastogenesis, lymphocyte-mediated cytotoxicity and migration inhibition assays[140–143]. All these techniques are subject to inhibition by blocking serum factors as shown in the studies of Hellström *et al.*[140,142,143]. Correlation of blocking serum factors with tumour growth or spread has not been well-established, despite previous claims to the contrary[144].

Numerous attempts at immunotherapy of breast carcinoma have been made. Non-specific immunostimulation (BCG), specific active immunization with tumour cells (often modified to increase antigenicity) and adoptive immunization with transfer factor (see Chapters 2 and 3) have all been tried[145,146] with variable effect. Attempts with immunostimulants alone to deter metastatic disease have fared poorly. Administration of xenogeneic (horse) immune antiserum putatively directed against breast carcinoma antigens has been abandoned, despite early claims of tumour regression in serum treated patients[147]. Immunization with autologous breast carcinoma cells has improved survival in one series[148]. Immunization with breast tumour cells coupled to rabbit gammaglobulin and administered with Freund's adjuvant has promoted antitumour antibody formation with temporary clinical tumour remission[149]. Women autografted with irradiated breast tumour following mastectomy and postoperative radiotherapy have demonstrated increased lymphocyte sensitization to allogeneic breast carcinoma antigens[150]. Of interest, such tumour autografting appeared to increase the radiosensitivity of residual tumour. Twelve of 16 patients with clinically unfavourable breast carcinoma who received autografts of irradiated tumour were alive 4 to 7 years later.

Quite obviously, immunotherapy must be combined with other forms of therapy. In this regard, several studies are now in progress for carcinoma of the breast in which treatment combines surgery, systemic chemotherapy or hormonal therapy, and non-specific adjuvant immunostimulation. Guttermann and colleagues[151] have found that a remission rate of 75% is possible with a chemotherapeutic combination of 5-fluorouracil, adriamycin and cyclophosphamide, with or without intermittent BCG scarification. Although remission rates were identical, the duration of remission for patients achieving partial remission was significantly longer than remissions for patients on chemotherapy alone. Survival of the chemo-immunotherapy treated group has been significantly longer than that of the group receiving chemotherapy alone[151]. If this report can be confirmed, a practical approach using combined systemic therapy following local resection will greatly augment the long-term prognosis for this disease. This is currently under investigation in randomized prospective trials.

Neuroblastoma

Neuroblastomas are unique, fascinating tumours with a clinical spectrum which includes frequent spontaneous regression and differentiation as well as stable and aggressive malignant disease. There is good evidence for immune interaction directed against neuroblastoma cells since infiltration of tumour by lymphocytes is common, circulating lymphocytes cytotoxic to autologous and allogeneic neuroblastoma cells are demonstrable, and circulating antibodies directed against neuroblastoma cells are easily found[152–156]. Both tumour lymphocytic infiltration and peripheral blood lymphocytosis have correlated with a favourable prognosis. Lymphocytes from neuroblastoma patients are toxic to both autologous and allogeneic tumour cells but do not correlate with clinical patient status. Cytolytic anti-neuroblastoma antibodies are demonstrable in the sera of the patients who are tumour-free and serum factors which block lymphocyte-mediated cytotoxicity to neuroblastoma cells are evident in the sera of patients with progressive tumours[157,158].

Choriocarcinoma

Choriocarcinomas are immunologically unusual tumours since they express both embryonic antigens and the histocompatibility antigens of the mother and father. They also produce chorionic gonadotrophin, are coated with unusual sialomucin and exhibit a wide range of neoplastic behaviour. Since they represent hemi-allogeneic tissue, their growth characteristics may be due to decreased display of paternal antigens, immunosuppression produced by chorionic gonadotrophin, normal or abnormal blocking serum factors or the increased sialomucin tumour coat[159,160]. Since trophoblastic tumours do bear lymphocytes of maternal origin, attempts have been made to grade lymphocyte reaction in choriocarcinomas with prognosis. In one study the majority of patients with minor lymphocytic infiltration of their tumours died and most patients with a heavy lymphocytic infiltration lived, although some lymphocytic reactivity is visible in normal placenta[160].

Immunotherapy of gestational choriocarcinoma has consisted of various schedules of immunization of the patient with paternal cells[161–163]. In Bagshawe's series[161], patients were given either intradermal BCG or husband leukocytes in Freund's complete adjuvant plus repeated husband skin allografts. Although second grafts from the husbands were rejected more rapidly than the initial grafts, the clinical value of immunotherapy in this condition awaits large, controlled trials.

Adenocarcinoma of the gastrointestinal tract

The embryonic antigen of colorectal malignancies (CEA), originally described by Gold and Freedman[164], has emerged as one of a group of antigens termed oncofetal antigens. The appearance of these in circulation after fetal life usually signifies the presence of a gastrointestinal malignancy or of disturbed or altered physiology (pregnancy, gut-associated inflammation or regeneration). The highest levels of such antigen are found in the blood of patients with carcinomas of colon and rectum, but elevated levels have been found in other gut adenocarcinomas, other malignant tumours and certain benign disease states. Because of this lack of specificity, the CEA test does not have a firm role in the diagnosis of colorectal carcinoma, although very few patients with such tumours do not have elevated levels of CEA. CEA levels, further, do not correlate well with tumour size or grade but tumour removal does result in a fall in CEA titre and subsequent regrowth is attended by a rising CEA titre[165–168]. The autologous tumour and mitogen reactivity of regional node lymphocytes in patients with colon carcinoma is extremely variable. Lymphocyte-mediated cytotoxicity to autologous and allogeneic tumour cells has been demonstrated, as have serum factors that inhibit these reactions. Cell-mediated immunity to carcinoembryonic antigens has been suggested by experiments with lymphocytes from patients with colon carcinomas which inhibit the growth of cultured fetal gut and liver cells (but not control fetal kidney) although the clinical relevance of this remains unclear.

Several controlled trials are underway to compare the effects of post-surgical 5-fluorouracil chemotherapy with chemotherapy plus non-specific immunotherapy with BCG, *C. parvum* or levamisole. Tumour-specific immunotherapy trials have implemented irradiated or neuraminidase-treated autologous or allogeneic tumour cells or transfer factor derivative of immune lymphocytes. Tabulated or statistically significant data are not yet available. Oral (and intraperitoneal) BCG administration for gastrointestinal adenocarcinoma has resulted in prolonged survival, with or without tumour regression as shown by Falk *et al.*[33,34] with the best results noted in patients with minimal residual disease. As already noted, side-effects with orally administered BCG are minimal. The cellular aspects of immunostimulation by this route remain incompletely defined, but present data suggest that increased B-cell activity, in the context of existing macrophage activation, perhaps promote antibody-dependent tumour cell lysis (Falk, in preparation). This concept requires definition since oral BCG appears to be the least toxic approach available for non-specific immunostimulation.

A further approach has involved intraperitoneal immunization with BCG at the time of laparotomy, or following surgery by dialysis catheter. Variable peritoneal inflammation is produced, subsiding in 2–5 days in 95% of cases. Vigorous delayed hypersensitivity reactions can be achieved, as assessed by tuberculin skin testing, even in patients with far advanced disease. Massive macrophage activation has been produced although this does not necessarily correlate with demonstrable regression. In the initial assessment of this route of administration combined with standard chemotherapy, an improvement in survival has been noted for stomach and colorectal, but not pancreatic carcinomas. Further long-term follow-up of these patients will be of considerable interest.

A large series of patients with gastrointestinal carcinomas was first cross-immunized with allogeneic tumour cells and later given putatively immune plasma and leukocytes[169–171]. Thirty-two patients with colorectal carcinomas were given intradermal killed allogeneic tumour cells or solubilized tumour cell antigens at weekly intervals for 5 weeks. Plasma and leukocytes were later exchanged between immunized patients. Twenty patients completed this programme and 12 showed a beneficial clinical or laboratory response. Seven of the responses were subjective, with diminished pain and nausea; five were objective, with a 50% or greater reduction in tumour cell mass or the development of tumouricidal antibodies. Antibody–toxin and antibody–enzyme conjugates have also been prepared for therapy in colorectal carcinoma. Antibody to surface antigens of human colonic carcinoma has been conjugated with glucose oxidase to produce more effective *in vitro* cytotoxicity than antibody alone[172]. Rosato *et al.*[173] treated patients with gastrointestinal tumours, melanomas, sarcomas and breast carcinomas by immunization with neuraminidase-treated autochthonous tumour cells. In immunized patients increased lymphocyte-mediated cytotoxicity without blocking factors was noted. Six of 25 patients experienced prolonged survival without progressive disease. Large gastrointestinal tumours not amenable to resection have been injected with live mumps virus in an effort to produce tumour cell death with, hopefully, enhanced immunity[174,175]. Viral injection of tumours has resulted in occasional tumour regression. One patient treated intranasally with Newcastle disease virus evidently showed regression of intrathoracic deposits of a rectal carcinoma.

In the comparatively large series from the M. D. Anderson Hospital, a total of 58 patients with colorectal cancer of the Dukes' C classification were entered into the study during a period of 21 months. Patients were randomized to receive BCG either alone or in combination with oral 5-fluorouracil postoperatively. Comparison of the two groups to date has shown a longer disease-free interval and survival among the patients treated with 5-fluorouracil plus BCG[176].

Bronchogenic carcinoma

In patients with bronchogenic carcinoma there has been clear demonstration of immunological suppression[177,178]. In large studies, those patients with lung carcinomas who have failed to respond to tuberculin and streptococcal antigens or to convert to positive DNCB reactivity have died significantly more quickly than those with maintained delayed hypersensitivity responses. In advanced bronchogenic carcinoma, lymphocyte mitogen-induced blastogenesis is diminished with a further diminution in reactivity notable following radiotherapy or chemotherapy[179]. A serum factor inhibitory to lymphocyte blastogenesis has also been documented in these patients' sera in high titres[180]. T lymphocytes are present in the circulation in patients with squamous cell carcinoma in significantly lower numbers[181,182]. T-cell levels of 'cured' patients show rapid restoration to normal levels. The nature of the serum inhibitor of lymphocyte blastogenesis is unknown, but may be an alpha-2-globulin or an antibody of as yet undetermined specificity.

An occasional complication of pneumonectomy for carcinoma of the lung, postoperative empyema, has been associated with a striking 50% 5-year survival, in contrast to only 18% of patients surviving 5 years without empyema[183,184]. This phenomenon has suggested that the non-specific immunostimulation produced by the infective process can produce tumour cell death. Such cytotoxicity is probably non-specific and dependent on macrophage activation in response to bacterial antigens. This 'accidental' immunotherapy is probably analogous to experimental stimulation of regional lymph nodes with BCG, or the treatment of skin tumours by delayed hypersensitivity reactions elicited to pertinent antigens. Bacterial toxins may also directly damage tumour cells, as postulated by Coley at the turn of the century.

Clinical trials with BCG immunostimulation post-resection for bronchogenic carcinoma have determined that certain immune responses may improve following treatment, and survival can be favourably influenced. Two centres have reported initial results of randomized, prospective trials with prolonged recurrence free intervals and longer survival. McNeally and co-workers have used intrapleural BCG following treatment with isoniazid (thus attempting to reduplicate a temporary and controlled empyema situation) to non-specifically stimulate the immune system[185]. The 3-year follow-up in their series shows a significant difference for patients with resected stage 1 disease. A second study by Stewart Harris and co-workers has employed combined chemoimmunotherapy with high dose methotrexate and citrovorum rescue followed, at the time of optimal immune recovery, by immunization with a purified lung tumour antigen in Freund's complete adjuvant[186]. A remarkable difference has been demonstrated in time to recurrence and survival time, with an even more impressive correlation of the patients' clinical course with skin test reactivity to the same tumour antigen preparation. Their results indicate that the best response is observed in patients with an HLA phenotype which includes A1 and B8[187], a phenotype associated with several types of autoaggressive disease. This phenotype is also associated with increased reactivity in a semi-quantitative mixed lymphocyte reaction (Osoba, D. and Falk, J. A. in press). If confirmed, this observation suggests that a type of 'autoaggressive reactivity' may be necessary if dramatic improvement in survival from neoplasia can be produced through immune mechanisms. This confirms an impression of the authors that the most effective results with immunostimulation to neoplasia may occur with concomitant symptoms of autoaggressive disease.

Carcinomas of the genitourinary tract

Kidney

Renal cell adenocarcinomas are among those tumours with a high rate of spontaneous remission[188–190]. Those few cases in which pulmonary metastases have regressed after surgical removal of primary tumour suggest an immunological host/tumour interaction[189,191]. In lymphocyte-mediated cytotoxicity assays, highly specific reactions to cultured autologous or allogeneic renal carcinomas have been reported[191,192]. However, other studies have been at variance with these findings and have not shown consistent cytotoxicity to renal carcinoma cells but have shown cytotoxicity towards unrelated cell lines and cytotoxic reactivity in normal or control patients[193]. Adenocarcinoma of the kidney has been treated with non-specific immunostimulation (Coley's toxins)[194] and with passive immunization using xenogeneic or homologous antitumour sera[195]. Both treatment modalities have caused or coincided with periods of long-term tumour regression. Present experimental use includes BCG, *C. parvum*, levamisole, active immunization with irradiated or polymerized autologous tumour cells or with viral oncolysates of autologous tumour, and cross-immunization/transfusion. At the time of writing no large or statistically significant results have been announced.

Urinary bladder

Patients with genitourinary carcinoma frequently fail to exhibit delayed hypersensitivity skin responses to either a sensitizing or challenge application of DNCB. In one study 98% of patients with local transitional cell carcinoma of the urinary bladder and 100% of patients with metastases were anergic or had subnormal reactivity, compared to patients with renal carcinomas who displayed more normal responses[195].

Transitional cell carcinoma of the urinary bladder is one of the human tumours against which specific lymphocyte-mediated cytotoxicity has been consistently demonstrated by several groups of investigators[196–204]. Transitional cell carcinomas of bladder and renal pelvis cross-react but no significant cross-reaction with carcinoma of the kidney, prostate or testis occurs. A much larger number of patients with localized carcinoma of the bladder have yielded lymphocytes cytotoxic to bladder carcinoma cells *in vitro* than lymphocytes harvested from patients with more advanced disease. Since lymphocyte-mediated cytotoxicity diminishes after surgical removal of tumour, continuing dispersal of tumour antigens may be required to maintain immunity. Patients with tumour-killing lymphocytes have longer survival times without recurrence than others without this ability. The work of O'Toole and colleagues[200] showed that a non-T-cell fraction of lymphocytes produced specific tumour cell death.

Specific bladder carcinoma antigens are difficult to detect, although specific protein has been found in the urine of such patients[205]. Non-specific immunostimulation and adoptive immunization with xenogeneic lymphocytes have been tried for the treatment of genitourinary carcinomas. In 19 patients with carcinomas of kidney, bladder, prostate or testis, monocyte function (as measured by the monocyte chemotaxis assay) has improved after immunostimulation with BCG, although skin test responses changed little[195]. Intracavity BCG plus scarification sensitization has produced long periods without tumour recurrence in patients treated thus after initial tumour fulguration[206].

Prostatic carcinoma

Prostatic carcinoma has not been studied extensively from an immunological point of view, although such a study would appear promising for several reasons. Such tumours are very common but lie dormant for long periods in their elderly hosts. The prostate does not have a known lymphatic vascular circulation[207], although tumour lymphocyte invasion does occur. Oncofetal antigens are released from prostatic tumours and several normal prostatic enzymes are produced in increased amounts. Alpha-2-globulins, which may be immunosuppressive, are also detectable in the blood of patients with prostatic carcinoma[208,209]. Blood group antigens are not expressed in prostatic carcinoma cells, suggesting antigenic loss[210,211]. Although circulating antibodies toxic to lymphocytes have been found in some patients with prostatic carcinoma, their importance remains obscure[212].

The immunotherapeutic approaches in prostatic carcinoma have included bacterial toxins, BCG and *C. parvum* administration[213,214], specific immunization with tumour cells coupled to rabbit gammaglobulin and cryotherapy[215]. BCG injection into the malignant prostate gland has produced tumour necrosis. Several patients treated with BCG have shown clinical remission, but others were not benefited when BCG was given by multiple puncture[214]. Since regression of pulmonary metastases has occurred in a small number of patients with prostatic carcinoma following local cryotherapy, it has been suggested that such treatments are, in fact, analogous to a specific tumour immunization protocol. Indeed, elevated serum globulins following such therapy do correlate with a good clinical response.

Ovary and testis

Testicular carcinoma has not been adequately investigated from the immunological point of view. The common infiltration of seminomas by lymphocytes appears to be related to prognosis[216]. Cytotoxic lymphocytes and blocking serum factors can be found in patients with testicular carcinoma and these do not cross-react with other genitourinary malignancies[217]. Bacterial toxin immunotherapy following surgery and radiotherapy has been termed successful in a large percentage of operable cases and in a smaller fraction of inoperable patients[218]. Patients with ovarian carcinoma have been shown to have lymphocytes cytotoxic to allogeneic ovarian (but not uterine) tumour cells, but blocking factors have not been demonstrated. Patients with ovarian carcinoma have been immunized with tumour or tumour extracts with occasional prolongation of life accredited to this therapy in uncontrolled trials[219,220]. Treatment of patients with mumps virus has failed to alter the clinical course of patients with embryonal cell carcinoma of testis, although this virus seeds selectively to testicular tissue[221].

Skin tumours

Clearance of primary or metastic skin tumours of various histological origins (e.g. melanoma, basal or squamous cell carcinoma, leukaemia or metastatic breast tumour, Kaposi's sarcoma) can occur within the area of delayed hypersensitivity reactions elicited by different agents (DNCB, triethylene iminobenzoquinone, PPD, BCG, streptokinase, streptodornase, etc.). To achieve this, following initial sensitization, subsequent challenge with antigen is applied in the area of the tumour. Once inflammation clears, complete resolution of tumour nodules is often noted without residual scarring[222,223]. The mechanism of this phenomenon is unknown, although it appears that macrophages and lymphocyte products effect tumour cell destruction, since direct injection of activated macrophages or lymphotoxins into tumour nodules can result in reduction in size or complete resolution of skin tumours. Amplification of pre-existing specific immunity could also occur in the tumour area following a delayed hypersensitivity response. In this regard, patients with squamous cell carcinoma of skin have demonstrable antibodies to membrane and cytoplasmic antigens as well as lymphocytes cytotoxic to autologous tumours[223]. Local immunotherapy by delayed hypersensitivity responses can be further improved with the addition of local chemotherapy[224].

Perspectives

The notion that immunosuppression precedes and/or accompanies cancer is often interpreted to suggest that immunosuppression is necessary for carcinogenesis. If one discounts patients with advanced cancer or patients who received extensive chemotherapy or radiotherapy, the association of extrinsic immunosuppression with cancer will not be applicable to the majority of patients who develop neoplasia. Other mechanisms must, therefore, facilitate the growth of tumours. Among several possible mechanisms, inappropriate host–tumour immune interactions and tumour immunoresistance deserve special consideration. The best documented of these is the inappropriate immune response, i.e. the blocking of lymphocyte-mediated tumour cell destruction in an immunologically specific fashion by serum factors. These serum factors are believed to be soluble tumour antigens, tumour antigen-directed antibodies or complexes of these factors. The tumour specificity of this phenomenon in man has been repeatedly demonstrated by lack of cross-blocking among unrelated tumours[140,143,225]. Antigen excess in the complex would pre-empt cytotoxic lymphocyte-function, while the antibody component of the complex is probably responsible in preventing lymphocyte–tumour interaction at the surface of the tumour cell. A large number of events may favour tumour growth. Immune defects, especially involving T lymphocytes, may occur on a genetic or developmental basis. Non-specific immunosuppression by such serum factors as α_2-globulins may also permit tumour cell growth. Then again, tumours may themselves release factors which non-specifically prevent effective lymphocyte function. Tumour-specific immunosuppression by blocking antibodies or complexes has already been mentioned. The same phenomenon may occur at a cellular level with the development of 'immunosuppressive' lymphocytes, notably suppressor T cells which may be specifically suppressive to a particular tumour[226,227] and may release specific, T cell-derived suppressor factors.

With regard to carcinogenesis and immune interactions in general, there is consensus regarding several concepts. Patients with early or localized tumours seldom show gross immune deficit. Such defects as may subsequently appear do so as an effect rather than a cause of the neoplasm. If remission can be obtained with conventional measures, clinical immune status will remain normal or improve. Certain tumours (sarcomas and melanomas) may maintain consistent and effective immune reactivity despite tumour progression. Other tumours cured by radiotherapy (most often head and neck squamous cell tumours) manifest demonstrable T-cell defects without tumour regrowth[228].

SUMMARY

Human tumours probably have specific antigens that are not present on normal cells and immune reactions to these antigens occur. From animal experimental work, it has been assumed that such immune reactions can destroy incipient tumours, although this has not been directly proven in man. Involvement of the immune system in tumour genesis in man is largely based on circumstantial evidence, such as spontaneous regression of cancer, infiltration of cancer by lymphocytes and macrophages, and an elevated incidence of cancer under certain conditions of immunosuppression. This is supported by abundant evidence in laboratory animals, in which tumour antigens and immune reactions to these antigens have been clearly documented. Such laboratory work has provided the enthusiasm for clinical immunotherapy.

Immunotherapy of human cancer has proved most successful locally in the form of agents that produce delayed hypersensitivity responses. Systemic administration of non-specific immunostimulants has reportedly prolonged survival in patients with cancer who have responded to chemotherapy; other reports note delayed recurrence rates in patients treated following elimination of tumour by other means. These reports remain largely anecdotal, however, and await confirmation in large controlled trials with suitable patient evaluation and simultaneous immunological measurement. The direction of relevant clinical work is clear from the data to date: immunotherapy is more likely to display benefit under optimal clinical circumstances (i.e. small tumour burden) than when used in patients with far advanced or disseminated disease.

The need for laboratory research is also apparent. Indeed, many tumours in laboratory animals are not measurably immunogenic. Emerging serological techniques, plus the ability to grow tumour cells *in vitro* for long periods, will permit classification and biochemical characterization of the surface antigens of the more common cancers and may provide clues as to their origin. This knowledge is most important, since tumour cells of laboratory animals seem to escape from immunological control by reduction of cell surface antigenicity. Immune mechanisms may provide an external pressure by which, from all the genetic variants of a rapidly growing tumour, those least antigenic are selected. Alternatively, a temporary, phenotypic adaptive change may occur under circumstances in which antibody to surface antigens causes their disappearance (antigenic modulation), permitting continued cell growth in the face of prior immunity. Recent immunogenetic research has also shown that the ability of the immune system to respond to certain antigenic determinants is controlled by immune response (Ir) genes[229]. Consideration of the tumour immune response from an immunogenetic standpoint promises to be an important field since genetic inability to react to a given tumour may mitigate against standard immunotherapies which would continue to be inept; such circumstances might benefit if tumour cell antigen were altered in some fashion, to put it within the realm of host reactivity.

Much has been said as well about the inhibition of cell-mediated immunity by circulating soluble antigen or antigen–antibody complexes, although the actual existence and relevance of such macromolecular structures has not been definitely established in man. If these complexes do exist and do block immune reactivity, laboratory work must establish the site and mechanism of such suppression. There is now evidence that the complexity of the T-cell system approaches that of humoral antibodies[230], with the various classes, subclasses and factors they release. Dissection of the role of T lymphocytes, non-T lymphocytes and macrophages is in an early phase. There are a number of factors which influence these cells directly (e.g. thymopoietin and T cells; lymphokines and macrophages) and selective control of the function of the cells of the immune system may one day be possible.

Under present circumstances it is evident that tumour immunotherapy is of minimal benefit when applied against a large tumour burden. Immunotherapy is potentially most effective when tumour cell load has been reduced to a minimum by an appropriate combination of surgery, chemotherapy and radiotherapy with immunotherapy instituted once the immune system has had opportunity to recover from the immunosuppressive nature of such prior treatment. If combined with chemotherapy, immunotherapy should be timed such that proliferating, functional lymphoid cells are readily available at the time of therapy. Although non-specific immunostimulation would appear to be the mainstay of immunotherapy for the near future, more specific and less hazardous agents will surely follow and these will probably be combined with tumour-specific active immunization. If this can be done with elimination of specific suppressor cells and humoral factors, it may be possible to control the neoplastic cell.

ACKNOWLEDGEMENT

The authors greatly appreciate the secretarial assistance of Miss Ethel Kerr and Miss Audrey Lock.

References

1. Coley, W. B. (1898). The treatment of inoperable sarcoma with the mixed toxins of erysipelas and *Bacillus prodigiosus*. *J. Am. Med. Assoc.*, **31**, 389, 456
2. Coley, W. B. (1908). The treatment of sarcoma by mixed toxins of erysipelas and *Bacillus prodigiosus*. *Boston Med. Surg. J.*, **58**, 175
3. Coley, W. B. (1911). A report of recent cases of inoperable sarcoma successfully treated with mixed toxins of erysipelas and *Bacillus fragiosus*. *Surg. Gynecol. Obstet.*, **13**, 174
4. Coley, W. B. (1929). Treatment of bone sarcoma. *Cancer Rev.*, **4**, 426
5. Foley, E. J. (1953). Antigenic properties of methylcholanthrene induced tumours in mice of the strain of origin. *Cancer Res.*, **13**, 835
6. Morton, D. L. (1974). Cancer immunotherapy: an overview. *Semin. Oncol.*, **1**, 297
7. Parker, C. W. (1973). The immunotherapy of cancer. *Pharmacol. Rev.*, **25**, 325
8. Crispen, R. G. (1974). BCG vaccine in perspective. *Semin. Oncol.*, **4**, 311
9. Gershon, R. K. and Kondo, K. (1971). Infectious immunological tolerance. *Immunology*, **21**, 903
10. Yu, A., Watts, H., Jaffe, N. and Parkman, R. (1977). Concomitant presence of tumour specific cytotoxic and inhibitor lymphocytes in patients with osteogenic sarcoma. *N. Eng. J. Med.*, **297**, 3, 121
11. Falk, R. E., Nossal, N. A. and Falk, J. A. (1978). Effective anti-tumour immunity following elimination of suppressor T cell function. *Surgery* (In press)
12. Unanue, E. R. (1975). Function of macrophages. *Fed. Proc.*, **34**, 1723
13. Rhodes, J. (1977). Altered expression of human monocyte Fc receptors in malignant disease. *Nature (Lond.)*, **265**, 253
14. Romans, D. G., Falk, J. A., Dorrington, K. J. and Falk, R. E. (1975). Studies on the Fc receptor of human peripheral blood monocytes and peritoneal macrophages: evidence for inducibility. *Proc. Canad. Fed. Biol. Soc.*, **18**, 84
15. Brent, L. and Holborow, J. (eds.) (1974). Mechanisms of immunological unresponsiveness. In: *Progress in Immunology I, Vol. III* (Amsterdam: North Holland Publishing Co.)
16. Möller, G. (ed.) (1972). Immunological tolerance—effect of antigen on different cell populations. *Transplant. Rev.*, **8**, 000
17. Nossal, G. J. V. (1973). The cellular and molecular basis of immunological tolerance. In: *Essays in Fundamental Immunology, I* (I. Roitt, ed.), p. 28 (Oxford: Blackwell)
18. Elkins, W. L., Hellström, I. and Hellström, K. E. (1974). Transplantation tolerance and enhancement, concepts and questions. *Transplantation*, **18**, 38
19. Falk, R. E. and MacGregor, A. B. (1976). Antigen reactive cells to tumour antigens in normal and tumour patients. *J. Surg. Res.*, **20**, 247
20. Guerin, C. (1957). The history of BCG. In: *BCG Vaccination against Tuberculosis* (S. R. Rosenthal, ed.), pp. 48–53 (Boston: Little, Brown)
21. Dubos, R. J. and Schaedler, R. W. (1957). Effects of cellular constituents of mycobacteria on the resistance of mice to heterologous infections. I. Protective effects. *J. Exp. Med.*, **105**, 703
22. Halpern, B. N. (1963). Role du systéme reticulo-endothelial dans l'immunité anti-bacterienne et antitumoral. *Coloque Int. Centre Nat. de la Recherche Scientifique*, **115**, 319

23. Halpern, B. N., Biozzi, G., Stiffel, C. *et al.* (1959). Effet de la stimulation du système reticulo-endothelial par l'inoculation du bacille de Calmette-Guerin sur le developpement l'epithelioma atypique T-8 Guerin chez le rat. *C. R. Soc. Biol. (Paris)*, **153**, 919
24. Old, L. J., Clarke, D. A. and Benacerraf, B. (1959). Effect of Bacillus Calmette-Guerin infection on transplanted tumours in the mouse. *Nature (Lond.)*, **184**, 291
25. Bast, R. C., Zbar, B., Borsos, T. and Rapp, H. J. (1974). BCG and cancer. *N. Engl. J. Med.*, **290**, 1413
26. Baldwin, R. W. and Pimm, M. V. (1973). BCG immunotherapy of pulmonary growths from intravenously transferred rat tumour cells. *Br. J. Cancer*, **27**, 48
27. Laucuis, J. F., Bodurtha, A. J., Mastrangel, M. J. and Creech, R. H. (1974). Bacillus Calmette-Guerin in the treatment of neoplastic disease. *J. Reticuloendothel. Soc.*, **16**, 347
28. Nathanson, L. (1974). Use of BCG in the treatment of human neoplasms: a review. *Semin. Oncol.*, **1**, 337
29. Pimm, M. V. and Baldwin, R. W. (1975). BCG immunotherapy of rat tumours in athymic nude mice. *Nature (Lond.)*, **254**, 77
30. Hanna, M. G. Jr. (1971). Immunologic aspects of BCG-mediated regression of established tumours and metastasis in guinea-pigs. *Semin. Oncol.*, **1**, 319, 714
31. Möller, G. (1975). One non-specific signal triggers B lymphocytes. *Transplant. Rev.*, **23**, 126
32. Aungst, C. W., Sokal, J. E. and Jager, B. V. (1975). Complications of BCG vaccination in neoplastic disease. *Ann. Int. Med.*, **82**, 666
33. Falk, R. E., MacGregor, A. B., Landi, S., Ambus, U. A. and Langer, B. (1976). Immunostimulation with intraperitoneally administered Bacille Calmette Guerin for advanced malignant tumours in the gastrointestinal tract. *Surg. Gynecol. Obstet.*, **142**, 363
34. Falk, R. E., MacGregor, A. B., Ambus, U., Landi, S., Miller, A. B., Samuel, E. S. S. and Langer, B. (1977). Combined treatment with BCG and chemotherapy in metastatic gastrointestinal cancer. *Dis. Colon Rectum*, **20**, No. 3
35. McKneally, M. R., Maver, C. and Kausel, H. W. (1976). Regional immunotherapy of lung cancer with intrapleural BCG. *Lancet*, **i**, 7956, 377
36. Falk, R. E., Landi, S., Cohen, Z. *et al.* (1975). Use of oral and intraperitoneal BCG in the treatment of malignant melanoma and adenocarcinoma. *Proc. of 1974 Chicago Symp: Neoplasm Immunity: Theory and Application*, University of Illinois. ITR 904 W. Adams, pp. 169–80
37. MacGregor, A. B., Falk, R. E., Landi, S. L. *et al.* (1975). Oral BCG immunostimulation in malignant melanoma. *Surg. Gynecol. Obstet.*, **141**, 747
38. Falk, R. E., Ambus, U., Landi, S. L. *et al.* (1977). Report of a randomized trial utilizing BCG and 5-fluorouracil to treat gastrointestinal cancer. Presented at the 1977 Chicago Symposium, *Immunotherapy of Solid Tumors*, February 24–25
39. Levy, N. L., Mahaley, M. S. and Day, E. D. (1972). Serum-mediated blocking of cell-mediated antitumour immunity in a melanoma patient: Association with BCG immunotherapy and clinical deterioration. *Int. J. Cancer*, **10**, 244
40. Lamoureux, G. and Poisson, R. (1974). BCG and immunological anergy. *Lancet*, **i**, 989
41. Scott, M. T. (1974). *Corynebacterium parvum* as an immunotherapeutic anti-cancer agent. *Semin. Oncol.*, **1**, 367
42. Woodruff, M. F. A. and Boak, J. L. (1966). Inhibitory effect of injection of *Corynebacterium parvum* on the growth of tumour transplants in isogeneic hosts. *Br. J. Cancer*, **20**, 345
43. Oettgen, H. F., Pinsky, C. M. and Delmonte, L. (1976). Treatment of cancer with immunomodulators. *Med. Clin. N. Amer.*, **60**, 511
44. Woodruff, M., Dunbar, N. and Ghaffar, A. (1973). The growth of tumours in T-cell deprived mice and their response to treatment with *Corynebacterium parvum*. *Proc. R. Soc. Lond. Ser. B*, **184**, 97
45. Howard, J. G., Christie, G. H. and Scott, M. T. (1973). Biological effects of *Corynebacterium parvum*. IV. Adjuvant and inhibitory effects on B lymphocytes. *Cell. Immunol.*, **7**, 290

46. Ghaffar, A., Cullen, R. T. and Woodruff, M. R. A. (1975). Further analysis of the anti-tumour effect *in vitro* of peritoneal eludate cells from mice treated with *Corynebacterium parvum*. *Br. J. Cancer*, **31**, 15
47. Klein, E. and Holtermann, O. A. (1972). Immunotherapeutic approaches to the management of neoplasms. *Nat. Cancer Inst. Monogr.*, **35**, 379
48. Klein, E., Holtermann, O. A., Milgrom, H. *et al.* (1976). Immunotherapy for accessible tumours utilizing delayed hypersensitivity reactions and separated components of the immune system. *Med. Clin. N. Amer.*, **60**, 389
49. Editorial (1975). Levamisole. *Lancet*, **i**, 151
50. Stewart, T. H. M. *et al.* (1977). Specific active immunochemotherapy in lung cancer: a survival study. *Can. J. Surg.*, **20**, No. 4, 370
51. Currie, G. A. (1972). Eighty years of immunotherapy: a review of immunological methods used for the treatment of human cancer. *Br. J. Cancer*, **26**, 141
52. Morton, D. L. (1973). Horizons in tumor immunology. *Surgery*, **74**, 69
53. Pilch, Y. H., Fritze, D. and Kern, D. H. (1976). Immune RNA in the immunotherapy of cancer. *Med. Clin. N. Amer.*, **60**, 567
54. Nauts, H. C. (1974). Ewing's sarcoma of bone: end results following immunotherapy (bacterial toxins) combined with surgery and/or radiation. New York Cancer Research Institute, Monograph No. 14
55. Mendoza, C. B., Moore, G. E., Watne, A. L. *et al.* (1968). Immunologic response following homologous transplantation of cultured human tumor cells in patients with malignancy. *Surgery*, **64**, 897
56. Currie, G. A. (1973). Effect of active immunization with irradiated tumour cells on specific serum inhibitors of cell-mediated immunity in patients with disseminated cancer. *Br. J. Cancer*, **28**, 25
57. Southam, C. M., Marcove, R. C., Levin, A. G. *et al.* (1972). Clinical trial of autologous tumor vaccine for treatment of osteogenic sarcoma. In: *Seventh National Cancer Conference Proceedings*, American Cancer Society and National Cancer Institute (Philadelphia: J. B. Lippincott Co.)
58. Marcove, R. C., Mike, V., Huvos, A. G. *et al.* (1973). Vaccine trials for osteogenic sarcoma. *Cancer*, **23**, 74
59. Townsend, C. M. and Eilber, F. R. (1975). Adjuvant immunotherapy for skeletal sarcomas. *Sci. Proc. Am. Soc. Clin. Oncol.*, **16**, 261 (Abstract No. 1162)
60. Gunnarson, A., McKhann, C. F., Simmons, R. L. *et al.* (1974). Metastatic sarcoma. Combined surgical and immunotherapeutic approach. Neuraminidase treated tumor cells a tumor vaccine. *Minn. Med.*, **57**, 558
61. Harris, J. E. and Sinkovics, J. G. (1976). Immunology and immunotherapy of human tumors. In: *The Immunology of Malignant Disease*. Second edition, p. 465 (St Louis: The C. V. Mosby Co.)
62. Williams, D. E., Romero, J. J., Sinkovics, J. G. *et al.* (1975). Assessing patient's sarcoma-specific immune responses during immunotherapy. *Tex. Med.*, **71**, 55
63. Green, A. A., Webster, R. G. and Smith, K. (1975). Autologous tumor cells modified by influenza virus generated immune responses in a patient with osteogenic sarcoma. *Sci. Proc. Am. Soc. Clin. Oncol.*, **16**, 271 (Abstract No. 1202)
64. Nesbit, M. E. Jr., Kersey, J. H., Leonard, A. S. *et al.* (1974). Role of immunotherapy and chemotherapy: humoral antagonism of cell-mediated immunity in a malignant tumor: reversal following immunotherapy. In: *Selected Topics of Cancer, Current Concepts* (K. K. N. Charyulu and A. Sudarsanam, eds.) (New York: Intercontinental Medical Book Corp.)
65. Humphrey, L. J., Murray, D. R. and Boehm, O. R. (1971). Effect of tumor vaccines in immunizing patients with cancer. *Surg. Gynecol. Obstet.*, **132**, 437

66. Nadler, S. H. and Moore, G. E. (1969). Immunotherapy of malignant disease. *Arch. Surg.*, **99**, 376
67. Krementz, E. T., Mansell, P. W. A., Hornung, M. O. *et al.* (1974). Immunotherapy of malignant disease: the use of viable sensitized lymphocytes or transfer factor prepared from sensitized lymphocytes. *Cancer*, **33**, 394
68. Yonemoto, R. H. and Terasaki, P. I. (1972). Cancer immunotherapy with HLA-compatible thoracic duct lymphocyte transplantation. *Cancer*, **30**, 1438
69. Neff, J. and Enneking, W. (1974). Adoptive immunotherapy in primary osteosarcoma. An interim report. In: *Interaction of Radiation and Host Immune Defense Mechanisms in Malignancy.* Brookhaven National Laboratory Symposium (Brookhaven, N.Y.: U.S. Atomic Energy Commission)
70. Morton, D. L., Malmgren, R. A., Holmes, E. C. *et al.* (1968). Demonstration of antibodies against human malignant melanoma by immunofluorescence. *Surgery*, **64**, 233
71. Lewis, M. G. and Phillips, T. M. (1972). Separation of two distinct tumor-associated antibodies in the serum of melanoma patients. *J. Nat. Cancer Inst.*, **49**, 915
72. Lewis, M. G. (1973). Mechanisms of humoral tumor immunity in malignant melanoma. In: *Proceedings of the Tenth Canadian Cancer Research Conference* (P. G. Scholefield, ed.) National Cancer Institute of Canada, Toronto. (Toronto: University of Toronto Press)
73. Wood, G. W. and Barth, R. F. (1974). Immunofluorescent studies of the serologic reactivity of patients with malignant melanoma against tumor-associated cytoplasmic antigens. *J. Nat. Cancer Inst.*, **53**, 309
74. Gupta, R. K. and Morton, D. L. (1975). Suggestive evidence for *in vivo* binding of specific antitumour antibodies of human melanomas. *Cancer Res.*, **35**, 58
75. Hartmann, D., Lewis, M. G., Proctor, J. W. *et al.* (1974). *In vitro* interactions between anti-tumour antibodies and anti-antibodies in malignancy. *Lancet*, **ii**, 1481
76. Nagel, G. A., Piessens, W. F., Stibmant, M. M. *et al.* (1971). Evidence for tumor-specific immunity in human malignant melanoma. *Eur. J. Cancer*, **7**, 41
77. Ambus, U., Mavligit, G. M., Gutterman, J. U. *et al.* (1974). Specific and non-specific immunologic reactivity of regional lymph node. Lymphocytes in human malignancy. *Int. J. Cancer*, **14**, 291
78. Mavligit, G., Gutterman, J. U., McBride, C. *et al.* (1974). Tumor-directed immune reactivity and immunotherapy in malignant melanoma. *Current Status, Prog. Exp. Tumor Res.*, **19**, 222
79. Spitler, L. E., Littooy, F., Sagbiel, R. W. *et al.* (1978). Malignant melanoma. I. Cellular immunity to melanoma antigens. (Submitted for publication)
80. Jehn, U. W., Nathanson, L., Schwartz, R. S. *et al.* (1970). *In vitro* lymphocyte stimulation by a soluble antigen from malignant melanoma. *N. Engl. J. Med.*, **282**, 329
81. Cochran, A. J., Jehn, U. W. and Gothoskar, B. P. (1972). Cell-mediated immunity in malignant melanoma. *Lancet*, **i**, 1340
82. Falk, R. E., Mann, P. and Langer, B. (1973). Cell-mediated immunity to human tumors: abrogation by serum factors and nonspecific effects of oral BCG therapy. *Arch. Surg.*, **107**, 261
83. Mavligit, G. M., Gutterman, J. U., McBride, C. M. *et al.* (1973). Cell-mediated immunity to human solid tumors. *In vitro* detection by lymphocyte blastogenic responses to cell-associated and solubilized tumor antigens. *Nat. Cancer Inst. Monogr.*, **37**, 167
84. Nairn, R. C., Nind, A. P., Guli, E. P. G. *et al.* (1972). Antitumor immunoreactivity in patients with malignant melanoma. *Med. J. Aust.*, **1**, 397
85. Hellström, I. and Hellström, K. E. (1973). Some recent studies on cellular immunity to human melanomas. *Fed. Proc.*, **32**, 156
86. Clark, D. A. and Nathanson, L. (1973). Cellular immunity in malignant melanoma. In: *Proceedings of the Eighth Pigment Cell Conference* (V. Riley, ed.) (Basel: S. Karger Ag.)

87. de Vries, J. E., Cornain, S. and Rümke, P. (1974). Cytotoxicity of non-T versus T-lymphocytes from melanoma patients and healthy donors on short- and long-term cultured melanoma cells. *Int. J. Cancer*, **14**, 427
88. Heppner, G. H., Stolbach, L., Byrne, M. *et al.* (1973). Cell-mediated and serum blocking reactivity to tumor antigens in patients with malignant melanoma. *Int. J. Cancer*, **11**, 245
89. Hellström, I., Hellström, K. E., Sjogren, H. O. *et al.* (1973). Destruction of cultivated melanoma cells by lymphocytes from healthy black (North American Negro) donors. *Int. J. Cancer*, **11**, 116
90. Currie, G. A. and Basham, C. (1972). Serum mediated inhibition of the immunologic reactions of the patient to his own tumour. A possible role for circulating antigen. *Br. J. Cancer*, **26**, 427
91. Pihl, E., Nind, A. P. P. and Nairn, R. C. (1974). Electron microscope observation of the *in vitro* interaction between human leukocytes and cancer cells. *Aust. J. Exp. Biol. Med. Sci.*, **52**, 737
92. The, T. H., Eibergen, R., Lamberts, H. B. *et al.* (1972). Immune phagocytosis *in vivo* of human malignant melanoma cells. *Acta Med. Scand.*, **192**, 141
93. Everson, T. C. and Cole, W. H. (1966). *Spontaneous Regression in Cancer* (Philadelphia: W. B. Saunders Co.)
94. Lewis, M. G. and Copeman, P. (1972). Halo naevus: a frustrated malignant melanoma? *Br. Med. J.*, **2**, 47
95. Cochran, A. J. (1969). Histology and prognosis in malignant melanoma. *J. Pathol.*, **97**, 459
96. Little, J. H. (1972). Histology and prognosis in cutaneous malignant melanoma and skin cancer. In: *Melanoma and Skin Cancer, Proceedings of the International Cancer Conference*, Sydney, Australia (W. H. McCarthy, ed.) (V. C. N. Blight, Government Printer)
97. Borsos, T. and Rapp, H. J. (1973). Antigenic relationship between *Mycobacterium bovis* (BCG) and guinea-pig hepatoma. *J. Nat. Cancer Inst.*, **51**, 1085
98. Faraci, R. P., Barone, J. and Schour, L. (1975). BCG-induced protection against malignant melanoma: possible immunospecific effect in a murine system. *Cancer*, **35**, 372
99. Bucana, C. and Hanna, M. Jr. (1974). Immuno-electron microscopic analysis of surface antigens common to *Mycobacterium bovis* and tumor cell. *J. Nat. Cancer Inst.*, **53**, 1313
100. Morton, D. L., Eilber, F. R., Holmes, E. C. *et al.* (1974). BCG immunotherapy of malignant melanoma: summary of a seven-year experience. In: *Neoplasm Immunity: BCG Vaccination* (R. G. Crispen, ed.) (Evanston, Ill.: Schori Press)
101. Smith, G. V., Morse, P. A., Deraps, G. D. *et al.* (1973). Immunotherapy of patients with cancer. *Surgery*, **74**, 59
102. Nathanson, L. (1973). Regression of intradermal melanoma after intralesional injection of *Mycobacterium bovis* strain BCG. *Cancer Chemother. Rep.*, **56**, 659
103. Pinsky, C. M., Hirshaut, Y. and Oettgen, H. F. (1973). Treatment of malignant melanoma by intratumoral injection of BCG. *Nat. Cancer Inst. Monogr.*, **39**, 225
104. Mastrangelo, M. J., Sulit, H. L., Prehn, L. M. *et al.* (1976). Intralesional BCG in the treatment of metastatic malignant melanoma. *Cancer*, **37**, 684
105. MacGregor, A. B., Falk, R. E., Landi, S. *et al.* (1977). Adjuvant immunostimulation in malignant melanoma with oral Bacille Calmette Guerin. *Can. J. Surg.*, **20**, 185
106. Littman, B., Zbar, B. and Rapp, H. J. (1972). Effects of *Mycobacterium bovis* (BCG) on tumour cell growth in muscle. *Proc. Am. Assoc. Cancer Res.*, **13**, 96 (Abstract 381)
107. Bornstein, R. S., Mastrangelo, M. J., Sulit, H. *et al.* (1973). Immunotherapy of melanoma with intralesional BCG. *Nat. Cancer Inst. Monogr.*, **39**, 213
108. Bluming, A. Z., Vogel, C. L., Ziegler, J. L. *et al.* (1972). Immunological effects of BCG in malignant melanoma: two modes of administration compared. *Ann. Int. Med.*, **76**, 405
109. McCulloch, P., Dent, P., Lui, V. *et al.* (1975). Improved survival in metastatic malignant melanoma with BCG therapy. *Proc. 66th Annu. Meet. Am. Assoc. Cancer Res.*, **16**, 174 (Abstract No. 693)

110. Gutterman, J., Mavligit, G., Kennedy, A. *et al.* (1975). Adjuvant BCG immunotherapy for minimal residual disease in malignant melanoma: a three-year experience. *Proc. 11th Annu. Meet. Am. Soc. Clin. Oncol.*, **16**, 245 (Abstract No. 1096)
111. de Wys, W. D. and Taylor, S. G. (1975). Chemoimmunotherapy of malignant melanoma. *N. Engl. J. Med.*, **292**, 159
112. Gutterman, J. U., Mavligit, G., Gottlieb, J. A. *et al.* (1974). Chemoimmunotherapy of disseminated malignant melanoma with dimethyl triazeno imidazole carboxamide and Bacillus Calmette Guerin. *N. Engl. J. Med.*, **291**, 592
113. Seigler, H. F., Shingleton, W. W., Metzger, R. S. *et al.* (1972). Non-specific and specific immunotherapy in patients with melanoma. *Surgery*, **72**, 162
114. Levy, N. L., Seigler, H. F. and Shingleton, W. W. (1974). A multiphase immunotherapy regimen for human melanoma: clinical and laboratory results. *Cancer*, **34**, 1548
115. Seigler, H. F., Shingleton, W. W., Metzgar, R. S. *et al.* (1973). Immunotherapy in patients with melanoma. *Ann. Surg.*, **178**, 352
116. Bodurtha, A., Kim, Y. H., Laucius, J. F. *et al.* (1974). Hepatic granulomas and other hepatic lesions associated with BCG immunotherapy for cancer. *Am. J. Clin. Pathol.*, **61**, 747
117. Hunt, J. S., Silverstein, M. J., Sparks, F. R. *et al.* (1973). Granulomatous hepatitis: a complication of BCG immunotherapy. *Lancet*, **ii**, 820
118. Sparks, F. C., Silverstein, M., Hunt, J. S. *et al.* (1973). Complications of BCG immunotherapy in patients with cancer. *N.Engl. J. Med.*, **289**, 827
119. McKhann, C. F., Hendrickson, C. G., Spitler, L. E. *et al.* (1975). Immunotherapy of melanoma with BCG: two fatalities following intralesional injection. *Cancer*, **35**, 514
120. Levy, N. L., Mahaley, M. S. Jr. and Day, E. D. (1972). Serum-mediated blocking of cell-mediated anti-tumor immunity in a melanoma patient: association with BCG immunotherapy and clinical deterioration. *Int. J. Cancer*, **10**, 244
121. Sparks, F. C. and Breeding, J. H. (1974). Tumor regression and enhancement resulting from immunotherapy with Bacillus Calmette-Guerin and neuraminidase. *Cancer Res.*, **34**, 3262
122. Summer, W. V. and Foraker, A. G. (1960). Spontaneous regression of human melanoma. Clinical and experimental studies. *Cancer*, **13**, 79
123. Teimoorian, B. and McCune, W. S. (1963). Surgical management of malignant melanoma. *Am. Surg.*, **29**, 515
124. Krementz, E. T. and Samuels, M. S. (1967). Tumor cross-transplantation and cross-transfusion in treatment of advanced malignant disease. *Bull. Tulane Univ. Med. Fac.*, **26**, 263
125. Humphrey, L. J., Jewell, W. R., Murray, D. R. *et al.* (1971). Immunotherapy for the patient with cancer. *Ann. Surg.*, **173**, 47
126. Humphrey, L. J., Lincoln, P. M. and Griffin, W. O. (1968). Immunologic response in patients with disseminated cancer. *Ann. Surg.*, **168**, 374
127. Gentile, J. M. and Flickinger, J. T. (1972). Isolation of a tumor-specific antigen from adenocarcinoma of the breast. *Surg. Gynecol. Obstet.*, **135**, 69
128. Silva, J. S. and Leonard, C. M. (1975). Cell-mediated immunity against allogeneic and autologous tumor cell extracts in breast cancer. *Proc. 66th Annu. Meet. Am. Assoc. Cancer Res.*, **16**, 148 (Abstract No. 592)
129. Nordquist, R. E., Lerner, M. P. and Anglin, J. H. (1976). Glycoprotein shedding from human mammary carcinoma cells. *Proc. 67th Annu. Meet. Am. Assoc. Cancer Res.*, **17**, 35 (Abstract No. 140)
130. Story, M. T., Pattillo, R. A., Ruckert, A. C. G. *et al.* (1974). On the isolation and characterization of soluble antigens from human breast tumor cells. *In Vitro*, **10**, 388
131. Humphrey, L. J., Estes, N. C., Morse, P. A. *et al.* (1974). Serum antibody in patients with mammary disease. *Cancer*, **34**, 1516

132. Estes, N. C., Morse, P. A. and Humphrey, L. J. (1974). Antibody studies of sera from patients with breast cancer. *Surg. Forum*, **25**, 121
133. Black, M. M. and Asire, A. J. (1969). Palpable axillary lymph nodes in cancer of the breast: structural and biologic considerations. *Cancer*, **23**, 251
134. Silverberg, S. G., Chitale, A. R., Hind, A. D. *et al.* (1970). Sinus histiocytosis and mammary carcinoma: study of 366 radical mastectomies and an historical review. *Cancer*, **26**, 1177
135. Friedell, G. H., Soto, E. A., Kumaoka, S. *et al.* (1974). Sinus histiocytosis in British and Japanese patients with breast cancer. *Lancet*, **ii**, 1228
136. Di Paola, M., Angelini, L., Bertolotti, A. *et al.* (1973). Histology of breast cancer and regional lymph nodes: immunological significance. *Int. Res. Commun. Syst.*, **1**, 29
137. Fisher, B., Saffer, E. and Fisher, E. (1972). Studies concerning the regional lymph node in cancer. *Cancer*, **30**, 1202
138. Ellis, R. J., Wernick, G., Zabriskie, J. B. *et al.* (1975). Immunologic competence of regional lymph nodes in patients with breast cancer. *Cancer*, **35**, 655
139. Hudson, M. J. K., Humphrey, L. J., Mantz, F. A. *et al.* (1974). Correlation of circulating serum antibody to the histological findings in breast cancer. *Am. J. Surg.*, **128**, 756
140. Sjogren, H. O., Hellström, I., Bansal, S. C. *et al.* (1972). Elution of 'blocking factors' from human tumors, capable of abrogating tumor cell-destruction by specifically immune lymphocytes. *Int. J. Cancer*, **9**, 274
141. Whittaker, M. G., Rees, K. and Clark, C. G. (1971). Reduced lymphocyte transformation in breast carcinoma. *Lancet*, **i**, 892
142. Hellström, I., Hellström, K. E. and Warner, G. A. (1973). Increase of lymphocyte-mediated tumor cell destruction by certain patient sera. *Int. J. Cancer*, **12**, 348
143. Hellström, I., Hellström, K. E., Sjogren, H. O. *et al.* (1971). Serum factors in tumor-free patients cancelling the blocking of cell-mediated tumor immunity. *Int. J. Cancer*, **8**, 185
144. Levin, A. C. (1975). Facilitation of lymphocytotoxicity using plasma from breast cancer patients and normal controls. *Proc. 66th Annu. Meet. Am. Assoc. Cancer Res.*, **16**, 150 (Abstract No. 631)
145. McCredie, J. A., Brown, E. R. and Cole, W. H. (1959). Immunological treatment of tumors. *Proc. Soc. Exp. Biol. Med.*, **100**, 31
146. Oettgen, H. F., Old, L. J., Farrow, J. H. *et al.* (1974). Effects of dialyzable transfer factor in patients with breast cancer. *Proc. Nat. Acad. Sci. USA*, **71**, 2319
147. Murray, G. (1958). Experiments in immunity in cancer. *J. Can. Med. Assoc.*, **79**, 249
148. Gorodilova, V. V., Silino, I. G. and Soraeva, Z. M. (1965). The first experience in vaccination against metastases in patients with breast cancer. *Vopr. Onkol.*, **2**, 22
149. Czajkowski, N. P., Rosenblatt, M., Wolf, P. I. *et al.* (1967). A new method of active immunization to autologous human tumor tissue. *Lancet*, **ii**, 905
150. Anderson, J. M., Kelly, F., Wood, S. E. *et al.* (1974). Stimulatory immunotherapy in mammary cancer. *Br. J. Surg.*, **61**, 778
151. Gutterman, J. U., Mavligit, G., Gottlieb, J. A. *et al.* (1974). Chemoimmunotherapy of disseminated malignant melanoma with dimethyl triazenoimidazole carboxamide and Bacille Calmette Guerin. *N. Engl. J. Med.*, **291**, 592
152. Martin, R. F. and Backwith, J. B. (1968). Lymphoid infiltrate in neuroblastomas: their occurrence and prognostic significance. *J. Pediatr. Surg.*, **3**, 161
153. Bill, A. H. and Morgan, A. (1970). Evidence for immune reactions to neuroblastoma and future possibilities for investigation. *J. Pediatr. Surg.*, **5**, 111
154. Kumar, S., Taylor, G., Steward, J. K. *et al.* (1972). Cellular immunity in Wilms' tumor and neuroblastoma. *Int. J. Cancer*, **10**, 36
155. Hellström, I., Hellström, K. E., Bill, A. H. *et al.* (1970). Studies on cellular immunity to human neuroblastoma cells. *Int. J. Cancer*, **6**, 172

156. Hellström, K. E. and Hellström, I. (1972). Immunity to neuroblastomas and melanomas. *Annu. Rev. Med.*, **23**, 19
157. Jose, D. G. and Skvarn, F. (1974). Serum inhibitors of cellular immunity in human neuroblastoma. IgG subclass of blocking activity. *Int. J. Cancer*, **13**, 173
158. Jose, D. G. and Seshadr, R. (1974). Circulating immune complexes in human neuroblastoma: direct assay and role in blocking specific cellular immunity. *Int. J. Cancer*, **13**, 824
159. Adcock, E. W., Teasdale, T., August, C. S. *et al.* (1973). Human chorionic gonadotrophin: its possible role in maternal lymphocyte suppression. *Science*, **181**, 845
160. Elston, C. E. (1969). Cellular reaction to choriocarcinoma. *J. Pathol.*, **97**, 261
161. Bagshawe, K. D. (1973). Recent observations related to the chemotherapy and immunology of gestational choriocarcinoma. *Adv. Cancer Res.*, **18**, 231
162. Donlach, I., Crookston, J. H. and Cope, T. I. (1958). Attempted treatment of a patient with choriocarcinoma by immunization with her husband's cells. *J. Obstet. Gynaecol. Br. Commonw.*, **65**, 588
163. Cinader, B., Hayley, M. A., Rider, W. D. *et al.* (1961). Immunotherapy of a patient with choriocarcinoma. *Can. Med. Assoc. J.*, **84**, 306
164. Gold, P. and Freedman, S. O. (1965). Specific carcinoembryonic antigens of the human digestive system. *J. Exp. Med.*, **122**, 467
165. Freedman, S. O. (1972). Carcinoembryonic antigen: current clinical applications. *J. Allergy Clin. Immunol.*, **50**, 384
166. Zamcheck, N. (1974). Carcinoembryonic antigen. In: *The Physiopathology of Cancer* (P. Shubik, ed.) (Basel: S. Karger Ag.)
167. Neville, A. M. and Laurence, D. J. R. (1974). The carcinoembryonic antigen (CEA). Present position and proposals for future investigation. *Int. Union Cancer Tech. Rep. Ser.*, **12**, 1
168. LoGerfo, P. and Herter, F. P. (1975). Carcinoembryonic antigen and prognosis in patients with colon cancer. *Ann. Surg.*, **181**, 81
169. Humphrey, L. J., Murray, D. R., Boehm, O. R. *et al.* (1971). Immunotherapy of cancer in man. VII. Studies of patients with cancer of the alimentary tract. *Am. J. Surg.*, **121**, 165
170. Griffen, W. O., Jewell, W. R., Meeker, W. R. *et al.* (1972). Newer concepts of cancer of the colon and rectum: immunotherapy for patients with cancer of the large intestine. *Dis. Colon Rectum*, **15**, 116
171. Griffen, W. O. Jr. and Meeker, W. R. (1972). Colon carcinoma and immunologic phenomena. *Surg. Clin. N. Amer.*, **52**, 839
172. Shearer, W. T., Turnbaugh, T. R., Coleman, W. E. *et al.* (1974). Cytotoxicity with antibody–glucose oxidase conjugates specific for a human colonic cancer and carcinoembryonic antigen. *Int. J. Cancer*, **14**, 539
173. Rosato, F. E., Brown, A. S., Miller, E. E. *et al.* (1974). Neuraminidase immunotherapy of tumors in man. *Surg. Gynecol. Obstet.*, **139**, 675
174. Asada, T. (1974). Treatment of human cancer with mumps virus. *Cancer*, **34**, 1907
175. Csatary, L. (1971). Viruses in the treatment of cancer. *Lancet*, **ii**, 825
176. Falk, R. E., Ambus, U., Langer, B. *et al.* (1977). Report of a randomized trial utilizing BCG and 5-fluorouracil to treat gastrointestinal cancer. Presented at the Chicago Symposium *Immunotherapy of Solid Tumors*, February 24–25
177. Krant, M. J., Manskopf, G., Brandrup, C. S. *et al.* (1968). Immunologic alterations in brochogenic cancer: sequential study. *Cancer*, **21**, 623
178. Han, T. and Takita, H. (1972). Immunologic impairment in bronchogenic carcinoma: a study of lymphocyte response to phytohemagglutinin. *Cancer*, **30**, 616
179. Thomas, J. W., Coy, P., Lewis, H. S. *et al.* (1971). Effect of therapeutic irradiation on lymphocyte transformation in lung cancer. *Cancer*, **27**, 1046

180. Silk, M. (1967). Effect of plasma from patients with carcinoma on *in vitro* lymphocyte transformation. *Cancer*, **20**, 2088
181. Dellon, A. L., Potvin, C. and Chretien, P. B. (1975). Thymus-dependent lymphocyte levels in bronchogenic carcinoma: correlations with histology, clinical stage, and clinical course after surgical treatment. *Cancer*, **35**, 687
182. Gross, R. L., Latty, A., Williams, E. A. *et al.* (1975). Abnormal spontaneous rosette formation and rosette inhibition in lung carcinoma. *N. Engl. J. Med.*, **292**, 439
183. Ruckdeschel, J. C., Codish, S. D., Stranahan, A. *et al.* (1972). Postoperative emphysema improves survival in lung cancer. *N. Engl. J. Med.*, **287**, 1013
184. Takita, H. (1970). Effect of postoperative emphysema on survival of patients with bronchogenic carcinoma. *J. Thorac. Cariovasc. Surg.*, **59**, 642
185. McKneally, M. F. (1977). Treatment of pulmonary tumors with BCG and isoniazid. Presented at the Chicago Symposium *Immunotherapy of Solid Tumors*, February 24–25
186. Stewart, T. H. M. (1977). Survival study of immunochemotherapy in lung cancer. Presented at the Chicago Symposium *Immunotherapy of Solid Tumors*, February 24–25
187. Sengar, D. P. S., McLeish, W. A., Stewart, T. H. M. *et al.* (1977). HLA antigens in bronchogenic cancer. *Oncology*, **34**, No. 4
188. Bloom, H. J. G. (1973). Hormone-induced and spontaneous regression of metastatic renal cancer. *Cancer*, **32**, 1066
189. Garfield, D. H. and Kennedy, B. J. (1972). Regression of metastatic renal cell carcinoma following nephrectomy. *Cancer*, **30**, 190
190. de Giorgi, L. S. (1972). Regression of pulmonary metastases during radiation to a hypernephroma: immunity and cancer. *Cancer*, **30**, 895
191. Bubenik, J., Jakoubkova, J., Krakova, P. *et al.* (1971). Cellular immunity to renal carcinomas in man. *Int. J. Cancer*, **8**, 503
192. Daly, J. J., Prout, G. R. Jr. and Ahl, C. A. (1974). Specificity of cellular immunity to renal cell carcinoma. *J. Urol.*, **111**, 448
193. Baldwin, R. W., Embleton, M. J., Jones, J. S. P. *et al.* (1973). Cell-mediated and humoral immune reactions to human tumors. *Int. J. Cancer*, **12**, 73
194. Nauts, H. C. (1973). Enhancement of natural resistance to renal cancer: beneficial effects of concurrent infections and immunotherapy with bacterial vaccines. (New York Cancer Research Institute, Monograph No. 12)
195. Brosman, S., Hausman, M. and Shacks, S. (1975). Studies on the immune status of patients with renal carcinoma. *J. Urol.*, **114**, 375
196. Bubenik, J., Baresova, M., Viklicky, V. *et al.* (1973). Established cell line of urinary bladder carcinoma (T24) containing tumor-specific antigen. *Int. J. Cancer*, **11**, 765
197. Bloom, E. T., Ossorio, R. C. and Brosman, S. A. (1971). Cell-mediated cytotoxicity against human bladder cancer. *Int. J. Cancer*, **14**, 326
198. Bean, M. A., Pees, H., Fogh, J. E. *et al.* (1974). Cytotoxicity of lymphocytes from patients with cancer of the urinary bladder: detection by a ^{3}H-proline microcytotoxicity test. *Int. J. Cancer*, **14**, 186
199. Elhilali, M. M. and Nayak, S. K. (1975). Immunologic evaluation of human bladder cancer: *in vitro* studies. *Cancer*, **35**, 419
200. O'Toole, C., Perlmann, P., Wigzell, H. *et al.* (1973). Lymphocyte cytotoxicity in bladder cancer: no requirement for thymus-derived effector cells? *Lancet*, **i**, 1085
201. O'Toole, C., Stejskal, V., Perlmann, P. *et al.* (1974). Lymphoid cells mediating tumor-specific cytotoxicity to carcinomas of the urinary bladder. Separation of the effector population using a surface marker. *J. Exp. Med.*, **139**, 457
202. Hakala, T. R. and Lange, P. H. (1974). Serum induced lymphoid cell mediated cytotoxicity to human transitional cell carcinomas of the genitourinary tract. *Science*, **184**, 795

203. Hakala, T. R., Lange, P. H., Castro, A. E. *et al.* (1971). Antibody induction of lymphocyte-mediated cytotoxicity against human transitional cell carcinomas of the urinary bladder. *N. Engl. J. Med.*, **291**, 637
204. Hakala, T. R., Lange, P. H., Castro, A. *et al.* (1974). Cell-mediated cytotoxicity against human transitional cell carcinomas of the genitourinary tract. *Cancer*, **34**, 1929
205. Monaco, A. P., Gozzo, J. J., Schlesinger, R. M. *et al.* (1975). Immunological detection of human bladder carcinoma. *Ann. Surg.*, **182**, 325
206. Eidinger, D. and Morales, A. (1978). Intracavitary BCG for bladder tumors. *Ann. N.Y. Acad. Sci.* (In press)
207. Gittes, R. F. and McCullough, P. L. (1974). Occult carcinoma of the prostate: an oversight of immune surveillance. A working hypothesis. *J. Urol.*, **112**, 241
208. Ablin, R. J. (1973). Interference of immunologic surveillance by immunoregulatory α-globulin: A hypothesis. *Neoplasma*, **20**, 159
209. Ablin, R. J. (1970). Immunologic studies of normal, benign and malignant prostatic tissue. *Cancer*, **29**, 1570
210. Davidson, I. (1972). Early immunologic diagnosis and prognosis of carcinoma. *Am. J. Clin. Pathol.*, **57**, 715
211. Gupta, R. K., Schuster, R. and Christian, W. D. (1973). Loss of isoantigens A, B and H in prostate. *Am. J. Pathol.*, **70**, 439
212. Ablin, R. J. and Baird, W. M. (1972). Cytotoxic antibodies to allogeneic lymphocytes in prostatic cancer. *J. Am. Med. Assoc.*, **219**, 87
213. Merrin, C., Han, T., Klein, E. *et al.* (1975). Immunotherapy of prostatic carcinoma with Bacillus Calmette-Guerin. *Cancer Chemother. Rep.*, **59**, 157
214. Guinan, P., John, T., Crispen, R. G. *et al.* (1974). BCG immunotherapy in carcinoma of the prostate. In: *Neoplasm Immunity: BCG Vaccination* (R. G. Crispen, ed.) (Evanston, Ill.: Schori Press)
215. Ablin, J. (1974). Immunological aspects of the development and advances of cryosurgery of the prostate. In: *Cryosurgery in Urology* (H. J. Reuter and R. H. Flocks, eds.) (Stuttgart: George Thieme Verlag Ag)
216. Thachray, A. C. (1964). Seminoma, the pathology of testicular tumors. *Br. J. Urol.*, **36**, 12
217. Hellström, I., Sjogren, H. O., Warner, G. *et al.* (1971). Blocking of cell-mediated tumor immunity by sera from patients with growing neoplasms. *Int. J. Cancer*, **7**, 266
218. Fowler, G. E. (1968). Testicular cancer treated by bacterial toxin therapy as a means of enhancing host resistance. New York Cancer Research Institute, Monograph No. 7
219. Graham, J. B. and Graham, R. M. (1962). Autogenous vaccine in cancer patients. *Surg. Gynecol. Obstet.*, **114**, 1
220. Willoughby, H., Latour, J. P. A., Tabah, E. J. *et al.* (1970). Cross-implantation of tumor tissue and cross-transfusion in patients with advanced cancer. *Am. J. Obstet. Gynecol.*, **108**, 889
221. Taylor, G. and Odili, J. L. I. (1972). Histological evidence of tumor rejection after active immunotherapy in human malignant disease. *Br. Med. J.*, **2**, 183
222. Stjernsward, J. and Levin, A. (1971). Delayed hypersensitivity-induced regression of human neoplasms. *Cancer*, **28**, 628
223. Nairn, R. C., Nina, A. P. P., Guli, E. P. G. *et al.* (1971). Specific immune response in human skin carcinoma. *Br. Med. J.*, **4**, 701
224. Klein, E., Holtermann, O. A., Case, R. W. *et al.* (1974). Responses of neoplasms to local immunotherapy. *Am. J. Clin. Pathol.*, **62**, 281
225. Hellström, I., Hellström, K. E., Sjogren, H. O. *et al.* (1971). Demonstration of cell-mediated immunity to human neoplasms of various histological types. *Int. J. Cancer*, **7**, 1
226. Falk, R. E., Nossal, N. A. and Falk, J. A. (1977). Effective antitumor immunity following depletion of T cell function. *Clin. Res.*, **25**, No. 5, 695

227. Greene, M. I., Dorf, M. E., Pierres, M. *et al.* (1977). Reduction of syngeneic tumor growth by an anti-I-J alloantiserum (tumor growth/H-2 complex/I region). *Proc. Nat. Acad. Sci. USA*, **74**, 11, 5118
228. Tarpley, J. L., Potvin, C. and Chretien, P. B. (1975). Prolonged depression of cellular immunity in cured laryngopharyngeal cancer patients treated with radiation therapy. *Cancer*, **35**, 638
229. Old, L. J. and Boyse, E. A. (1972). Current enigmas in cancer research. *Harvey Lect.*, **67**, 273
230. Shiku, A., Takahashi, T., Bean, M. A. *et al.* (1976). Ly phenotype of cytotoxic T cells for syngeneic tumor. *J. Exp. Med.*, **144**, 1116

Index